HEALTHY IMMUNITY

Scientifically Proven Natural Treatments for Conditions from A–Z

Allergies • Autoimmunity • Cancer • Heart Disease • Menopause • Thyroid and More

HEALTHY IMMUNITY

Scientifically Proven Natural Treatments for Conditions from A–Z

Allergies • Autoimmunity • Cancer • Heart Disease • Menopause • Thyroid and More

LORNA VANDERHAEGHE

Macmillan Canada
Toronto

First published in Canada in 2001 by
Macmillan Canada, an imprint of John Wiley & Sons Canada, Ltd.

National Library of Canada Cataloguing in Publication Data

Vanderhaeghe, Lorna R.
    Healthy immunity : scientifically proven natural treatments for conditions from A–Z :
    allergies, autoimmunity, cancer, heart disease, menopause, thyroid and more

Includes bibliographical references and index.

ISBN 1-55335-010-3

1. Immunity—Popular works. 2. Immunity—Nutritional aspects.
3. Natural immunity. I. Title.

R733.V35 2001   616.07'9   C2001-901529-1

This book is available for bulk purchases by your group or organizations for sales promotions,
premiums, fundraising, and seminars. For details, contact: John Wiley & Sons Canada, Ltd.,
22 Worcester Road, Etobicoke, ON, M9W 1L1. Tel: 416-236-4433.
Toll Free: 1-800-567-4797. Fax: 416-236-4448. Web site: www.wiley.ca.

 3 4 5 TRANS 05 04 03 02

Cover design by Sputnik Art + Design Inc.
Cover photograph/illustration by Jesse Koppel/Stone
Author photograph by David Brooks
Text design and typesetting by Susan Thomas/Digital Zone

Macmillan Canada
An imprint of John Wiley & Sons Canada, Ltd.
Toronto

Printed in Canada

This book is dedicated to the health of our children. Each child deserves the best possible chance for optimal health: excellent nutrition, clean water, and plenty of love and understanding.

For my children, Crystal, Kevin, Kyle, and Caitlyn, and my grandsons, Matthew and Hayden

TABLE OF CONTENTS

A TO Z LIST OF DISEASES

(Names in bold indicate autoimmune diseases)

Addison's Disease
Acne
Allergies
Alopecia (Hair Loss)
Anemia
Arthritis (Osteoarthritis and Rheumatoid
   Arthritis)
Asthma
**Autoimmune Diseases
   (see Chapter 3)**
Bladder Infection (see Urinary Tract Infection)
Bowel Disease
Breast Cysts (see Fibrocystic Breast Syndrome)
Bronchitis
Cancer
Candidiasis
Carpel Tunnel Syndrome
Celiac Disease
Cervical Dysplasia (see Warts)
Cholesterol (High)
Chronic Fatigue Syndrome
Cold Sores (see Herpes Virus Infection)
Constipation
Crohn's Disease (see Bowel Disease)
Depression
Diabetes
Diarrhea
Diverticulitis
Eczema
Endometriosis
Estrogen Dominance (see Chapter 4)
Fever (see Influenza)
Fibrocystic Breast Syndrome
Fibroids
Fibromyalgia
Fungal Infections
Gallstones and Gallbladder Disease
Gingivitis
Goiter (see Thyroid)
Gout
Graves' Disease
Guillain-Barré Syndrome
Hair Loss (see Alopecia)
Halitosis (see Gingivitis)
Hashimoto's Thyroiditis
Hay Fever (see Allergies)
Headache (and Migraine)
Heart Disease
Heart Palpitations (see also High Blood
   Pressure)
Hemorrhoids
Hepatitis
Herpes Virus Infection (Genital,
   Shingles/Zoster, Simplex)
High Blood Pressure (Hypertension)

Hives (see Allergies)
HIV (Human Immunodeficiency Virus)
Hypoglycemia
Hypertension (see High Blood Pressure)
Idiopathic Thrombocytopenia Purpura
Immune System (see Chapter 3)
Inflammatory Bowel Disease (see Bowel
   Disease)
Influenza
Interstitial Cystitis (see Urinary Tract
   Problems)
Joints (see Arthritis)
Leaky Gut Syndrome
Malabsorption Syndrome (see Leaky Gut
   Syndrome)
Menopause
Migraines (see Headache)
Mononucleosis
Multiple Sclerosis
Myasthenia Gravis
Nausea
Osteoporosis
Ovarian Cysts
Pain (see Headache)
Parasite Infection
Parkinson's Disease
Pernicious Anemia (see Anemia)
Polyps
Prostate Problems
Psoriasis
Raynaud's Disease/Phenomenon
Reiter's Syndrome
Restless Leg Syndrome
Rheumatoid Arthritis (see Arthritis)
Rosacea
Scleroderma
Seasonal Affective Disorder
Shingles (see Herpes Virus Infection)
Sjogren's Syndrome
Sinusitis (Bacterial)
Snoring
Sore Throat
Systemic Lupus Erythematosus
Thyroid (Hypo/Hyper Thyroid)
Tinnitus
Toxic Metal Poisoning
Ulcers (Stomach and Intestinal)
Urinary Tract Problems (Bladder Infections,
   Interstitial Cystitis)
Vaginal Yeast Infections (see Candidiasis)
Varicose Veins
Vasculitis
Vitiligo
Warts (Cervical Dysplasia, HPV)

ACKNOWLEDGMENTS

Thank you to the thousands of people who have written to me via the Web site and after reading my first book, *The Immune System Cure*. Your requests for simple step-by-step information on how to reverse disease conditions provided the encouragement and enthusiasm to write this book. To my children—Crystal, Kevin, Kyle, and Caitlyn—and grandsons, Matthew and Hayden, you have given me so much joy. You are the reason I continue to research disease prevention and treatment. Mom, thank you for providing me with a strong genetic constitution and the drive to succeed. To my husband, John, for your love and support while I spend hours writing. Thank you to Tanja Hutter for your months of labor in helping to compile this book. Special regards to the late Emanuel Cheraskin, MD, DMD, for taking me under your wing more than a decade ago and encouraging me to soar. Rose and Abram Hoffer, I must thank you for all your encouragement when I worked and studied at the *Journal of Orthomolecular Medicine*. Thank you to the late Linus Pauling, Ph.D., for sharing his stories of his wife's determination to succeed at a time when women were not given the recognition they deserved—you inspired me to defy conventional doctrine. Richard Kunin, MD, Russell Jaffe, MD, Ph.D., and Melvyn Werbach, MD, your work has inspired me. I am grateful to John Morgenthaler for your kindred spirit and respect. To Anthony Almada, MSc, Michael Wilson, ND, Ronald Reichert, ND, and Jim Chan, ND, thank you for the hours of discussion regarding human biochemistry and nutrition. Also special thanks to Deane Parkes, Terry Duffield, Nancy Cheeseman and Claire Farr for your long friendship and continued support. To the Chapmans and Liebenbergs for providing a forum for me to educate the public. To Rolof Liebenberg for sharing your life's work with me, and to Patrick for your expertise in immunology, your research, and the camaraderie we have shared. To Robert Harris and Susan Girvan at Macmillan for publishing this book. Special thanks go to the orthomolecular pioneers who broke new ground, enabling health educators to provide the latest information to those who are sick and in need. To those whose research and concepts I am sharing with the world, thank you.

FOREWORD

This book is truly a labor of love for Lorna Vanderhaeghe. Lorna has been an editor, writer, and health researcher for over twenty years. She has always practiced what she preaches, and brought up four children using a philosophy of natural healing and wholesome nutrition. She has been one of the pioneer educators in the natural health world.

After the outstanding success of her first book, *The Immune System Cure*, which she co-authored with Professor Patrick Bouic, a leading immunologist at Stellenbosch University, she received emails from hundreds of thousands of people from around the world. Many were testimonials about how her immune support program had greatly improved their health. And many more were desperate appeals for help from people suffering from serious and challenging health problems.

Lorna has written this book to address the need for clear and concise health information. Drawing from a wide variety of sources, and a solid background of scientific data, Lorna has distilled this information into a comprehensive manual for health maintenance and restoration.

The book is divided into eight chapters, including an A to Z listing of conditions. The first chapter deals with the digestive system, which is critical to immune function as well as to hormone function, a fact of which few are aware. The second chapter provides information on the cardiovascular system, and the third is an elegant explanation of the intricacies of the immune system.

Immune system abnormalities can involve either a depressed or an overactive immune response. When the immune system reacts against the body's own tissues, this is known as an autoimmune reaction. There are few popular books available on autoimmune diseases.

Lorna has delved deeply into this whole area, studying the mechanisms by which autoimmune diseases have taken hold in the body and illuminating the specific ways that natural remedies can correct faulty pathways.

She explains the specific actions of plant sterols in modulating or balancing the immune system, and documents the research behind them. She has made a major contribution to our understanding of autoimmune diseases.

In addition, Lorna devotes three chapters to mini-courses on nutrition, supplements, herbal remedies, healthy cooking, stress reduction, and exercise. She breaks down a large amount of information into highly digestible bite-size formats useful both for the beginner and for the expert.

Finally, the book gives specific and practical protocols for over 100 conditions, neatly summarized in tables. Conditions include thyroid disease, chronic fatigue syndrome, bowel disease, diabetes, asthma, arthritis, all the autoimmune diseases, as well as multiple sclerosis and Parkinson's disease.

Parkinson's and other degenerative neurological diseases are now affecting a younger population. Lorna gives the latest nutritional data as well as highlighting the exciting work of Dr. David Perlemetter, who has been getting excellent results using intravenous glutathione.

A topic I find fascinating is the link between stress and osteoporosis. Lorna found new research indicating that calcium and vitamin D won't halt osteoporosis if your immune system is dysfunctional. The research showed that under sustained stress, our immune cells release certain types of interleukins that deplete calcium from the bones, thus contributing to osteoporosis.

Lorna has been meticulous in presenting treatments that are backed by scientific evidence, with preference given to human studies. Each nutritional prescription is backed by recent references from the scientific literature published in the last ten years.

These days, family doctors are much more interested in natural medicine, although their education is often lacking in many areas. This is a handy book to take along to your doctor so they can become more informed and check out the journal articles for themselves.

The recommendations in this book can also be used along with more conventional treatments. Any possible drug interaction with either herbs or supplements is carefully described.

In today's world, the public as well as the professional caregiver can be overwhelmed with information on the newest and latest natural cures. It is difficult to separate fact from fantasy and hype. In this book, Lorna has provided a solid basis of evidence based both on suggestions and on common sense advice stemming from her personal experiences.

— Carolyn DeMarco, M.D.
Author of *Take Charge of Your Body* and
Dr. DeMarco Answers Your Questions
(content of both books available at demarcomd.com)

INTRODUCTION

As little as two decades ago, those seeking medical treatments using herbs, homeopathy, detoxification, vitamins, and minerals would have had a hard time locating a general practitioner who would even discuss these types of treatments, let alone recommend their use. The term given to this non-drug approach to disease elimination was "alternative." People sought this type of treatment after exhausting what conventional medicine had to give. Only a handful of medical doctors would offer "alternative" medical care to their patients for fear of being threatened by their medical boards or ostracized by their peers. Anyone seeking an alternative approach to drug therapies had to educate themselves by reading books and other materials. Or they enlisted the help of health food store owners, herbalists, homeopaths, traditional Chinese medicine doctors, acupuncturists, and the rare naturopath.

In twenty years much has changed. A dramatic shift in our health consciousness has taken place. Pharmacists are being trained in herbal and homeopathic medicine. Thousands of medical practitioners are prescribing to the principles of natural medicine. Many more medical doctors practice "integrative" medicine, where they combine research-backed alternative medical treatments with the best of allopathic medicine. And several hundred licensed naturopathic doctors are offering excellent patient care. In addition, medical universities now offer courses on alternative medicine. The University of British Columbia, McMaster University in Ontario, and the University of Alberta offer complementary medicine programs for medical students. Post-graduate degrees are available in homeopathy and naturopathy at Bastyr University in Seattle. The University of Maryland at Baltimore offers a two-year fellowship in Integrative and Complementary Medicine. Harvard Medical School Center for Alternative Medicine Research provides post-secondary education for doctors. Stanford Medical School, the University of Arizona, and the University of Berkeley, California, also offer such programs.

Thousands of research studies on plant nutrients and vitamins and minerals have been performed in university laboratories and clinical settings. These studies are confirming the effectiveness of alternative treatments, giving validation to decades of traditional use. Recognized journals worldwide, including *The Lancet* and *The New England Journal of Medicine*, among others, regularly publish the promising results of nutritional medicine. Physicians are reading these scientific reports and the validation is clear. Science is confirming what traditional healers and pioneers in alternative medicine have known since the beginning of time—Mother Nature provides us with what we need to be well.

Many people are becoming disenchanted with conventional medicine's drugs and the cut and burn approach to disease. Illnesses that are caused by inadequate nutrition, too much stress, and environmental toxins—many of which are dealt with in this book—do not respond well to prescription drug therapies. Strange diseases not seen several decades ago now plague our society: fibromyalgia and autoimmune diseases such as lupus, MS, scleroderma, as well as HIV. Diabetes and arthritis are rampant. These diseases are caused by lifestyle and environmental problems, not by a lack of prescription drugs. Moreover, the rise of antibiotic-resistant bacteria, and viruses that mutate so fast that current treatments quickly become ineffective, have also made people realize that there must be a better way. People are looking for solutions, and starting to understand that preventing disease and taking charge of their family's health makes sense. Our medical doctors also now recognize conventional medicine's shortcomings.

Healthy Immunity: Scientifically proven natural treatments for conditions from A–Z provides you with the most up-to-date, research-backed recommendations for treatment of the top 100 modern diseases, with special emphasis on over 25 autoimmune disorders. Wherever possible, the treatments recommended throughout the book are scientifically backed with research using human subjects.

When using this book you can go directly to the disease that affects you and then read the associated chapters. *If you are currently taking medication, consult your physician before embarking on any new health care program.*

A healthy immune system is the basis for the prescription for health treatment suggestions. Your immune system is your body's internal healing machine. When in prime condition, you are well. When the immune system fails, you become ill. Optimal immunity is the key to good health and longevity.

CHAPTER 1

THE DIGESTIVE SYSTEM:
TAMING TUMMY TROUBLES

The American College of Gastroenterology states that over 50 million Americans are suffering with irritable bowel syndrome (IBS), 20 million have stomach ulcers, and 60 million suffer from heartburn. More than one in three are plagued with common digestive problems. The International Foundation for Bowel Dysfunction says that IBS is second only to the common cold as a cause of absenteeism from work.

Greasy fried foods, a lack of fiber-rich foods, enzyme-depleted processed foods, and just too much food period make up our diet. We are often in such a hurry when we eat that we barely chew our food before we swallow it. Treating our stomach like a human garburator has negative consequences. Dietary inadequacies are directly linked to the development of gastrointestinal diseases, even cancer.

We have all experienced the odd bout of heartburn, nausea, diarrhea, gas, bloating, burping, abdominal cramps, and constipation. Ignoring these complaints may lead to more serious intestinal distress. Go to any pharmacy section and view the large selection of antacids, laxatives, and gas-relieving over-the-counter medications sold today and you will realize that tummy troubles are commonplace. In her book *No More Heartburn,* Sherry Rogers, MD, says 90 percent of symptoms can be alleviated with simple dietary changes, the elimination of allergy-causing foods and *Candida albicans*, stress reduction, and immune enhancement.

In this chapter we will look at the digestive process, some causes of digestive upset, and what we can do to alleviate it.

FROM MOUTH TO BUTT: THE DIGESTIVE SYSTEM

Digestion begins with our eyes and nose. When we see food in a beautiful presentation or smell the aroma of freshly baked bread, savory sauces, or roasting vegetables, our saliva production increases and digestive enzymes are secreted in anticipation of the food about to enter our mouths.

Once the food is in our mouth, chewing is extremely important because it releases the enzyme that decomposes maltose and dextrin, thus facilitating digestion. If you gulp your food—by chewing only once or twice before swallowing—you bypass the beginning of the digestive process and leave the food in much bigger pieces that may not be broken down sufficiently before they pass through the intestines. The longer we chew our food, the more enzymes are secreted. Start chewing your food at least 20 times before swallowing. The saliva also lubricates the food so that it is easier to swallow. Think of the last time you gulped down a sandwich—even soft bread feels raw going down if it hasn't been properly lubricated.

The digestive system is a 30-foot long, winding passageway situated in the center of your body. It is the food transport system that breaks down mouthfuls of food into simpler chemical forms known as nutrients. Macronutrients such as fats, proteins, and carbohydrates must be broken down into micronutrients (vitamins and minerals) in order to be absorbed and utilized by the body.

Digestion and absorption are so important that even if we eat healthily and avoid fast foods, we can become vulnerable to disease if we do not digest our food or eliminate it from our bodies at an appropriate pace. A healthy digestive system is where it all starts. No other system of the body, neither the cardiovascular nor the immune system, can operate at peak performance if the digestive system is not providing the fuel to make the body run.

Once food is chewed, it is pushed past the pharynx down to the esophagus by the reflexive motion of swallowing, which is activated when food reaches the back of the tongue. Through a wave of contractions around the esophagus, food is sent down toward the cardiac sphincter—the circular muscle that governs entry to the stomach. (This is also the valve that is often damaged by gas and bloating, causing acid reflux.) Once in the stomach, pieces of semisolid food are churned up along with gastric hydrochloric acid (HCl) and digestive enzymes (most importantly, pepsin, rennin, and gastric lipase). Water and mucin (mucoproteins) are secreted to protect the stomach lining from the enzymes and hydrochloric acid. The stomach secretions destroy bacteria and regulate the levels of intestinal flora at the same time.

If your meal was made up of mostly solids, it will take three to four hours to digest the contents during this stage. The amount of time foods spend in the stomach varies. Liquids are the most easily passed; of the solid foods, carbohydrates are broken down first, then protein, and finally fats.

Hydrochloric acid is important because it stimulates hormone production in the stomach, destroys some of the bacteria present in the foods ingested, and promotes the uptake of minerals, coenzymes, and trace elements. See page 141 to discover if you have enough HCl. The intestinal juice contains more digestive enzymes that break down the nutrients even further to free single amino acids, split disaccharides into monosaccharides, break down lipids further, and convert nucleic acid into nucleosides and phosphoric acid.

Another hormone signals the gallbladder to contract, releasing bile into the small intestine. Bile neutralizes acids, emulsifies fats, and participates in the absorption of fat-soluble vitamins. Vitamins and minerals, the final products of the decomposed macronutrients, are released as complex molecules to be broken down and dispersed, allowing them to be absorbed into the bloodstream.

Any food or fluid that has not been used passes through to the large intestine. This reservoir uses "friendly" bacteria to decompose some of the undigested matter. The kind of bacteria, or intestinal flora, that we have depends on the diet we follow. High-protein diets call for a greater amount of bacterial flora. High-carbohydrate diets increase the fermentative flora in our gut, which can cause gas and bloating. Our intestinal bacteria manufacture some essential and non-essential nutrients as well.

Undigested plant fiber, along with cellular waste from the gastrointestinal tract, bacteria, and intestinal secretions and excretions, make up the feces that are discharged via the rectum. Insoluble plant fiber acts as a bulking agent that encourages easy and frequent elimination. Without it, constipation develops, allowing toxins and "unfriendly" bacteria to proliferate and disease to take hold.

How Nutrients Are Absorbed

Now that you understand how your digestion system works, let's back up a bit. Remember how, in the small intestine, the vitamins and minerals became complex molecules and were broken down again so that they could be transported to the bloodstream? That process is called absorption and is the key to good health.

With the exception of alcohol (which is absorbed by the stomach), all nutrient absorption takes place at specific sites along the small intestine. The ability of the intestine to absorb the nutrients depends on many conditions. Damage to the intestinal lining from allergies or inflammation, upset due to stress, or eating nutrient-poor food will all inhibit the absorption of nutrients.

By the time carbohydrates enter the bloodstream, they have been reduced to glucose, galactose, and fructose. The liver converts galactose and fructose into glucose as well, so that it can be used for fuel or stored for later use as glycogen. Protein has been reduced to water-soluble amino acids that are quickly sent to the bloodstream. Amino acids build and repair body tissue and are essential to the immune system for forming the antibodies that fight infection. Fats become water-soluble triglycerides, easily entering the bloodstream, while the less water-soluble monoglycerides, diglycerides, and long-chain fatty acids get help from bile salts to facilitate their entry into the bloodstream.

Once in the bloodstream, the nutrients are carried to the liver and then on to the tissues. If your liver is congested with residues from prescription drugs, toxins, and/or alcohol, it will not be able to facilitate this transfer of nutrients to the cells that require them. Glutathione, an amino acid peptide manufactured in the body and available in supplement form is one nutrient that is important for detoxifying the liver of the toxins mentioned above. It along with other liver detoxifiers will be mentioned throughout the book.

DETRIMENTS TO DIGESTION

The immune system and the digestive system are mutually dependent. The immune system relies on digestion to provide it with an optimal amount of nutrients to carry out its many functions. The digestive system, in turn, is inextricably linked to the immune system as it carries out some of its functions. The intestinal barrier contains cytotoxic T-cells and T-helper cells that destroy viruses and bacteria, B-cells and antibodies that neutralize toxins, and macrophages that ingest foreign matter and present antigens for destruction.

Our ability to absorb the most nutrients from our food depends on our rate of gastric emptying, that is, how quickly our stomach empties its contents into the small intestine, which depends on several variables. If medication is ingested with food, then the rate of absorption could be altered depending on the compound. When food or supplements that are metabolized quickly are eaten with something that is metabolized more slowly, the therapeutic value of the food or supplement may be lost because it was not digested appropriately in the digestive tract. The digestive system may be unable to break down nutrients because it lacks enzymes, stomach acid, intestinal flora, or any combination of the three.

The following are the usual suspects in digestive distress.

Bacterial Infections: Over 60 percent of our immune system is actively working around the gut to keep parasites, bacteria, *Candida albicans*, and other organisms under control. By regulating our immune system to destroy invaders more effectively, we can protect our digestive tract. Parasites, bacteria, *Candida albicans*, and viruses have been implicated in many digestive disturbances. *Helicobacter pylori* (*H. pylori*) bacteria is now an accepted cause of stomach ulcers. Untreated *H. pylori* is also implicated in the development of gastric cancers. Crohn's disease (see "Crohn's Sufferers Watch Out," page 7) may be caused by bacterial infections.

Viruses can cause stomach flu, and parasites have been known to keep many tropical vacationers locked in the bathroom.

Candida Albicans: *Candida albicans* overgrowth plays a large role in digestive disease. It is a harmless yeast that, when allowed to overgrow, mimics many diseases in the body. Small amounts of this yeast are found naturally in your intestines. A stool analysis diagnostic test can confirm if candida overgrowth is at the root of your digestive problems. Candida mimics most digestive problems, including gas, bloating, indigestion, pain, and heartburn. Allergies and chronic fatigue can result from candida overgrowth. (See Candidiasis, page 185, for specific treatment strategies.)

Crohn's Sufferers Watch Out— Milk May Not Do the Body Good!

Crusaders in the battle against Crohn's disease have discovered that a bacterium found in milk—even pasteurized milk—may be causing this difficult-to-treat disease. Crohn's is an inflammatory bowel disease that is very common in Europe and North America. Canada has the highest incidence rates of Crohn's in the world. It may affect all parts of the gastrointestinal tract, causing inflammation, pain, destruction of the tissues, and blockages requiring surgery. According to the Crohn's and Colitis Foundation of America, almost 1 million people suffer from this disease.

John Hermon-Taylor, of St. George's Medical School near London, claims that 55 percent of dairy herds in western Europe and America are infected with a bacterium called *Mycobacterium paratuberculosis* (MAP), which can survive the pasteurization process currently used to sterilize milk. Water supplies can also become infected from cow manure that seeps into the soil and contaminates well water. The normal pasteurization process heats milk to 72°C for 15 seconds. In order to kill the MAP bacterium, milk would need to be heated for 30 seconds. Although no definitive study has proven that *Mycobacterium paratuberculosis* causes Crohn's, specialists believe that there is increasing scientific evidence to support the role of an infectious agent, and that Crohn's treatments should focus on eliminating milk and treating bacteria.

Food Allergies: While diet or poor food choices are the main factor in aggravating intestinal distress, food allergy is another. Allergy is also a cause of nausea. Foods (especially wheat, eggs, and dairy products), dusts, molds, pollens, and environmental chemicals are common triggers. Celiac disease is the most serious form of food allergy to grains that contain gluten. Many months or years of food allergies, inflammation caused by intestinal invaders, or allergy and *Candida albicans* overgrowth can cause leaky gut syndrome (LGS). Crohn's disease, chronic fatigue, fibromyalgia, and arthritis may develop from leaky gut syndrome.

Improper Eating Habits: If you rush to finish eating, chances are you didn't chew enough, which means you didn't allow enough time for the enzymes to break down all the nutrients properly. Not only are you cheating yourself of valuable nutrients, you are allowing food to accumulate and putrefy in your intestines. Shoveling down food as you stand over the sink instead of sitting down while you eat increases tension, which in turn can constrict blood flow and impede nutrient delivery to the bloodstream.

Insufficient Intestinal-Friendly Flora: Poor nutritional choices and excessive use of antibiotics may have weakened the body's ability to attack and destroy potential disease-causing bacteria, parasites, and viruses. (See "Antibiotic Overuse and Misuse" on page 55.) Bad bacteria can flourish in the intestines if friendly bacteria, which facilitate digestion, are insufficient or absent.

Insufficient Water Intake: If you aren't drinking at least eight glasses of pure water daily, your stool will become hard and it will be that much more difficult to transport through the intestines. You will find yourself straining to have a bowel movement and it will become more painful over time as hard stools tear at the mucous membranes of the anus and put pressure on sluggish veins. (Straining does not mean that you are constipated. It means you are not getting enough water. Constipation is not having regular daily bowel movements.) If the situation continues, you will become susceptible to anal fissures or hemorrhoids.

Irritable Bowel Syndrome: Irritable bowel syndrome, also called spastic colon, is a disturbance of the colon or large intestine in which alternating bouts of chronic diarrhea or constipation occur. (See treatment for this condition on page 169.) Often IBS is confused with a much more serious group of bowel diseases called inflammatory bowel disease (IBD), a general term used for Crohn's and ulcerative colitis in which inflammation of the bowel causes anemia, fever, and weight loss.

Leaky Gut Syndrome: Once the gut lining is damaged or inflamed, bacteria, parasites, and undigested food enter the bloodstream, causing the immune system to mount an assault on the invaders, which leads to an inflammatory and allergic response. In food allergies, the injured gut lining opens or leaks and allows large food particles into the bloodstream. A leaky gut must be healed quickly to quell aggressive immune responses that promote an overproduction of antibodies leading to autoimmune and other disorders. Toxins from the intestinal tract escape through a leaky gut into areas that normally don't have to deal with them. Also, a leaky gut will not secrete digestive enzymes to break down foods, so malabsorption and nutritional deficiencies can occur.

Avoiding foods that aggravate your condition will allow your gut time to heal. To help you link the foods you eat with your digestive symptoms, write down everything you eat for a couple of weeks in a diet diary. As Sherry Rogers, MD, says, we have to get the "CRAP" out of our lifestyle: cigarettes, coffee, refined sugars, alcohol, aspirin, pop, and processed foods.

Low Fiber/Highly Refined Food Diets: Diets that are low in fiber and high in refined foods lower the body's need for hydrochloric acid and do not contain enzymes to aid digestion. The digestive system becomes very sluggish because it is not getting enough nutritional value from the food that is being eaten; what is being eaten isn't being digested properly and does not move very quickly through the intestines because there is not enough bulk to push it along.

Low Stomach Acid and Insufficient Digestive Enzymes: Many people think they have too much stomach acid and take Rolaids™, Tums™, and more powerful antacids. In reality, their digestive problems began with low stomach acid, very few digestive enzymes, and huge meals that were not chewed thoroughly, all causing food to sit in the digestive tract longer than it should. When food is not digested properly, it ferments, causing gas and bloating. As the gases rise, they distend the esophagus, which causes the pain in the chest that some of us say feels like a heart attack. Too much gas causes the valve that keeps the stomach contents out of the esophagus to stretch, spilling the contents of the stomach, acid and all, into the esophagus, causing that stinging heartburn. Taking an antacid may temporarily quell that burning feeling, but it also reduces the stomach acid, again causing improper digestion of food, which ferments and starts the whole problem all over again. It has been shown that when you try and control stomach acid with antacid medications, the stomach compensates by providing more acid. If you suspect that your stomach acid is low, you can ask your doctor to test you for hydrochloric acid (HCl) deficiency. Doctors once believed that only the elderly suffered from low stomach acid, but it is now evident that even children can be affected. You can take betaine HCl with your meal to improve your stomach's ability to digest foods. See page 141 to find out how to test for HCl deficiency.

Sedentary Lifestyle: Sedentary lifestyle causes digestive system dysfunction. Occupations that necessitate many hours of sitting or standing, a bustling family life of chauffeuring kids to appointments and games, or coping with an illness that is fatiguing make it harder to motivate us to be active, yet that would be the best medicine. When we are not physically active, many systems become sluggish. Our circulation slows down, our muscles tire easily, and our digestive system is impaired.

Upsetting Emotions/Stress: There is no question that emotions affect digestion. Your gastric rate slows down when you experience fear or depression. In contrast, hostility and anxiety will speed it up, promoting diarrhea.

When good nutrients are left undigested and pass straight on to the large intestine or when the value of our nutrient intake is not high enough, our body becomes malnourished. When the body does not get enough nutrients from food, it thinks it is starving and it tells us to eat more food, leading to overeating and ultimately weight gain. The same could be said when our intestinal capillaries are constricted because of tension and impede the absorption of nutrients into the bloodstream, or when digestive hormones don't secrete at the proper time in the proper amount because our emotions work against them.

RELIEF FOR TUMMY TROUBLES

Relief from digestive troubles is often sought in the form of antacids, antidiarrhea medications, laxatives, and much stronger prescription medications. The good news is that natural remedies provide safe, effective relief for gut complaints.

Diet Is Everything

Eat seven to ten half-cup servings of organic fruits and vegetables every day. If you don't eat raw vegetables regularly, start by steaming your vegetables. Eat a half cup of acidophilus-rich yogurt every day unless you are lactose intolerant. Lactose intolerance is a common cause of tummy troubles. Stop all dairy products for six weeks and see if your gut distress is relieved. Drink soymilk instead. Cut out the white pasta, white rice, and white flour.

Tea and Lemon: Get your digestive juices flowing with 1 tsp of fresh-squeezed lemon juice in a cup of herbal tea 15 minutes before your breakfast. Herbal tea is a healthy alternative to coffee, which aggravates gut problems. Drink peppermint, fennel, or ginger tea to soothe a troubled tummy. Ross Pelton, pharmacist, clinical nutritionist, and coauthor of *The Nutritional Cost of Prescription Drugs,* states that "Peppermint tea has been used in treating children's digestive problems such as colic, gas, and upset stomach. The oil of peppermint is used routinely in Europe to reduce cramping, to relieve gas and to increase bile, with its most prevalent use in irritable bowel syndrome."

Digestive Enzymes

Enzymes are catalysts, meaning they help to accelerate certain tasks or make things work faster. Thousands of enzymes and enzymatic reactions keep us alive. They are involved in coagulation, immune function, repair to damaged tissues, removal of toxins, control of excessive inflammation, and more. Enzymes work constantly in the body like an orchestra playing a symphony with perfect mastery. In the case of digestion, enzymes are essential to breaking down our food.

In the book *Enzymes: The Fountain of Life*, authors D.A. Lopez, MD, R. Michael Williams, MD, Ph.D, and Klaus Meihlke, MD, state that the three basic food materials—proteins, carbohydrates, and fats—need three groups of enzymes:

- Protease enzymes can degrade up to 300 g of protein per hour.
- Lipase enzymes can degrade 175 g of fat per hour. Lipase must mix with bile from the gallbladder to be broken down.
- Amylase enzymes can degrade 300 g of carbohydrates per hour.

The fresh, live fruits and vegetables we eat also provide enzymes that help digest our food. Bromelain, found in naturally ripened pineapples, is an example. Asian cultures have eaten enzymatically alive foods for generations. Tamari or soy sauce and Worcestershire sauce are some of the oldest, enzymatically alive foods. Choose foods rich in natural enzymes, and take digestive enzymes, such as betain hydrochloride supplements, in capsule form with each meal to aid digestion. Gas and bloating will be reduced, and bowel movements will improve.

Eat Small Meals

Big meals are hard to digest. Eating small meals throughout the day will not only help heal stomach problems but keep your blood sugar in a healthy range and enhance your immune system.

Fiber Does the Body Good

Fiber is the bulky substance that pushes waste through the intestines at the appropriate rate—not too fast, not too slow. Combat constipation and control diarrhea by adding ground flaxseeds, psyllium powder, guar gum, or pectin to your daily regimen. Drink six to ten glasses of purified water every day, especially if you are taking fiber supplements.

There are two types of fiber: soluble and insoluble. Soluble fiber (found in apples in the form of pectin, the gooey stuff in cooked oatmeal and the slippery substance surrounding flaxseeds that have been soaked) binds to excess cholesterol, allowing it to be eliminated. Insoluble fiber, found in bran and psyllium, acts as a bulking agent, speeding elimination of bowel toxins. Fiber-rich foods also make you feel full and can help with weight management. Fiber also regulates blood sugar levels, which is important for diabetics. (See recipe section on page 377.)

Adding whole, unrefined foods to your diet will add fiber, but be sure to include a digestive enzyme supplement if you are not used to eating whole foods. Eating more fiber without preparing your malfunctioning digestive system first can cause a different set of problems. Don't eat too much fiber; more than 1.5 oz (40 g) per day can cause a cranky colon and is not recommended for diabetics.

Halt Heartburn

Heartburn is anything but harmless. Heartburn sufferers carry a 43 percent higher risk of developing esophagus cancer compared to those who do not suffer from heartburn or indigestion. To reduce heartburn, loosen your belt a couple of notches, raise the head of your bed a few inches from the foot, chew your food, stop smoking and drinking caffeinated beverages, don't drink fluids with your meals, and lose a few pounds.

Immune Regulation

New evidence has found that inflammatory factors (also called cytokines) secreted by the immune system are associated with damage to the intestinal wall and increased inflammation in bowel disease. Several studies have shown that large doses of omega-3-rich fish oils reduce inflammation. As well, research published in the *International Journal of Immunopharmacology* found that plant sterols and sterolins were effective in lowering the inflammatory factors associated with inflammation in the body. By normalizing immune function and halting autoantibody production, the intestinal tract of those with gut problems will have time to heal. Promising treatments that combine halting inflammatory cytokines and killing bacteria may put an end to inflammatory bowel diseases.

Increase Your Exercise

Exercise is the best cure for a lethargic digestive system as it stimulates the digestion of nutrients and moves waste through the intestines more quickly, thus encouraging optimal absorption of nutrients into the bloodstream. Walking half an hour per day is very beneficial.

No NSAIDs

Using non-steroidal anti-inflammatory drugs increases your risk of upper gastrointestinal ulcer, bleeding, and digestive difficulties. *Nature's Pain Killers* by William Cabot, MD, and Carl Germano, RD, recommends willow bark, boswellia, turmeric, pycnogenol, and other safe alternatives to NSAIDs.

Nutrients Are Essential

Nutrient deficiencies are commonplace among those with gastrointestinal disorders. A multivitamin with minerals, an antioxidant supplement, and extra zinc should be taken to replenish nutrient stores. Iron deficiency anemia is often present in those with bowel disorders. You should have a blood test to determine your iron status. Damage to the surface cells of the digestive tract often impairs vitamin B_{12} absorption. B_{12} injections may be required to ensure optimal absorption. Look up the appropriate condition for specific nutrient recommendations for each digestive disease.

Probiotics

Friendly bacteria, or probiotics such as acidophilus, bifidus, and bulgaricus, aid the digestive system by preventing bad bacteria from flourishing in the intestines. Found in fermented foods and in supplement form, probiotics improve nutrient absorption, help produce B vitamins, boost the immune system, and metabolize cholesterol. Probiotics increase gamma-interferon, an important immune-enhancing protein that prevents viruses from replicating. These friendly bacteria also cause a reduction in inflammatory responses of the gut.

Another important immune protein called immunoglobulin E (IgE) is very effective in destroying parasites. Its action is significantly enhanced when lactobacillus bulgaricus-rich yogurt is added to the diet. Probiotics are a must for anyone who is taking antibiotics. Antibiotics cannot distinguish between good and bad bacteria and destroy them all, thereby leaving the intestines vulnerable to attack from disease-causing bacteria.

Reduce Stress and Relax

What we choose to eat and drink, and the environment we choose to do it in, can either aid the digestive process or impede it. Our immune system and digestive system work in concert to protect the body from outside invaders. Enzymes produced by the body and provided in the healthy fresh foods we eat, act together to destroy viruses, bacteria, parasites, and other intestinal invaders.

Intestinal flare-ups, colitis, Crohn's disease, and excess acid production are often associated with increased stress. The connection between stress, the immune system, and inflammation is now clear. Do whatever it takes to reduce your stress levels. Meditation, yoga, breathing exercises, and/or a walk in the park can help reduce the intestinal effects of stress.

Try making your eating environment pleasant to alleviate a negative mood. Put flowers on the table, use the "good" dishes, play light or soothing music, and adjust the lighting to making it bright during the day or provide candlelight at night. (See Chapter 6 for a discussion on how emotions affect our digestion.)

It is also important to take time to enjoy your meals. When was the last time you sat down to dinner at the table without the TV/computer in front of you, without balancing your checkbook, or multitasking of some sort?

Use a Healthy Sweetener

Look for the herbal sweetener stevia at your health food store. Sorbitol and other artificial sweeteners can create gas, bloating, and increased diarrhea. White sugar has been found to reduce the activity of certain immune cells that fight bacteria, viruses, parasites, and cancer. As little as 1 tsp (5 mL) of white sugar inactivates these important immune cells for up to six hours.

Water, Mother Nature's Elixir

Water and fiber work together to regulate the passage of fecal matter. Although you should drink plenty of water throughout the day, you should *not* drink during a meal or else you will dilute your digestive enzymes. (See Chapter 4 for a fascinating new theory on water consumption.)

If you have a digestive problem, look up the condition for specific treatment strategies. Most digestive problems are not serious, but if you have rectal bleeding, fever, sharp abdominal pain, or intestinal obstruction, consult your physician immediately. If not, adopt as many of the tips for repairing your digestive tract and enjoy freedom from intestinal distress.

CHAPTER 2

THE CARDIOVASCULAR SYSTEM:
THE BEAT GOES ON

North Americans have attempted to reduce fat and cholesterol in their diets for more than 30 years, but cardiovascular disease still causes over 40 percent of all deaths.

The cardiovascular system—comprising a heart, veins, arteries, some blood vessels, and blood—sounds simple enough. But when you discover a few facts—such as that the heart never rests or that in the course of an average lifetime, it could fill 100 swimming pools full of blood and will beat over 2 billion times—simple is not the adjective that comes to mind ... amazing would be more appropriate.

Sixty thousand miles (96,000 km) of blood vessels course through our anatomical landscape—that's two and a half times the circumference of the Earth at the equator—and is likened to a "river of health." The name is appropriate provided that the river can flow unhindered to bring food-stuffs to the cells (nutrients and oxygen) and haul away the trash (toxins and cellular wastes). However, if any routes along the river become jammed, the cells starve and die or mutate into abnormal or toxic cells and promote atherosclerosis (hardening of the arteries), and ultimately death.

As the transporter of our infection-fighting white blood cells, the cardiovascular system is crucial to the immune system. Without the nutrients delivered by blood, the immune system doesn't have the components to mount an adequate defense against invaders. If the toxins and wastes are not removed, the immune system will be over-worked in fighting deformed or abnormal cell growth in the body, in addition to its regular surveillance of external invaders. To have opti-mal immunity, the health and vitality of the cardiovascular system is paramount, with new research confirming a direct connection between immunity and cardiovascular disease.

A team of Canadian researchers discovered that an error in the regulation of certain immune cells that fight bacterial infections might be implicated in heart attacks and strokes. Josef M. Penninger, MD, Ph.D, an immunologist at the Amgen Institute and the Ontario Cancer Institute at Princess Margaret Hospital, and the department of Medical Biophysics at the University of Toronto, found that in some people the bacteria chlamydia causes the body's immune system to target the heart, causing inflammation and arterial plaque buildup, which leads to heart disease and myocardial infarctions (MI), commonly called heart attacks.

THE HEART AND THE RIVER OF HEALTH

The heart is roughly the size of a fist. When at rest, it pumps an average of 1.5 gal (5–6 L) of blood per minute. The heart is a hollow muscle consisting of two top chambers called the atria and two bottom chambers called the ventricles. The heart muscle is extremely active and contains a high number of mitochondria cellular powerhouses that produce ATP or energy, which keeps our heart pumping.

Five types of blood vessels transport blood between the heart and cells: arteries, arterioles, capillaries, venules, and veins. High cholesterol and bacterial infections can clog up and damage the blood vessel system. Keeping this system clear of debris is essential to longevity.

Arteries are large blood vessels that bring oxygen-rich blood from the ventricles. They are wide in diameter and have thick, elastic walls that are well suited to carrying blood at forceful pressures. There are two types of coronary arteries carrying blood throughout the body: the pulmonary circuit, which carries blood from the heart to the lungs then back to the heart, and the systemic circuit, which is the network of vessels from the heart to all areas of the body.

Before arteries reach the capillaries, they subdivide into smaller, thinner vessels called arterioles, which are thinner because as they disperse throughout the body, they don't have to accommodate the same level of pressure as the arteries. Their declining size works as a medium for linking the arteries to the capillaries.

The capillaries are the smallest vessels in the body. They connect arterioles to the venules. Capillaries have very thin walls that transfer nutrients and oxygen to the blood and tissues, and also remove carbon dioxide. Because different tissues require varying amounts of nutrients and oxygen, the number of capillaries they have varies accordingly. Muscle needs plenty of oxygen, so its capillary network is immense. The cornea and the skin do not require as much oxygen, so they have a smaller capillary network.

The venules are the tiny vessels that act as the medium between the capillaries and the veins. Veins are larger vessels that run alongside arteries, bringing oxygen-poor blood back to the heart. In contrast to the arteries, the venous walls are not under as much pressure in their circulation so they are thinner, less muscular, and less elastic.

Blood pressure is simply the force or the push against the walls of arteries as blood courses through them. Every heartbeat pumps out blood, so the pressure inside the arteries increases; as the heart relaxes between beats, the pressure drops. Two readings are required to evaluate your blood pressure. The first and larger figure is the systolic pressure—when the heart beats. The second and smaller figure is the diastolic pressure—when the heart is at rest. A normal range for systolic pressure is between 100 and 140 and between 60 and 90 for diastolic pressure.

Blood *Is* Thicker Than Water

Blood is composed of liquid and solid constituents. The liquid in blood is called plasma and the solids are made up of red blood cells, white blood cells, and platelets. An average adult has roughly 4–5 qts (over 4 L) of blood in his or her body. Plasma, which is 92 percent water, is a mixture of hormones, proteins, and vitamins. It holds the platelets and blood cells in suspension.

Ninety-nine percent of your blood cells are red blood cells. Their color is attributed to the protein hemoglobin, which transports oxygen to the cells of the body. A red blood cell count is the amount of red blood cells per cubic millimeter of blood. Healthy adults can have a red blood cell count of anywhere from 4 to 6 million cells.

White blood cells are created in bone marrow and are the warriors of your immune system. They eat bacteria and can produce the antibodies that destroy infectious invaders. The cells transport immune cells via the blood to the infected area. A white blood cell count for a healthy adult is only 4000 to 10,000 cells per cubic millimeter of blood. This is the cell count that doctors monitor for signs of illness. (To learn more about the immune system, see Chapter 3.)

Platelets are cell fragments that are less than half the size of red blood cells. They repair vessels by sticking to damaged walls and causing the blood to clot (coagulation) to prevent the blood from escaping the blood vessel, but this can also be a safety mechanism that turns disastrous when excessive stickiness occurs and promotes heart disease and stroke.

CARDIOVASCULAR CORRUPTION

As the intermediary between the digestive system and the immune system, a healthy cardiovascular system is integral to the body and its immunity. How do many people discover they have heart disease? Often the first sign of heart disease is death.

Heart disease is referred to as the "silent killer" because unless people have regular checkups to monitor their blood pressure and cholesterol levels, some people will not know they have a diseased heart until it is too late. If you have a family history of heart disease, or if you are overweight, have a stressful lifestyle, eat an inadequate diet, and have poor immunity, the strategies mentioned in this book will help you ameliorate these factors. The following are causes of heart disease.

High Cholesterol and Triglycerides

According to the Heart and Lung Association, 40 percent of adults have high cholesterol levels, the leading risk factor for heart disease. There are two types of cholesterol: low-density lipoprotein (LDL) cholesterol and high-density lipoprotein (HDL) cholesterol. When LDL, known as the "bad" cholesterol, gets too high, a slow buildup of plaque occurs on the walls of blood vessels, narrowing the arteries and making the heart work harder to force the blood through. If too much plaque accumulates, blood flow and oxygen to the heart is impeded, causing chest pain. If a blood clot forms and obstructs the artery, a heart attack may occur.

HDL cholesterol is called the "good" cholesterol because it sweeps away LDL cholesterol, carrying it back to the liver and protecting against hardening of the arteries. HDL also helps break down cholesterol into fatty acids, which are essential for cell membrane integrity. Keeping the correct balance of LDL to HDL (see "Are You at Risk?" below) is essential to heart health.

LDL cholesterol is not the only "bad" cholesterol. Lipoprotein(a), a plasma lipoprotein, is the worst cholesterol of all. A high level of lipoprotein(a) increases your risk of heart disease by 10 times that of LDL cholesterol. Lipoprotein(a) contains a sticky molecule called apolipoprotein(a), which makes this dangerous cholesterol stick to artery walls. Levels of lipoprotein(a) that are higher than 20 mg/dL are associated with a higher risk of heart disease.

As part of your annual physical exam, your doctor may check your triglyceride levels along with your cholesterol levels. Triglycerides are the most common form of fat in the body, and high levels of triglycerides may be a better predictor of heart disease than high cholesterol. Excess triglycerides are highly destructive to artery walls, further promoting arteriosclerosis. Normal triglyceride levels are 140–160 mg/dL and the ideal level is 140.

Are You at Risk? The National Heart, Lung, and Blood Institute offers these guidelines on total blood cholesterol in adults.

CHOLESTEROL
Desirable: Less than 200 mg/dL (milligrams per deciliter)
Borderline high: 200–239 mg/dL
High: 240 mg/dL or greater

HDL
Greater than 35 mg/dL

LDL
Desirable: Less than 130 mg/dL
Borderline high: 130–159 mg/dL
High Risk: 160 mg/dL or greater

TRIGLYCERIDE LEVELS
Less than 150 mg/dL

Diets High in "Bad" Fats and Low in Fiber

Fast food, junk food, and processed food are laden with bad fats, particularly trans fatty acids, which are toxic to our bodies. Margarine and hydrogenated vegetable oils raise the bad LDL cholesterol and lower the protective HDL cholesterol. Good health is derived from eating good fats, the essential fatty acids omega-3 and omega-6. These fatty acids break down to protect the body from infection, bacteria, and abnormal cell growth.

Obesity

Although North American culture is obsessed with consuming less fat, heart disease and obesity are on the rise. Just being overweight works against your health and increases risk of heart disease. Scientists have observed that where you carry the weight may be more important in determining your risk of heart disease. Pear-shaped bodies carry the bulk of their weight in the hips and thighs, whereas apple-shaped bodies hold the weight in front of their stomachs. The excess stores of fat around the stomach are associated with an increased risk of high cholesterol, high blood pressure, Type II diabetes, and resistance to insulin—all factors that increase the risk of heart disease.

Sedentary Lifestyle

Those who follow a sedentary lifestyle may get much more than a body that is out of shape. If you do not take part in some form of physical exercise that increases your heart rate every day, then you risk stroke, high cholesterol and high blood pressure, diabetes, depression, obesity, osteoporosis, and more.

Smoking

Heart disease is the leading cause of death in people who smoke. Smokers are less likely to survive heart attacks than non-smokers.

The nicotine in tobacco affects hypertension by raising the smoker's heartbeat. The heart needs more oxygen, while at the same time the blood's capacity for carrying oxygen is lowered by the carbon monoxide in the tobacco. In addition, smoking also squeezes the arteries, further reducing the blood supply to the oxygen-hungry heart. In a nutshell, smoking forces the heart to work harder with less oxygen. When people experience angina pectoris (chest pains), it is because the heart's blood supply has been restricted.

Unfortunately, non-smokers are also at risk if they socialize or are near smokers because they are exposed to the smoke from the lit end of the cigarette, which is not filtered and contains twice as much tar and nicotine, five times as much carbon monoxide, and over 4000 chemicals, 50 of which have been labeled true carcinogens (meaning cancer causing).

Diabetes

According to North American Diabetic Associations, diabetics have a threefold risk of premature death due to atherosclerosis. In diabetics, an elevated insulin level damages certain receptors on the bad LDL cholesterol and, as a result, the feedback system that stops cholesterol from being produced when it is no longer needed does not work. All this excess LDL cholesterol promotes hardening of the arteries.

Diabetics have also been found to have very low levels of dehydro-epiandrosterone (DHEA), the immune and anti-aging hormone. Physicians know that people with low levels of DHEA have higher rates of arteriosclerosis. In a study published in the *International Journal of Sports Medicine*, researchers reported that participants taking plant sterols and sterolins had an increase in DHEA and a decrease in cortisol. Scientists believe that plant sterols and sterolins may be used by the body to make DHEA, thereby protecting us from hardening of the arteries. As well, when cortisol, our stress hormone, is high, our DHEA levels drop, promoting clogged arteries.

Prescription Medication

In 1998, the statin cholesterol-lowering drugs were the third largest category of prescription drugs prescribed in the United States, according to the authors of *The Nutritional Cost of Prescription Drugs*. Statin drugs reduce your body's production of coenzyme Q10. Coenzyme Q10 is essential for energy production for your heart muscle, so a deficiency in coenzyme Q10 increases your risk of heart attack. Statin drugs also increase your need for the vitamins A, D, and E, and are implicated in increasing your risk of cataracts.

Low Levels of Antioxidants, Essential Fats, Magnesium, and Tension, Stress, and Personality

Early studies on the connection between heart disease and Type A personality found that those people have a predisposition to heart attacks. Later research discovered that it is not having a Type A personality, but rather particular negative elements of that behavior that trigger an increased risk of heart disease. The research described that Type A persons were often high achievers who are very aware of time, work hard, and hate standing in lines, but it was the associated feelings of hostility, distrust, and anger that affected these persons' susceptibility to heart disease.

People who dwell on the negative or who are under stress all the time overwork their nervous system by constantly secreting hormones like cortisol, epinephrine, and norepinephrine. These are the same stress hormones that are released when we believe we are in mortal danger and must decide to fight or run away. These hormones can damage the body when secreted continually. Elevated blood pressure, suppressed immunity, osteoporosis, rapid aging, and heart disease are some of the diseases associated with higher-than-normal cortisol levels.

Excessively Sticky Platelets

As we learned earlier, excessively sticky platelets promote heart disease and stroke. Platelets become a problem when we eat trans fatty acids and processed oils, margarines, and spreads. By adding omega-3 fats from flax and fish we can reduce the stickiness of our platelets and prevent heart disease. Garlic has also been shown to reduce sticky platelets, one aspect of its powerful heart protective ability. (See "Idiopathic Thrombocytopenia Purpura," an autoimmune disease of the platelets on page 276.)

High Blood Pressure and Low Thyroid

Blood pressure can vary dramatically depending on the activity performed at the time, but a continual pressure above 140/90 is an indicator of hypertension, commonly called high blood pressure. A person can have hypertension for years without any symptoms. Some symptoms, such as headaches, dizziness, fatigue, or weakness, are often mistaken as symptoms of other diseases. The Framingham study, which evaluated more than 5000 men and women for their cardiovascular health, found that the risk of stroke was five times higher in people with moderately elevated 160/95 levels of blood pressure. Congestive heart failure can also result when the heart's ability to pump is impaired. Severe hypertension leads to inadequate circulation, so the kidneys, lungs, and other organs suffer.

Poor diet, too much stress, kidney dysfunction, and tumors in the adrenal

> ### Barnes Basal Temperature Test
>
> Many people have subclinical low thyroid and yet are diagnosed with normal thyroid based on the current blood tests. This simple temperature test can determine if you have low thyroid. Men and non-menstruating women can take the test on any day, but women should take the test on the second or third day of their menstrual period. Put a standard thermometer on the nightstand before bed. Make sure you shake it down before going to sleep. Immediately upon awakening, place the thermometer snugly in the armpit for 10 minutes. Do not get up and move around; it is important to lie there fairly still and relax. A reading below the normal range of 97.8–98.2°F suggests low thyroid function. If it is above the normal range, then infection or an overactive thyroid may be the cause of the higher temperature.

gland have been implicated in high blood pressure, yet most cases of hypertension have no definite physical cause. According to the late Broda Barnes, MD, "Low thyroid function may promote elevation of blood pressure." Dr. Barnes studied goiter patients who had partial thyroid removals to prevent the choking threatened by their greatly enlarged glands. They experienced an increase in blood pressure with each successive operation and, furthermore, the more thyroid gland that was removed, the higher the blood pressure became. If you have tried many treatments to lower your blood pressure without success, an underactive thyroid may be the source of your problem.

Thyroid medication may be an appropriate medication for high blood pressure. Dr. Barnes also noted that in cases of kidney dysfunction, thyroid medication did *not* lower blood pressure. Have your thyroid checked by your doctor and do the Barnes basal temperature test.

Hypothyroidism (low thyroid) is very common in North America. People living in the northern hemisphere often do not expose their skin to at least 20 minutes of sunshine per day, and as a result do not get adequate amounts of vitamin D, which are required to help make thyroxin, a thyroid hormone. Low thyroid can also be due to a lack of trace elements and minerals in the diet. These elements are used to make thyroid hormone, so a poor diet and a lack of vitamin and mineral supplements may lead to thyroid dysfunction.

If hypertension is not treated, the heart may enlarge to pump against the increased pressure, causing the heart muscle to weaken and irregular heartbeat to develop. The excess pressure caused by high blood pressure can weaken or damage the artery walls, thus promoting atherosclerosis.

Atherosclerosis, hardening of the arteries, is the most common cause of blockage and is responsible for over 40 percent of all deaths in North America. A buildup of cholesterol, fatty material, high triglycerides, injury to arteriole walls, and inflammation caused by bacteria are all implicated in the deadly narrowing of our arteries. Diet and lifestyle changes could reduce a large percentage of these deaths. Angina, a pain or squeezing feeling in the chest, is often the result of a thickening of the arteries due to atherosclerosis, thus causing a reduction in oxygen to the heart. If you are experiencing angina, be sure you get immediate medical attention.

High Levels of Homocysteine

Scientists believe that elevated homocysteine levels may promote heart disease by damaging artery walls. Homocysteine is produced by the body during the conversion of certain amino acids. Without adequate levels of vitamins B_{12}, B_6, and folic acid, homocysteine levels can become dangerously elevated. A high homocysteine level is a risk factor for heart attack, stroke, and osteoporosis. It also contributes to atherosclerosis by damaging artery walls and disrupting collagen formation (collagen disruption also results in poor bone development, an increased risk factor for osteoporosis). Almost 40 percent of patients with heart disease will have elevated homocysteine levels. By simply taking a high potency B-complex supplement containing 400 mcg of folic acid with 50 mg of vitamin B_6 and 500 mcg of vitamin B_{12}, homocysteine levels will normalize, thus reducing the risk of heart attack, stroke, and atherosclerosis. A vitamin B-complex daily is also essential for protecting against osteoporosis.

HOW TO KEEP YOUR HEART HEALTHY

Lower Your Cholesterol

There is no substance as controversial or as confusing as cholesterol. Cholesterol has truly gotten a bad rap. Produced by the liver and found in many foods we eat, cholesterol is essential to our health. We require it for repair mechanisms in the body; it insulates our nerves, makes up cell membranes, and is involved in the production of certain sex hormones. In most people a protective feedback mechanism ensures that if they consume an abundance of cholesterol-containing foods, a decrease in the production of cholesterol from the liver will occur. For others, cholesterol levels must be kept in balance with simple dietary changes and nutritional supplements. It is a fact that 999 out of 1000 people can control their cholesterol levels with just simple dietary changes. Lowering LDL blood cholesterol and triglycerides and increasing HDL cholesterol has an enormous impact on reducing your risk of heart disease and stroke. The Heart and Stroke Foundation states that "for every 1 percent drop in LDL cholesterol a 2 percent reduction in risk of heart attack occurs and for every 1 percent increase in HDL levels, the risk of heart attack drops 3 to 4 percent." Scottish researchers have found that eating two medium-size raw carrots every day can reduce your cholesterol by 50 points in a little as 21 days. Supplementing your diet with vitamin B_3 or non-flushing niacin (inositol hexanicotinate), folic acid, vitamin B_{12}, and pyridoxal-5-phosphate (the active form of vitamin B_6) can help lower heart attack risk by 75 percent.

Plant sterols are nature's cholesterol-lowering superstars. Sterols are an essential component of cell membranes, and both animals and plants produce them. Over 40 plant sterols (or phytosterols) have been identified, but beta-sitosterol, campesterol, and stigmasterol are the most abundant. These three sterols are structurally similar to cholesterol and are therefore powerful cholesterol-lowering agents. They reduce the absorption of cholesterol from the gut by competing for the limited space for cholesterol in the intestinal lumen, which delivers mixtures of lipids for absorption into the mucosal cells. About 0.25 g of plant sterols and 0.3 g of cholesterol occur naturally in the daily diet; the amount of plant sterols consumed daily is twice as high in a vegetarian diet. By simply adding plant sterols to your diet, you can reduce the absorption of cholesterol in the gut—both dietary and endogenous (that is, excreted in bile)—by about half to one quarter. This reduced absorption lowers serum cholesterol despite the compensatory increase in cholesterol manufactured by the liver. By the 1980s it was recognized that as naturally occurring substances, plant sterols could be added to foods or taken as nutritional supplements with very effective cholesterol-lowering action. Over 400 published clinical trials to date have shown that sterols have excellent cholesterol-lowering action without the side effects associated with taking standard cholesterol-lowering drugs. In September 2000 the U.S. Food and Drug Administration gave phytosterols a recognized health claim for reducing the risk of coronary heart disease. In the future you will see plenty of new phytosterol-based supplements for the treatment of heart disease.

A Healthy Heart Diet

Simple diet changes alone can reduce cholesterol by 20 percent. A rainbow of fruits and vegetables, plenty of soluble fiber (oats, legumes, beans, and apples) and lots of water is all it takes. A review article that appeared in Volume 94 (1994) of the *Journal of the American Dietetic Association* reported that the higher the dietary intake of fiber, the greater the decrease in cholesterol levels. Oat bran and oatmeal were responsible for some of the greatest drops in serum cholesterol. (Dietary changes are more effective in preventing heart disease and reducing the recurrence of heart attacks than aspirin. Aspirin is not without its own risks. Side effects of aspirin use include gastrointestinal bleeding due to peptic ulcer.)

Fiber is usually thought of in terms of correcting digestive disorders, but it has its place in preventing heart disease as well. The mortality rate due to heart disease is lower in people who follow high-fiber diets (like vegetarians). Studies show that some types of fiber (not wheat bran) are linked to lowering cholesterol. Initial studies of pectin, the dietary fiber in fruit (especially apples), show that it selectively lowers LDL cholesterol (the "bad" cholesterol) and serum cholesterol levels. Fiber binds to excess cholesterol and removes it in our daily bowel movements.

Oat fiber is linked to lowering serum cholesterol levels, while increasing bile salt excretion. Excreting bile salts is important in inhibiting the reabsorption of cholesterol. Saponin in beans and alfalfa also reduces serum cholesterol levels by increasing bile salt excretion.

Fish are rich in heart-protective good fats. Use "better" butter sparingly instead of margarine (see recipe for better butter on page 407), and avoid sugar, trans fatty acids, and hydrogenated oils. Reduce saturated fat (lard, animal fats) and decrease your egg consumption to one a day (each egg contains approximately 200 mg of cholesterol).

Saturated fats and cholesterol always get the blame, but a century or two ago American farmers ate fresh dairy products, including homemade butter and eggs, as staples. Fatty meat, cured bacon and hams, pork sausages fried in lard, and thick cream skimmed off the top of the milk were eaten every day, yet heart attacks were not the problem they are today. Sugar consumption, trans fatty acids, and hydrogenated oils are the culprits. The recipes I recommend in the back of this book are free of all of these heart-damaging anti-foods.

Don't skip breakfast! A national survey evaluating the nutritional practices of Americans found that those who ate whole grain cereal for breakfast had the lowest serum cholesterol levels. Those who ate cholesterol-laden breakfast foods still had lower total cholesterol than those who skipped breakfast altogether.

Eat these foods for lowering cholesterol: vegetables (plenty of salads), fruits, whole-grain bread, herbal tea, vegetable juices, sodium-free herbal salt, cold-pressed vegetable oils (extra-virgin olive oil), fish, and skinless, boneless chicken or turkey.

Avoid these foods: all margarine, salt, cakes, cookies, biscuits, candy, white foods (including bread, flour, sugar, rice, pasta), artificial sweeteners (aspartame), fake fats, and fake coffee creamers.

Remember, diet is everything. Adopt these diet recommendations, drink plenty of water, and eat lots of fiber.

Get into the Groove

Regular exercise, specifically aerobic activity, combats heart disease on many levels. It burns fat, helping to maintain or reduce weight; it improves the circulation of blood and provides more oxygen to the heart; and it helps relieve stress by reducing tension in the body. For people who have been diagnosed with borderline hypertension, studies have shown that regular exercise can return their blood pressure to normal. Other research has indicated that exercise improves insulin sensitivity for several hours afterwards. Yoga and tai chi are highly recommended because they double as exercise and as emotional stress-reducers. Move your body, and get your blood flowing and your heart pumping. Start an exercise program even if it means walking to the corner of your street and back.

Emotions in Motion

An adjustment in attitude is imperative in reducing the risk of disease. When events occur and you find yourself in a negative spiral, stop your thoughts and make a mental note of the positive aspects. Keep running that list in your head until the negativity goes away. (See Chapter 6 for discussion of emotions and stress-reduction techniques.)

Nutrients to the Rescue

Carnitine Heart Fuel: Carnitine is another important nutrient for the heart that provides mitochondria cells with increased energy. Without adequate carnitine, the heart will not get enough oxygen, thus causing angina, high blood pressure, and congestive heart failure. A heart without enough carnitine is like a computer without memory; it will work until it is overloaded and then it crashes. Carnitine has been used in doses of 200–300 mg three times a day. It has been shown in many double-blind, placebo-controlled studies to improve cardiac output in those with congestive heart failure.

Coenzyme Q10: Coenzyme Q10 is the spark for our mitochondria and important to heart health. When our heart mitochondria become deficient in coenzyme Q10, they cannot fire the sparks that make our hearts beat and angina, high blood pressure, mitral valve prolapse, and eventually congestive heart failure occur. Coenzyme Q10 is so essential that every person should take 30 mg per day to prevent heart disease and much more to treat specific heart conditions.

Garlic: Garlic is a vampire's enemy and the heart's best friend. Fresh, raw garlic is protective against all types of heart disease. One to four cloves per day will reduce the risk of stroke and heart attack and lower cholesterol and high blood pressure. If you want the heart benefits of garlic but not the aftertaste and smell, then choose a garlic supplement, such as Kyolic garlic.

Gugulipid: Native to India and commonly used in ayurvedic medicine to lower cholesterol, gugulipid is the standardized extract of the mukul myrrh tree (*Commiphora mukul*). Several clinical studies have confirmed gugulipid's ability to lower both cholesterol and triglyceride levels. It increases the liver's metabolism of LDL cholesterol. Gugulipids have been shown to be free of side effects and have a similar action to cholesterol- and triglyceride-lowering medications. In his book *Heart Disease and High Blood Pressure*, Michael Murray, ND, reports that "typically total cholesterol levels will drop from 14 percent to 27 percent in a 4 to 12 week period, while LDL cholesterol and triglyceride levels will drop from 25 to 35 percent and 22 to 30 percent respectively. HDL cholesterol levels will increase by 16 to 20 percent."

Heart Healthy Hawthorn: Hawthorn has been used in European cardio-vascular protocols for centuries. Hawthorn berry (*Crataegus monogyna*) has been shown to reduce angina attacks, lower blood pressure and cholesterol, and enhance general heart health. Look for hawthorn extracts that are standardized and take 100–300 mg per day. Hawthorn works synergistically with vitamin E as an overall heart tonic.

Marvelous Magnesium: Arrhythmias or irregular heartbeat can be treated easily using magnesium. The heart muscle is rich in magnesium and potassium, which are required to spark heart muscle contractions. A deficiency in magnesium will also cause a drop in potassium. Over the last six decades, dozens of studies have shown that magnesium is an effective agent in treating arrhythmias.

In one study researchers compared digoxin (a prescribed drug for arrhythmias) with magnesium in controlling arrhythmias. Two groups were compared. One group received digoxin plus placebo (a fake pill) and one group receiving digoxin plus magnesium sulfate intravenously. In the group receiving magnesium the heart rate dropped dramatically to 80 beats per minute, whereas in the digoxin-only group the heart rate averaged 105. Magnesium is obviously a better, safer, and more effective treatment for arrhythmias. A dose of 350 mg three times per day should help normalize arrhythmias. (See Magnesium on page 98 for more information.)

Vitamins: Vitamins B_3, B_6, B_{12}, and folic acid have been shown to lower blood homocysteine levels, thereby reducing heart attack risk.

Renowned medical doctor Abram Hoffer was the pioneer in niacin (vitamin B_3) research. Early in the 1950s he realized that niacin was an effective agent in lowering high cholesterol. Since then hundreds of studies have verified its effectiveness at not only lowering LDL cholesterol but also triglycerides while raising HDL cholesterol. The Coronary Drug Project published in 1986 in the Journal of the American College of Cardiology found that niacin was the only lipid-lowering substance to reduce mortality. In 1994 niacin's lipid-lowering effects were compared to Lovastatin (a commonly prescribed lipid-lowering drug) in the *Annals of Internal Medicine*. Participants who were given 1.5 g of niacin had a 33 percent increase in HDL, whereas Lovastatin increased HDL by 7 percent. Some people do not like the discomforts of the accompanying harmless "niacin flush" and nausea, and dosages must be increased gradually. Those who dislike the side effects of niacin can take inositol hexanicotinate, commonly sold in health food stores as non-flushing niacin. If you are taking pure niacin, have your physician check your liver enzymes (niacin is not recommended for those with liver disease or diabetes unless you are under the care of a physician) and cholesterol levels every three or six months while on niacin and reduce your niacin intake to a maintenance dose when your cholesterol and triglycerides get in the healthy range (see chart for optimal cholesterol and triglyceride levels on page 18).

Fortunately, heart disease is easy to prevent. Reversing it requires a commitment to the recommendations made in this book, but it *is* possible to reverse heart disease.

HAND IN HAND

Once the digestive system has absorbed the nutrients we ingest, it is up to the cardiovascular system to deliver them. This teamwork is the foundational support for immunity and any breakdown in this delivery system is ominous for the immune system. In the short term, the immune system can cope by finding ways to adapt. However, if the digestive system and/or the cardiovascular system are compromised for long periods of time, the immune system cannot provide adequate protection and disease sets in. As you read the next chapter, you will understand the complex nature of the immune system.

THE IMMUNE SYSTEM:
BALANCE = HEALTH

If you have already read my first book, *The Immune System Cure*, you probably have a good understanding of the immune system. This chapter provides more information on the developments and new discoveries in how the immune system functions and exciting new research on stress and immunity, autoimmune disease, pain and the immune system, and the dangers of routine vaccines.

Life is all about balance. Those who have discovered the joys of physical and emotional health have perfected the art of juggling work and play, exercise and relaxation, good food and junk food. On a smaller scale, even certain body functions are programmed for balance—our hormones need to be in the right ratios for optimal health, the acidity or alkalinity of the body is carefully controlled, and microscopic cells of the immune system must be in harmony or disease results.

The key to optimal health lies with our immune system. Returning balance and strength to the immune system in the face of daunting diseases like AIDS and cancer may seem very challenging. Allergies, autoimmune disease, viral infections (including herpes and human papilloma virus, the virus that causes warts and that is implicated in cervical cancer), HIV, cancer, and even heart disease are linked to a dysfunctional or imbalanced immune system. Media reports would have us believe that boosting the immune system is the key to correcting all deficiencies, but scientists are learning that many common diseases are caused by overactive or misdirected immunity. Autoimmune disease, allergies, and inflammatory conditions like fibromyalgia and osteoarthritis are a few of the diseases where balancing immune function is more appropriate. Immune modulation is the medical term for balancing your immune system and this is the concept that you will be continually revisiting throughout the book. Intricate processes must occur in our immune system to ensure optimal function.

Little evidence is required to demonstrate how crucial the immune system is to our survival. Researchers noted that once people had recovered from some types of illness (like measles or mumps), they usually would not become infected again. It was discovered that if people survived, they developed lifelong protection against that specific illness. Childhood is looked upon as immunity's training ground, the time when this important defense system learns to recognize and fight against harmful organisms. If an infant is born with a defective immune system, the baby's only chance of survival is to be protected in a completely sterile environment from germs of all types.

Immunity to diseases like chicken pox, measles, smallpox, and other infectious organisms is based on the production of antibodies, Y-shaped glycoproteins produced by white blood cells. This protein is programmed to kill a specific intruder or antigen (foreign matter that provokes a response from the immune system). Antigens are attached to the surface of a virus or bacteria and form a unique structure that can be recognized only by an antibody specifically designed to identify that structure. When a different antigen is presented, its specific antibody must be produced each and every time. As we gain more and more antibodies, we develop resistance. Resistance to a specific antigen is called immunity. However, the immune system provides several methods of defense to protect us from foreign invaders.

When a foreign organ is transplanted, patients must take immunosuppressants to prevent organ rejection because the immune system is so vigilant about anything foreign in the body that it will destroy the newly transplanted organ. Immunosuppressant drugs prevent rejection, but make a person highly susceptible to infections and more serious conditions such as cancer and osteoporosis. Withdrawing the immunosuppressants can reverse the conditions, but only by sacrificing the transplanted organ.

The appearance of acquired immune deficiency syndrome (AIDS) has sparked a flurry of interest in immunology not seen since the smallpox epidemics. AIDS, a devastating disease brought about by the human immunodeficiency virus (HIV), suppresses the immune system and leaves a person so vulnerable to opportunistic infections that even minor infections can become fatal.

AN IMMUNE SYSTEM OVERVIEW

Healthy babies inherently benefit from the natural immunity they get from their mothers as their own immune systems mature. This innate immunity or resistance to disease begins with a response against a broad range of foreign infiltrators. The response is so subtle that you are not even aware that it is going on. The perimeter of defense begins with the physical barrier of the skin and mucous membranes. The skin keeps bacteria and foreign particles out, excretes toxins and waste from within the body by sweating, and regulates body temperature. Mucous membranes of exposed body cavities—such as nasal passages, the eyes, the vagina, and the mouth—are vigilant in neutralizing potential invaders before they can enter. Saliva, tears, and vaginal secretions are the weapons that enable them to dilute and wash away microbes.

Think about how many times a day you touch your finger to the side of your nose, eyes, or mouth. Each time we do this we provide invaders direct entry into the inner body. The immune system protects us by making sure that all of our body fluids are rich in immune factors that destroy bacteria, viruses, parasites, and more, but what if we are dehydrated? Water is essential. It ensures that we have fluid-rich areas that are full of potent immune factors. If we are dehydrated, those fluids and their immune factors around the eyes, nose, and mouth shrink and invaders have an open door to our bodies. Water is the least expensive and most effective virus fighter. Ensure that you drink eight glasses a day, especially in the winter when you are in your centrally heated home and the viruses are just waiting for an opportunity to gain hold.

If an invader gets past our physical barriers, then our immune system is waiting with a powerful arsenal of cells and immune factors. Have you ever gotten a piece of a thorn from a raspberry bush or rose stuck in your finger? Within a few hours the place where the thorn damaged the skin will become red and inflamed or swollen. This means that your innate immunity has launched an attack and is repairing the broken skin. In the tissues of your skin, macrophages are defending you against infection. A full-blown inflammatory response is now occurring in your finger.

Your immune system is made up of organs including the thymus, spleen, bone marrow, lymph glands and microscopic cells that communicate with one another through chemical messengers called cytokines and they regulate many other systems of the body. The main cells include natural killer (NK) cells, T-helper cells, cytotoxic T-cells, B cells, and macrophages.

Macrophages

Macrophages are the cells that eat and digest foreign matter (macrophage literally means "big eater"). They are like Pac-Man cells that go throughout the body, eating and digesting invaders and waste products and taking pieces of those invaders and presenting them to other immune cells so they can be recognized for destruction. When an infection occurs, the macrophages patrolling the area trap, break up, and destroy the foreigner, a process called phagocytosis. As well, macrophages release certain immune factors or chemical messengers to alert the rest of the immune system. Unlike some immune cells that are very limited as to which microbes they can destroy, macrophages are not very picky, so they will attack a wide variety of viruses, bacteria, and old and dead cells. Although not all invaders are destroyed, this method is very effective. Some microbes, including *staphylococci* and *tubercle bacillus*, can actually kill macrophages or remain dormant for months or even years as they wait for the immune system to weaken and become vulnerable to attack. A healthy immune system, however, can stop these troublemakers in their tracks or leave them waiting dormant for their "big break" as long as we live.

Fever

Fever is another method of preventing bacteria and viruses from taking hold. Elevating the body's temperature, even by two degrees, can hinder an invader's progress or kill it. The phagocytes release pyrogens (a fever-producing substance released by phagocytes) to induce fever. If the fever goes too high (just a few degrees or more), it can be deadly to the host. Because the window of opportunity to destroy viruses is so narrow and the ill-fated consequences lethal (death of the individual or the brain cells), immunologists are beginning to hypothesize that fever is an outmoded method of immune system defense, and that if humans survive another several thousand years, we may evolve in such a way that fever may no longer be used to kill invaders.

Inflammation

Inflammation is also a way for the body to defend itself and can be activated within seconds of an injury or invasion. The pain, redness, swelling, and heat that we feel destroys microbes, toxins, and other foreign material at the site of penetration. The blood vessels are constricted to repair damages and prevent the infection from spreading further. Following the activation of several different immune cells—including mast cells, macrophages, and T-cells—the lipids in the cell membranes are converted into inflammatory mediators that have potent effects. There are three inflammation promoters: prostaglandin D2 (PGD2, derived from arachidonic acid), leukotrienes (also from arachidonic acid), and platelet-activating factor (PAF, produced by mast cells). Certain nutrients, such as essential fatty acids, control these inflammation promoters. For example, PAF released as a result of the immune response, has a profound effect on smooth muscle tissue in the lung, causing bronchial constriction, tightness in the chest, and wheezing, all of which are symptoms of asthma. Remember that inflammation is necessary to heal tissues or eject an invader and becomes a problem only when it is chronic or long term. We don't want to totally eliminate inflammation in the body or we will stop the immune system from healing damaged tissues. The problem with some of the strong anti-inflammatory medications is that they can slow the inflammatory response to the point where the immune system cannot do proper healing or eliminate invaders. (See the sections on NSAIDs and COX-2 inhibitors on page 43.)

Complement

Complement, another agent of the immune system, is a combination of 20 proteins (enzymes) that circulate in the blood acting as catalysts in antibody reactions. When an invader appears, complement releases a protein (enzyme), then another enzyme, and another in a cascade until all 20 proteins have been set in motion. Each one of the 20 steps in the complement reaction has a particular function that happens at an appropriate phase in the process of killing invaders. The end result is that complement proteins call in a cavalry of phagocytes to the site of the inflammation and turn them into voracious eaters of the invaders.

Powerful Cancer-Fighting Cells

Natural killer cells (NK cells) are like assassins or professional hit men in that they have a little more finesse in the way they operate compared to macrophages. They destroy their attacker by penetrating its surface and releasing toxic enzymes into it. Like phagocytes, NK cells assume their own command and do not need to be told to kill invaders. However unlike antibodies, they do not have memory, so each confrontation is a new battle.

NK cells target parasites, viruses, bacteria, and fungi, but they have an extra assignment. They seek out and destroy cancerous cells on contact before they attach and develop into a tumor—in effect, they are the first strike against cancer. NK cells also attack cells infected by pathogens other than viruses. Studies evaluating cancer patients' immune status have shown that their numbers of NK cells are drastically reduced; the lower the number of NK cells, the more severe the cancer.

An interesting characteristic of NK cells is that they release interferons, the chemical messengers or immune factors that prevent virus replication. Interferons incite aggression in NK cells and call more NK cells to join the fight, thus improving their overall killing ability.

Our immune system is incredibly intricate and sensitive to subtle changes, but it runs like a well-tuned orchestra and keeps us healthy as long as we provide it with all the tools it needs: good nutrition, supplements, relaxation, and exercise. If we have been neglectful by not getting enough nutrients or are under an excessive amount of stress, we put a dent in the armor, so when a particularly strong or determined microbe beats our immune system, we get sick.

The Thymus, a Superhero

The thymus is a flat, soft, pinkish-gray gland that sits behind the breast-bone. At birth, it is bigger than the heart. Physicians in the 1950s mistakenly believed that a large thymus was a defect in infants and used radiation to shrink it. Thankfully, this practice was stopped when they realized that a strong healthy immune system required a healthy-sized thymus gland. The gland continues to grow until puberty when it reaches approximately 1.2 oz (34 g). As we age, it gradually shrinks, resulting in a corresponding decline in immunity. Doctors have told patients that this is a normal aging process, yet vitamins A, C, and E and the minerals zinc and selenium can enlarge even the most immune-compromised and shrunken thymus gland.

Conventional wisdom of the past dictated that a loss of immunity was to be expected through the course of aging. Aging decreases production of the hormone thymulin, which in turn decreases the production of T-cells and prevents the immune system from maturing.

We now know that the thymus is not doomed to shrink. Tarzan really knew what he was doing when he was pounding his chest. Find the curved bone in the center of your chest and gently pound it about a dozen times. Do this when you think about it throughout the day. This is a form of acupressure that stimulates the thymus gland to maintain size and the secretion of thyroid hormones.

Not Just Lymphing Along

The lymphatic system is made up of lymph fluid, lymphatic vessels, bone marrow, lymph nodes, the spleen, and the tonsils. It is involved in the elimination of toxic waste from tissues and is a crucial component of the immune system. Muscles, not the heart, pump fluid through this system. A sluggish lymphatic system is usually attributed to a lack of exercise. If the battle against an infection is underway, the lymph glands become swollen and tender as they try to clear and clean the system. One of the best methods of cleaning the sludge out of your lymphatic system is to use a rebounder. A rebounder is a small trampoline that you bounce on for 10–20 minutes per day to get your lymphatics draining properly. It is also great exercise. Look for a rebounder at local department or fitness stores.

Immune Cells, the Last Line of Defense

Red cells and white cells reside in the blood, but only white cells are immune cells. Lymphocytes are one type of white blood cell that is born in the marrow of the long bones of the body. Upon maturity, white blood cells have two options: they can remain in the marrow to evolve into B-cells, or circulate throughout the body via the blood to the lymph until they reach the thymus gland, where they develop as T-cells.

When T-cells mature, they can differentiate between invading cells ("non-self") and our own cells ("self"). Under normal circumstances, the immune system attacks only foreign substances or pathogens, whether they invade from outside the body or are made from within, like cancer cells. However, there are times when the immune system may become confused and attack healthy body cells.

T-cells are in charge of the cell-mediated responses to infection. Cell-mediated immunity is very important in fighting bacteria, yeast, viruses, fungi, and parasites (especially those pathogens residing within cells) by moving around the body on a seek-and-destroy mission. When they find invaders, the T-cells adhere to the cells and kill them. There are three main types of T-cells: T-helper cells, cytotoxic T-cells, and suppressor T-cells.

T-Helper Cells: T-helper cells, also known as T4 cells or CD4 cells, sound the sirens that an invasion has occurred and help the cytotoxic T-cells prepare for battle. They secrete protein messengers to initiate the growth, proliferation, and destructive ability of other immune cells. They also secrete proteins to raise the inflammatory response and the killing action of macrophages and NK cells. T-helper cells must signal the cytotoxic T-cells or other immune cells or else those cells cannot do their job. T-helper cells also send signals to the B-cells to produce antibodies.

Less than a decade ago immunologists discovered that we have two types of T-helper cells. T-helper cells are subdivided into T-helper-1 (Th-1) or T-helper-2 (Th-2), and each produces very different chemical messengers. A healthy immune system needs a balance of both Th-1 and Th-2 cells to be able to respond to different kinds of situations in the body.

T-helper-1 cells are the good guys. They prime the immune system by producing interleukin-2, which stimulates the cytotoxic T-cells to kill the infected cells. Interleukin-2, in turn, notifies the macrophages and NK cells to become aggressive and abundant. Th-1 cells also release gamma-interferon, a potent cancer and virus-fighting factor. Most importantly, Th-1 cells regulate the Th-2 cells. A failure of the Th-1 arm of the immune system to control an overactive Th-2 is implicated in a wide variety of chronic illnesses. These include AIDS, allergies, cancer, autoimmune disorders, and more to be discussed later. In HIV's progression to AIDS, there is a shift from Th-1 dominance to Th-2, exacerbating the disease.

Th-2 cells are involved in the inflammatory, allergic, and antibody responses. Antibody production increases when Th-2 responds and if Th-2 is un-regulated, it can cause the destruction of the "self" cells. Several of the immune factors (cytokines, the chemical messengers) released by T-helper-2 cells are involved in promoting inflammation and pain.

The Th-2 arm of the immune system becomes "bad" only when it is chronically overactive and when the Th-1 arm is suppressed. What causes our immune system to function inappropriately or to switch to "bad" immunity? Chronic stress, environmental toxins, and inadequate nutrition are the top three reasons.

If the two arms of your immune system could be balanced by enhancing Th-1 cells and decreasing the activity of Th-2 cells, many chronic diseases would disappear. Immunologists are searching for a drug that does exactly that, yet nature already supplies us with some powerful plant nutrients and nutritional supplements that accomplish the job very effectively. For optimal immunity, we want to keep our immune system in a Th-1 or "good" state while regulating Th-2 function.

Cytotoxic T-Cells: Cytotoxic T-cells (also known as killer T-cells, but I will refer to them as cytotoxic so as not to cause confusion with natural killer cells) rush to the site of the invasion and hook onto abnormal, malignant (cancerous), or infected cells. The surface receptors on cytotoxic T-cells are customized to identify specific invaders and then kill the invader directly by injecting a lethal cytokine. They also release another substance that improves the macrophages' appetite and digestion, entices more macrophages to the site of infection, and encourages those macrophages to remain there.

Cytotoxic T-cells are similar to natural killer cells in that they discharge a toxic enzyme, but they are not the voracious eaters that NK cells are. Like NK cells, cytotoxic T-cells secrete interferons, immune factors that prevent the reproduction of viruses and enhance the killing action of the T-cells themselves. Cytotoxic T-cells are also effective against cancer cells and slow-growing bacteria such as tuberculosis.

Suppressor T-Cells: After an infection, suppressor T-cells close down some of the immune response operations. They stop the release of cytokines from cytotoxic T-cells and the production of antibodies. Suppressor T-cells help maintain the immune system's balance until the next invasion begins. A healthy ratio of T-helper cells to suppressor T-cells is 2:1. When there are not enough suppressor T-cells, B-cells continue to produce antibodies in an unregulated fashion and throw the body into distress.

Thousands of microscopic reactions occur on a daily basis. They are quick and accurate and take place prior to any appearance of symptoms. The communication between these billions of T-cells allows us to function optimally.

Cytokines

Cytokines, or immunoregulating factors, are protein messengers with very important immune functions. They act as biochemical messengers and elicit many different responses from immune cells.

Researchers have focused on immune system enhancement to win the war on cancer. They have synthesized cytokines—such as interleukin-2, interferon, and tumor necrosis factor (TNF)—and made them available as prescription drugs. When used in very large doses as immunotherapies to treat certain cancers, these cytokines have shown some positive results. Kaposi's sarcoma, hairy cell leukemia, and renal cell carcinoma reacted well, but unfortunately not without serious side effects, which included the suppression of bone marrow, severe weight loss, and liver damage. Nutritional science has made progress in the field of immunotherapy, and discovered that many natural substances can increase the body's ability to produce these cytokines without side effects.

Interleukins

At this stage of research, more than 30 interleukins (IL) have been identified. I will discuss the most common: IL-1, IL-2, IL-4, IL-6, IL-8, IL-10, and IL-12.

Interleukin-1: Interleukin-1 is a cytokine that induces fever, which, as discussed earlier, slows down pathogens or kills them. Raising the temperature only two or three degrees can be enough to do the job. Macrophages are the greatest producers of IL-1, which encourages T-cells to increase IL-2 production. Yet if macrophages are continually stimulated by using agents classified as "immune boosters," the IL-1 that is released will eventually promote too much IL-6, which is a potent inflammatory interleukin; excessive amounts of IL-6 are implicated in many diseases.

Scientists have discovered that excessive IL-1 is associated with depression, arthritis, and many other inflammatory diseases, including fibromyalgia. IL-1 breaks down collagen and increases the bad prostaglandins, thus causing pain.

Interleukin-2: Interleukin-2, secreted mainly by T-helper-1 cells, signals natural killer cells to attack and also increases the NK cells' killing action. It also sends a message to all T-cells to release more IL-2 as required, thus increasing their efforts to kill even more invaders. It is especially effective in enhancing immune responses against tumors. Interleukin-2 is an extremely powerful immunomodulator because it promotes the production of more T-helper-1 cells and controls overactive T-helper-2 cells.

Interleukin-4: Interleukin-4, secreted by T-helper-2 cells, optimizes the antibody production of B-cells, specifically the immunoglobulins IgG and IgE (they will be discussed a little later). IL-4 promotes the allergic response and inhibits the effect of macrophages. Research on the effects of lowering IL-4 shows that IgE antibody activity was suppressed, thus reducing allergic responses. In response to an allergen, T-helper-2 cells secrete IL-4 and then B-cells mature into plasma cells and secrete IgE antibodies. IgE then attaches to mast cells and they release histamine. Histamine causes the itchy skin, red eyes, runny nose, clogged mucous membranes, and more.

Interleukin-6: Interleukin-6 is secreted by T-helper-2 cells and stimulates antibody production in B-cells. Inflammation, allergic conditions (especially eczema), and autoimmune disorders are related to abnormal production of IL-6. In asthmatics IL-6 causes lung tissue damage that, if not controlled, can lead to reliance on steroid medications and puffers. IL-6, a powerful pro-inflammatory messenger that causes pain and massive inflammation in rheumatoid arthritis and other autoimmune disorders, is also involved in promoting osteoporosis. Certain nutrients control the action of IL-6, including plant sterols and sterolins, vitamins D and E, fish oils, glutathione, and magnesium. (See the actions of each nutrient in Chapter 5.)

IL-6 can also be overstimulated by excessive use of echinacea. Research performed at Bastyr University in Seattle, Washington, in 2000 set out to prove that if we took echinacea every day, we would be able to prevent or dramatically reduce the occur-

> **Colds and Stress**
>
> Scientists have found a link between the cause of the common cold and stress. When we are under stress, interleukin-6 is secreted by our immune system. IL-6 is known to suppress our immune function, allowing viruses a chance to replicate and cause illness. Sheldon Cohen, MD, of Carnegie Mellon University in Pittsburgh, says the connection between psychological stress (the mind-body connection) and infection by respiratory viruses is clear. Cohen and his colleagues had established in earlier studies that stress was a risk factor for colds and flu, but could not find the direct link. Now with the confirmation that IL-6 causes immune suppression, they are confident that stress reduction will reduce the occurrence of respiratory illness.

rence of colds and flu. Two groups were studied; one group received echinacea while the other group received a fake pill known as a placebo. After many months the research was evaluated. To the researchers' surprise, the group that received echinacea every day had more colds and flu than the group that received the fake pill. Shocking? No. Echinacea stimulates macrophages that then release IL-1, which in the short term has a positive effect of making more immune cells respond to invaders and makes them better killing machines. But when echinacea is given every day over a long term, it may promote IL-1 to then promote the secretion of IL-6 from Th-2 cells. IL-6, when overstimulated, promotes a cascade of inflammatory responses, the activation of antibodies, and more. Some viruses actually use IL-6 to replicate and we do not want to enhance IL-6 in many viral infections. The German Commission E, the bible for herbs, states that echinacea should not be taken over the long term and it is contraindicated (meaning we should not take it) for autoimmune diseases and HIV. Echinacea was designed to be taken at the onset of a cold or flu or to jump-start the immune system. Take it for the duration of a cold.

Interleukin-8: Interleukin-8 is a pro-inflammatory messenger secreted by the endothelium (cells lining the internal cavities of the body), T-cells, and macrophages. When calcium is low in the blood, IL-8 acts as a translator in the communication between the parathyroid hormone and osteoclasts, telling the osteoclasts to release calcium from the bone to the blood. The secretion of too much Interleukin-8 can promote osteoporosis.

Interleukin-10: Interleukin-10 has an immunosuppressant action on T-cells, decreasing the rate of Th-1 proliferation in localized environments when the body deems that Th-2 would be more appropriate in the area. In tandem with IL-4, it influences the switch from the good Th-1 to the inflammatory Th-2. IL-10 stimulates B-cell activity.

Interleukin-12: Interleukin-12 is secreted by macrophages in retaliation against viruses or bacteria. IL-12 influences virgin T-cells to become Th-1, which is more beneficial in fighting bacteria and viruses than Th-2, which is more effective on parasites. IL-12 also encourages NK cells to release gamma-interferon and stimulate killing activity.

Interferons, the Virus Killer

Interferons are the first strike against most viruses and a very powerful one at that. There are three kinds of interferons: alpha, beta, and gamma. The alpha and beta interferons send a signal to nearby cells that a virus is in the area and if the cells become infected, they must commit suicide (called apoptosis). This act prevents the virus from replicating itself within the cell and then infecting the surrounding cells. Gamma-interferon, secreted by T-cells and NK cells, revs up the macrophages for duty and the B-cells for production of antibody IgG. As mentioned earlier, it also stimulates aggression in NK cells. Attempts to synthesize interferon have not been very successful. Synthetic prescription interferon is used in cancer, hepatitis C, and autoimmune disorders, often with poor results and severe side effects.

Tumor Necrosis Factor

When macrophages become hyperactive, they make and release the cytokine tumor necrosis factor (TNF). It induces fever, can kill some tumors and virus-infected cells, and sparks other immune cells into action. TNF can also bind to tumors that have TNF receptors on their surface and can cause a tumor to commit suicide. Overproduction of TNF by macrophages can aggravate the joint inflammation experienced by rheumatoid arthritis sufferers. Patients in recent clinical studies who were given an antibody to deactivate the TNF showed improvement. In addition to interferon, scientists have synthesized tumor necrosis factor.

MORE IMMUNE HEROES

B-Cells

Every day the body creates about a billion B-cells. Born in the bone marrow, they eventually take up residence in the lymph nodes; unlike T-cells, they are unaffected by the thymus and they do not travel around in the blood. The role of the B-cell is to produce and secrete antibodies, and each B-cell is specific to one unique antigen or invader. With a little help from T-cells, B-cells maintain antibody production against antigens. They introduce or present antigens to the T-cells, a necessary step before T-cells can do their work.

Upon finding an intruder, T-cells signal B-cells to begin producing antibodies. B-cells evolve into plasma cells, and produce millions of antibodies unique to that intruder. As antibodies are completed, they are released into the bloodstream to find an antigen and hook onto it, thereby tagging it for destruction. More than one antibody can latch onto an antigen. This can either completely inactivate the invader or at least delay it long enough for other immune cells to arrive and kill it.

Some plasma cells become the historians that memorize the invader's antigens. These memory B-cells will live a long life so as to be available in case another invasion arises that requires the same set of antibodies. The next time around, the memory B-cells will make antibodies more quickly and will attack the invader more forcefully. The plasma cells that are not destined to become memory B-cells will die in about four or five days. During that short-lived time, however, antibodies will be released at an astounding rate of 2000 per second. Once an antigen has triggered an immune response, it is marked for life because memory cells are like elephants—they never forget.

Antibodies: The B-cells produce five classes of antibodies known as immunoglobulins (Ig): IgA, IgE, IgG, IgM, and IgD. IgD is rare and as yet its activity is not clear, so we will discuss only the first four.

IgA is ill equipped for tagging invaders in the blood, so most IgA is found in the mucous membranes, sweat, saliva, tears, and milk. It acts like a bouncer, pushing invaders completely out of the body or preventing them from entering in the first place. When babies receive IgA from their mothers' breast milk, it goes directly to the mucosal lining of their intestines. It is needed there to fight the germs that babies ingest when they explore their world by putting things in their mouths. People with immune deficiency usually have low amounts of IgA in the gastrointestinal tract.

IgE is identified in allergic reactions. Large cells in the connective tissue called mast cells secrete histamine, a substance that facilitates allergic reactions. IgE releases the histamine and if too much histamine enters the system, as during a severe allergic reaction, it may induce anaphylactic shock that can be fatal. IgE's protective mechanism also entails inflammatory reactions that can combat parasitic infections. Histamine is a powerful parasite-killing agent. Other inflammatory responses such as hay fever are also intended to be protective.

IgG is the most prolific antibody. It is exceptional at hooking onto pathogens and making them more appetizing for phagocytes. IgG covers microorganisms and is specifically trained to kill certain bacteria and viruses. IgG combats intracellular viruses by boring holes through cell membranes and accessing the cell's internal contents. There are four subclasses of IgG, each with its own special abilities, so if one of them is depleted, it can seriously impair immune function. IgG is also the antibody that a mother passes on to her fetus through the placenta. This supply of IgG is enough to last until several months after birth when the baby is able to produce its own.

IgM is the antibody that B-cells make the most of when they first start out. IgM accelerates the chain reaction that complement requires to spur on the phagocytes and it also neutralizes pathogens by hooking onto them, which prevents them from infecting a host cell. IgM is a large antibody, so it can operate only in the bloodstream

If something goes haywire in the production of these chemical messengers, it may lead to serious immune dysfunction and in some cases the production of autoantibodies. Autoantibodies identify and attack the body's "self" cells. The inflammation that results is usually specific to particular areas in the body. A few of the disorders that arise from autoantibody production include rheumatoid arthritis, which affects the joints; Sjogren's syndrome, where the exocrine glands malfunction and are eventually destroyed; multiple sclerosis, in which the myelin sheath surrounding nerves are destroyed; Crohn's disease, whereby the colon cells are attacked; systemic lupus erythematosus, which affects connective tissue; pernicious anemia, a vitamin B_{12} deficiency brought about by autoimmune gastritis; and Type I diabetes mellitus, which involves the destruction of beta cells of the pancreas.

SIGNS THAT YOUR IMMUNE SYSTEM IS DYSFUNCTIONAL

- allergies, asthma
- cancer, autoimmune disease, and chronic infections
- candida yeast overgrowth, bad breath, smelly feet, and fungal infections
- continual fatigue
- frequent colds and flus (anything more than one occurrence per year)
- heart disease
- herpes (cold sores) outbreaks
- painful joints and muscles
- parasite infections
- psoriasis, eczema, hives, and acne

The immune system is the commanding general that stands guard over the body, preparing to send its troops to do battle at the least sign of provocation. It has trillions upon trillions of soldiers embodied as phagocytes, complement, natural killer cells, T-cells, B-cells, and antibodies, all working together to prevent an invasion from outside pathogens and to destroy those that lurk within. Through regular surveillance, intruders are identified and expelled or marked for execution. The historians (called memory B-cells) will remember each unique invader, enabling a more rapid retaliation if the unlucky intruder makes repeated attempts at an invasion.

When the body's immune system is working optimally, it is a powerful force to be reckoned with and very few bacteria, viruses, fungi, and parasites can gain any ground. Sometimes, though, the immune system is too active in seeking and destroying cells and the result is friendly fire or the annihilation of the body's own cells—called autoimmune disease—which will be discussed later in the chapter and throughout the book.

THE IMMUNE SYSTEM AND PAIN

The immune system is involved in promoting pain and inflammation. If the body is injured or has arthritis, for example, several chemicals and immune factors send signals to the brain that cause us to feel pain and create inflammation. If we could inhibit the release of these chemicals and factors, we would be able to control pain and inflammation.

The immune factors associated with pain and inflammation include IL-1, IL-6, IL-8, and IL-12. Carl Germano and William Cabot, in their book *Nature's Pain Killers,* state that "IL-1 is directly responsible for breaking down collagen and other connective tissue increasing prostaglandin production and dilating blood vessels—all actions that create pain. IL-6 is a powerful pro-inflammatory factor that contributes to the symptoms in many painful and inflammatory conditions."

Things That Promote the Switch to "Bad" Immunity

- sugar suppresses certain immune cells, mainly macrophages and NK cells
- fats containing trans fatty acids; fried foods and certain margarines suppress immunity
- stress causes high cortisol levels, low DHEA, suppresses immunity, and/or causes overactive immunity
- environmental toxins, including pesticides, lead, mercury, and other heavy metals, suppress immunity and promote inflammation
- tobacco and alcohol suppress immunity and promote high cortisol and inflammation

---

COX-2

Some "bad" prostaglandins also cause pain and are made from an enzyme called cyclooxygenase-2, or COX-2. The COX enzyme is actually two enzymes. COX-1 provides the very important function of regulating the balance of the environments in the stomach and kidneys, a type of housekeeping for the body. COX-2 creates prostaglandins from arachidonic acid. Those prostaglandins generate the inflammation that causes pain. The challenge facing researchers is neutralizing the COX-2 enzyme activity without suppressing the beneficial COX-1 enzyme. While there are new COX-2 medications available that may do a good job of decreasing the inflammation and pain, they are not without side effects, such as preventing gastric ulcers from healing, inflaming colitis, and being ineffective in soothing the gastric indigestion associated with non-steroidal anti-inflammatory drug use.

Serious Side Effects from NSAIDs

Nonsteroidal anti-inflammatory drugs (NSAIDs), including Motrin, Ansaid, Clinoril, Neproxen, and others, are prescribed to control the pain associated with arthritis. Individuals taking NSAIDs may not be aware of the side effects. Over 20 percent will get an ulcer or gastrointestinal bleeding or even kidney and liver damage. Over 120,000 people per year are hospitalized and 18,000 die from the side effects of NSAIDs.

Joint damage is another side effect from long-term use of NSAIDs. Yes, you read it correctly! NSAIDs cause joint destruction. Doesn't it seem strange that you may be taking these painkillers for the pain associated with the joint destruction caused by your arthritis, but the NSAIDs prescribed by your doctor actually *cause* joint destruction? It is very clear in the published research. One study found that the hip joints of patients taking NSAIDs had greater joint destruction than those patients not taking NSAIDs.

New COX-2 Inhibitor Not So Safe: Celebrex, a new type of NSAID that is touted as much safer than the NSAIDs mentioned above, may not be so safe. Research performed at the University of Pennsylvania Medical Center has found that Celebrex may increase the risk of heart attack and/or stroke. Celebrex is a sulfa drug, like some antibiotics and oral diabetes drugs, so those with sulfa allergies must avoid it. Sulfa allergies affect 5 percent of the population. Many arthritis sufferers taking Celebrex have found that the gastrointestinal problems they had with NSAIDs still occur when taking Celebrex. Simon Huang, MD, a Vancouver rheumatologist who led local clinical trials on Celebrex, stated in the *Vancouver Sun* that "although Celebrex has been found to reduce ulcers in the upper GI tract the effects on the lower GI tract are unknown."

Prednisone Has Long-Term Side Effects

Prednisone is reserved for the most serious inflammatory, allergic, and autoimmune reactions. Steroid medications like Prednisone can increase your risk of heart disease, diabetes, eye damage, severe osteoporosis, poor wound healing, weight gain, and even cancer. Use steroids as the absolute last resort.

Acetaminophen Dangers

Acetaminophen, which is used to relieve pain and is commonly sold as Tylenol, also has dangerous side effects. Unintentional overdoses are very common. If you are in severe pain, you may be tempted to take too many acetaminophen tablets. Follow the dosing recommendations carefully. Liver toxicity can occur when taking only an extra couple of doses per day. Mixing acetaminophen with alcohol causes acute liver failure. The number one reason for liver transplants in the United States is acetaminophen overdose and misuse.

Thankfully, nature provides some exciting remedies that treat the cause of pain and inflammation, as I will discuss in Chapter 8.

THE IMMUNE SYSTEM AND STRESS

When we are exposed to stressors, our adrenal glands secrete the stress hormone cortisol, causing a corresponding drop in our antiaging and immune-enhancing hormone dehydroepiandrosterone (DHEA). A tremendous body of research has shown that when our level of cortisol goes up, DHEA drops, and when DHEA is normal, cortisol also normalizes. Low DHEA levels are seen in those who are immune compromised, have arteriosclerosis (hardening of the arteries), diabetes, and lupus. If you have one of these diseases, ask your doctor to test your DHEAs and cortisol levels.

Cortisol helps the body maintain homeostasis (equilibrium) in the face of stressors, counteracts inflammatory and allergic reactions, and controls the metabolism of protein and carbohydrates. Cortisol is a very misunderstood hormone. Balance is the key. In naturally low doses, it stimulates the immune system, and in high doses (as prescribed in synthetic drug form) it can be immune suppressing. Remember that cortisol plays a role in counteracting inflammatory responses in the immune system, so when cortisol is not available because the adrenal glands have become exhausted from too much stress, inflammation is allowed to continue unchecked.

The immune system also responds to stressors and the secretion of cortisol by causing certain immune cells to secrete the pro-inflammatory cytokines interleukin-1 (IL-1) and interleukin-6 (IL-6). These cytokines are both involved in inflammation and IL-6 in particular is thought to worsen the symptoms of autoimmune diseases and fibromyalgia. Interleukin-6 has been found to act as a growth factor in several tumors and cause calcium to be released from bone, thus promoting osteoporosis. Some viruses also use IL-6 to replicate. We must control the release of these cytokines if we want to enhance immunity and reduce degenerative diseases.

In the presence of stressors, the immune system and endocrine system work as an integrated circuit. Deficiencies in the immune system and abnormalities in the cross talk with the endocrine system can make a

Early Risers and High Cortisol

According to a study published in *New Scientist*, British researchers have discovered that people who wake between 5:22 a.m. and 7:21 a.m. have higher levels of the stress hormone cortisol than do those who wake later, regardless of when they went to bed. The early risers' levels remained high all day. If you are trying to keep your cortisol level normal, do not rise too early. If your schedule requires you to get up before 7:21 a.m., you can take sterols and sterolins, which regulate cortisol. Remember—perpetually high cortisol levels are associated with weaker immune systems.

person more susceptible to developing chronic inflammatory disease, auto-immune disease like lupus, rheumatoid arthritis, a reduced ability to fight infections, osteoporosis, muscle atrophy, rapid aging, poor antibody production against vaccines, and more. Modulating or keeping cortisol levels in balance through a healthy diet, nutritional supplements, and stress reduction are key to disease prevention.

THE DANGERS OF VACCINATION

What Is Autoimmunity?

Autoimmune disorders occur when the immune system begins to attack the body. Autoimmune diseases can involve any system in the body, although some organs and tissues appear to be more susceptible than others. There are over 80 different autoimmune diseases, including anky-losing spondylitis, rheumatoid arthritis, systemic lupus erythematosus, myasthenia gravis, Graves' disease, Crohn's or celiac disease, insulin-dependent diabetes mellitus, idiopathic thrombocytopenic purpura, psori-asis, pernicious anemia, and autoimmune hemolytic anemia, to name a few. Five percent of our adult population is afflicted with one or more auto-immune diseases and two-thirds of those are women. Not even children are safe from the devastation of certain childhood autoimmune disorders such as juvenile diabetes, juvenile arthritis, lupus, alopecia, and colitis.

Autoimmune diseases are usually diagnosed in early adulthood, gener-ally after a bout of illness or severe stress. Remember that stress and illness cause imbalances in your immune system and are causally linked to the diseases of today. Often people affected by autoimmune disorders will experience periods of remission when the symptoms disappear alternat-ing with periods of acute episodes when symptoms flare up. Others will see their symptoms progressively worsen and their condition deteriorate.

Hereditary factors are involved in your predisposition to the disease, but as is found in studies involving twins, if one twin is diagnosed with an autoimmune disease, the other has a higher risk but does not neces-sarily acquire the disease. Many other factors are involved in the immune system turning upon the body.

Several hypotheses of the cause of autoimmunity have been postulated, including viral or bacterial infection, stress, and genetic susceptibility. Infection is considered the main culprit as scientists have realized that it often precedes the onset of an autoimmune diagnosis. Viruses and bacte-ria have devised methods to avoid detection, thereby allowing themselves access to the body. Certain viruses provide the immune system with strings of amino acids that are so similar to those of the body that they are thought of as "self" cells until some anomaly tells the body otherwise. As a result, the immune system can become confused and think it is attacking an invader when it is actually attacking itself. This is called molecular mimicry.

So why is it that everyone who is exposed to a virus does not acquire an autoimmune disease? Many factors have to be in place for the immune system to become disrupted. Our genetic makeup and a weakened immune system due to stress, poor diet, or exposure to environmental toxins all determine whether or not our immunity is affected and the body damaged by itself.

Lack of Tolerance

To some degree, autoimmunity is present in all of us. Scientists have hypothesized that autoantibodies function to remove "self" waste, for example, removing broken-down DNA with anti-DNA antibodies. However, why is it that one person with active autoimmunity is the picture of health, while another person becomes ill and may die?

When autoimmunity functions as it should to keep the body free of debris and waste products, it is called tolerance. T-cells with a propensity to kill "self" cells are usually deleted in the thymus during maturation. B-cells, which would normally attack the remaining T-cells that have anti-self receptors, receive a signal that prevents them from activating and destroying the ones left over. When tolerance breaks down, autoimmune disorders appear, but tolerance does not break down overnight. The immune system has layer upon layer of checks and balances to prevent breaches in the system. All or several of the "security checkpoints" must be neutralized for tolerance to be jeopardized and result in disease.

This explanation fits with certain characteristics of autoimmune disease. First, there is usually exposure to more than one environmental factor (poisons or toxins, severe stress, viral or bacterial infections) and there is often a hereditary factor. Second, most autoimmune diseases generally advance at a slower rate compared to the rate at which the immune system fights foreign microbes. This characteristic may indicate that some of the security checkpoints are still trying to do their job until they can no longer do so. Third, there are characteristic periods of remission and relapse throughout the illnesses that may indicate tolerance is back in control for a while.

Traces of Origin

Often the onset of an autoimmune disorder can be traced back to a viral or bacterial infection, although some researchers believe a faulty or permissive gene must still be present. Salmonella, chlamydia, yersinia, and mycobacterium tuberculosis have all been linked to immune dysfunction. Plucky viruses and bacteria can devise ways of hiding in the body by looking like they belong there. Viruses (like the adenovirus type 2) have amino acid sequences that are very much like the myelin proteins that shield nerves. During the body's attack on the virus, it gets confused and is unable to distinguish between the myelin and the virus. Eventually the immune cells destroy the myelin by mistake. This is what happens in those with multiple sclerosis.

Invaders Wreak Havoc: Coxsakie virus and other enteroviruses are now thought to be responsible for the majority of cases of human myocarditis. Rheumatoid arthritis is thought to have a strong association with mycobacterial infection and often tetracycline antibiotics have been able to destroy the bacterium. In Sjogren's syndrome, epithelial cells from a majority of patients were reported to be heavily infected with the Epstein-Barr virus compared to normal controls. Viruses or bacteria alone cannot cause autoimmune disease, but they are a factor to consider. Autoimmune specialists also state that dysfunction in the first line of defense against infection in the innate immune system is likely a large contributing factor, allowing viruses to gain entry and take hold in the first place.

Drug-Induced Autoimmunity: Drug- or chemical-induced autoimmune disease has been studied in lupus in which isoniazid and hydralazine have induced a lupus-like syndrome. Autoimmune thyroiditis can be initiated by taking too much supplemental iodine. Monkeys that were fed alfalfa seeds developed a type of systemic lupus erythematosus-like syndrome.

Metal Poisoning: Metals have also been studied as a possible initiator of autoimmune disease. Researchers have found that high concentrations of copper might be implicated in scleroderma. Interestingly, when scleroderma patients were given D-penicillamine, a metal chelator that removes copper, their disease responded positively. Mercury is a heavy metal that also plays a role in promoting autoimmunity. One example of this is heavy metal poisoning, which some physicians and health researchers think is a causal factor in autoimmune diseases. It has been suggested that thimersol, a mercury derivate and preservative added to some vaccines, may be implicated in autoimmune disease that develops after vaccination. Autoimmune diseases are more frequent in countries where vaccination is widespread.

Excessive Stress: Extreme or unrelenting stress increases the secretion of cortisol and inflammatory immune factors and activates B-cells to produce antibodies. Many people with an autoimmune disorder will claim that their disease began after the death of a loved one or a seriously stressful event. (See Chapter 6, page 125, for more on stress and autoimmune diseases.)

A COMPREHENSIVE BUT NOT DEFINITIVE LIST
OF AUTOIMMUNE DISEASES

Autoimmune Diseases

Addison's Disease (adrenal glands)

Alopecia Areata (hair follicles)

Ankylosing Spondylitis (joints of the spine)

Antiphospholipid Syndrome (phospholipids that surround the cell)

Autoimmune Hemolytic Anemia (red blood cell membranes)

Autoimmune Hepatitis (liver)

Behcet's Disease (blood vessels)

Bullous Pemphigoid (skin)

Celiac Sprue-Dermatitis (bowel)

Cystitis (Interstitial) (bladder)

Chronic Inflammatory Demyelinating Polyneuropathy (nerve roots and myelin sheaths)

Churg-Strauss Syndrome (blood vessels, white blood cells, many organs)

Cicatricial Pemphigoid (mucous membranes, skin, eyes, throat, genitalia)

CREST Syndrome (nervous system, skin, connective tissues, organs)

Cold Agglutinin Disease (red blood cells)

Crohn's Disease (bowel)

Discoid Lupus (skin)

Fibromyalgia-Fibromyositis (muscles)

Graves' Disease (thyroid)

Guillain-Barré (nervous system)

Hashimoto's Thyroiditis (thyroid)

Idiopathic Pulmonary Fibrosis (lungs)

Idiopathic Thrombocytopenia Purpura (ITP) (platelets)

IgA Nephropathy (kidneys)

Insulin-Dependent Diabetes (pancreatic beta-cells)

Juvenile Arthritis (joints)

Lichen Planus (mucous membranes of mouth, eyes, skin, genitalia)

Lupus (DNA, platelets, most tissues)

Ménière's Disease (inner ear)

Mixed Connective Tissue Disease (connective tissues)

Multiple Sclerosis (brain and spinal cord)

Myasthenia Gravis (nerves and muscles)

Pemphigus Vulgaris (skin and mucous membranes)

Pernicious Anemia (gastric parietal cells)

Polyarteritis Nodosa (arteries)

Polychondritis (cartilage)

Polyglandular Syndromes (glands)

Polymyalgia Rheumatica (muscles)

Polymyositis and Dermatomyositis (connective tissues and muscles)

Primary Biliary Cirrhosis (bile ducts)

Psoriasis (skin)

Raynaud's Phenomenon (arteries)

Reiter's Syndrome (eyes, joints, urethra)

Rheumatic Fever (group A beta-hemolytic streptococcal infection)

Rheumatoid Arthritis (cartilage and synovial joint linings)

Sarcoidosis (many body systems)

Scleroderma (skin, connective tissues, organs)

Sjogren's Syndrome (eyes and moisture-producing glands)

Stiff-Man Syndrome (central nervous system)

Takayasu Arteritis (arteries)

Temporal Arteritis/Giant Cell Arteritis (arteries)

Urticaria (mast cell disease)

Uveitis (eyes)

Vasculitis (blood vessels)

Vitiligo (melanocytes-skin pigmentation-containing cells)

Wegener's Granulomatosis (blood vessels and tissues)

This list, compiled from *The Autoimmune Diseases,* illustrates how diverse and varied autoimmune diseases can be, yet regardless which organs or tissue systems are attacked, the process is basically the same—autoantibodies and inflammatory cytokines are attacking certain tissues.

The Th-1/Th-2 Balance and Autoimmune Disease: Much research is underway to determine the role that T-helper-1 (Th-1) and T-helper-2 (Th-2) cells and their chemical messengers play in the development, maintenance, and the remission of the disease. T-helper-1-dominated responses are excellent at killing infectious organisms, including those that are living inside our cells. However, if the T-helper-1 response is not effective or if it responds continually it can become dangerous to our health because our macrophages and cytotoxic T-cells would not be controlled. As mentioned earlier, when macrophages are continually stimulated, they can have a negative effect, especially in relation to autoimmune disease. In contrast, T-helper-2 responses are not very effective at fighting infectious agents, but they are protective against gastrointestinal invaders and they down-regulate T-helper-1 mechanisms. As a result, T-helper-2 cells have a positive role in protecting us against excessive virus fighting. Yet, when T-helper-2 cells are overactive, they promote autoimmunity. Researchers have been trying to clearly pinpoint which side of the T-helper cells is responsible for promoting autoimmune disease. So far, they have discovered that a balance between these two helper cells is crucial in preventing and treating autoimmune disease.

Only a few of the autoimmune diseases have been extensively studied to determine which T-helper cell is involved in the initiation of the disease. Researchers have found that several organ-specific autoimmune diseases are promoted by overactive T-helper-1 cells and their cytokines; they include multiple sclerosis, Hashimoto's thyroiditis, Crohn's disease, and insulin-dependent diabetes mellitus. Whereas Graves' disease, rheumatoid arthritis, Sjogren's syndrome, systemic lupus erythematosus, systemic sclerosis, and idiopathic pulmonary fibrosis are clearly related to overactive T-helper-2 cells and their respective cytokines. By encouraging our immune system to switch from one type of T-helper cell dominance to the other, researchers have been able to control many autoimmune diseases. Chronic autoimmune diseases especially are related to the promotion of T-helper-2 cells. Noel Rose and Ian Mackay, the authors of *The Autoimmune Diseases*, state that "these findings suggest that by modulating the Th-1 or Th-2 cells' cytokines to stop the development of autoimmune disease new therapeutic strategies can be found." Immune modulation (balance) is the basis for all the treatment recommendations for each autoimmune disorder.

Vaccination and Autoimmunity: "Vaccinosis," a Dangerous Liaison?

There is growing concern about the general safety of vaccines and the connection between the development of autoimmune disease and vaccination. In 1976, 45 million adults received an influenza vaccination (swine-flu virus) as part of a government-sponsored program. The incidence rate of Guillain-Barré syndrome (a neurological disorder characterized by motor paralysis with mild sensory disturbances) jumped from a factor of four to eight. Vaccines have also been evaluated for their possible risk of arthritis and rheumatoid arthritis. The following vaccines have been associated with the initiation of arthritis: polio, mumps, rubella, typhoid, tetanus, hepatitis B and C, smallpox, and diphtheria. There have also been many documented cases of systemic lupus erythematosus developing after the injection of recombinant hepatitis B vaccine.

There has been much debate over the hepatitis B vaccine and its association with multiple sclerosis. In France over 600 people reported feeling ill after their inoculation. Their symptoms covered a range of illnesses, but many were related to autoimmune disorders or the nervous system. Some cases had definite documentation that showed demyelinization in the central nervous system appearing days or weeks after a hepatitis B shot.

The February 2000, volume 14 issue of *The Journal of Autoimmunity* has several articles evaluating the link between autoimmune disease and vaccination. Most authors, after reporting all of the potential risks and documented cases of vaccine-induced autoimmune disease, state that the risk-benefit equation is still in favor of vaccination, yet after reading all of the often-not-discussed risks in Catherine J.M Diodati's book *Immunization: History, Ethics, Law and Health*, I don't agree. You should read her book to ensure that if you vaccinate, you understand the risks involved.

Catherine was so kind as to let me reprint a section of her book that looks at the difference between natural and artificial immunity. You can purchase her book on Amazon.com or directly from her (see below).

We have discussed the cells and organs of the immune system, the cytokines they release, and the different environmental issues that affect immunity, but what about the type of immunity that is induced when we vaccinate our children? How does that differ from natural immunity?

Natural Versus Artificial Immunity:
Differences Affecting the Immune Response

Catherine Diodati, MA

When a disease is encountered naturally, the body reacts quickly by initiating an immune response at the point of entry as well as throughout the body where the various elements of the immune system become primed. Essentially, as the pathogens attempt to overtake the cells they are continually weakened and eliminated as they pass through a series of interdependent protective levels. In most cases, excluding tetanus and rabies among the "vaccine preventable diseases," the respiratory and gastrointestinal systems (secretory IgA systems) encounter the pathogens first. As soon as the body recognizes their presence, the immune response is initiated. This immediate response reduces the impact of infection, often eliminating disease even before symptoms become manifest. In the case of natural infection, "it has been estimated that the frequency of asymptomatic infections outnumber clinical illnesses by at least one hundred-fold," testifying to the efficacy and importance of the secretory/mucosal immune response.

Vaccines, on the other hand, bypass many of the body's initial immune defenses. This may be likened to a Trojan horse, wherein the "invaders" have been allowed to bypass the usual primary defensive mechanisms to initiate an internal "surprise attack," causing the defensive players to scramble into action. Unlike natural infection, which immediately functions to weaken the pathogen and simultaneously send out chemical "messages" to activate other immune system elements, there is no opportunity to "prime" the immune system as a whole. In this way, vaccines do not elicit an immune response that can be considered comparable to natural immunity. In fact, the immune system is so hard pressed to respond to the internal "attack" that it compensates by utilizing far more immune cells than it normally would during natural infection.

The differences in immune response demands are particularly significant for infants and young children, whose immune systems will not be fully developed until about age 12. Theoretically speaking, during the course of a typical childhood infection (e.g., chickenpox), approximately 3–7% of the body's immune capacity (e.g., plasma cells or lymphocytes) are utilized in eliminating disease whereas the immune response to immunization could utilize approximately 30–70% of that same child's immune capacity.

It should be emphasized that, once an immune body (plasma cell or lymphocyte) becomes committed to a given antigen, it becomes incapable of responding to other antigens or challenges.

For the infant, or young child, this means that an enormous percentage of his or her immune cells have been committed to the specific antigens introduced by the vaccine(s). The pathogens that are introduced through immunization are derived from 3–5 different viruses and/or bacteria and unlike natural infection, multiple diseases, chemicals, drugs and additives are introduced into the body simultaneously. The immune system must recognize and act upon a variety of pathogens all at once. The long-term potential consequences may be a greater susceptibility to infections, allergies, diabetes, cancers and various mental and behavioral disorders because the maturing immune system has been overwhelmed.

In most cases, vaccination series are initiated when a child reaches two months of age, long before the immune system has matured. In the developed world, it is rare that infants and very young children would encounter the diseases against which they are vaccinated: most endemic childhood diseases tend to demonstrate a marked increase as children enter school and they are exposed to many other people. When they do encounter pathogens naturally, they have the advantage of a secretory immune response, which is bypassed during immunization. Recent studies have also indicated that natural infections actually assist the immune system to mature while vaccines tend to depress cellular (e.g., T cell) immunity. In one study examining the tetanus vaccine, 11 healthy adults were found to have experienced a significant, albeit temporary, drop in helper T cells; in four of the subjects studied, "the T-helper cells dropped to levels seen in active AIDS patients." Natural infections, on the other hand, appear to stimulate and strengthen the immune system.

Furthermore, it is extremely unlikely that such young children would normally meet with the challenges presented by toxic and carcinogenic (e.g., formaldehyde) vaccine components; these simply are not present during natural infection and they add an additional burden to the immune system. It seems counter-productive to interfere with an immature immune system by unnecessarily challenging it with numerous pathogens and chemicals and, in so doing, threatening its normal development. The small amount of the immune bodies utilized during natural infection ensures that there are sufficient stores retained to respond to the various challenges presented throughout one's lifetime. The vast amounts of immune bodies utilized because the many neutralizing levels of the immune system are bypassed during vaccination have the potential to leave the body vulnerable and ultimately less capable of responding to future challenges. It is clearly unreasonable to expect that introducing disease and toxic chemicals into a body, and particularly into a body whose immune system is not completely developed, should result in improved health.

Degrees of Permanence

Both critics and proponents of immunization recognize that vaccines are indeed imperfect. A single dose of vaccine rarely, if ever, confers life-long immunity. Most vaccines are administered in a specified series, depending upon the type of vaccine and upon the recipient's age and locale, and usually booster doses are required to maintain sufficient immunity to prevent infection. Although standard vaccine schedules have been recommended for the maintenance of adequate immunity for the general populace, "there is no way of knowing how long this partial or temporary immunity will last in any given individual." If artificial immunity wanes during adolescence or adulthood, older individuals become susceptible to childhood diseases, when they present greater health risks. Even if the adult escapes infection, there remains yet another disadvantage of artificial immunity: individuals cannot confer passive immunity to their children. Natural immunity, on the other hand, provides permanent immunity and, as an added bonus, passive immunity can be passed onto one's progeny.

Diodati citing Harold E. Buttram and John Chriss Hoffman, *Vaccinations and Immune Malfunction* (Quakertown, PA: The Humanitarian Publishing Company, 1985), 50f.

Contact Catherine Diodati at Integral Aspects Incorporated, 110 Eugenie Street West, Suite 439, Windsor, Ontario N8X 4Y6, Tel (519) 972-9567, Fax (519) 966-3392

email: diodati@mnsi.net

BACTERIA: FRIEND OR FOE?

Our illogical fear of bacteria is putting the human race at risk for "superbugs" that will be able to survive no matter what agent we use to destroy them. Stuart Levy at Tufts University in Boston says that "not only will people have to stop over-using and abusing antibiotic prescriptions but they should also stop buying antibacterial soaps and detergents." Our quest to annihilate all bacteria is just plain dangerous.

Bacteria are the oldest forms of life on Earth. We need certain types of bacteria to survive. People cannot digest food without several kinds of bacteria that live in the gut. Levy says, "We should be kind to bacteria. They are our friends."

Antibacterial Agents Create Superbugs

We must understand that bacteria are necessary. By using antibacterial agents, we help to create super-bacteria that will be immune to even the strongest antibiotics. Antibacterial agents are now added to dishwashing and laundry detergents, hand soaps, infants' plastic toys, and even high chair trays. Levy's laboratory at Tufts found that E. coli bacteria can develop resistance to triclosan, one of the common antibacterial ingredients in commercial soaps. Triclosan works by acting on a single gene to kill the E. coli bacteria. They also found that tuberculosis has a similar gene. They believe it is possible that an overuse of triclosan could lead to a new antibiotic-resistant strain of tuberculosis. Creams and ointments, along with soaps, are now loaded with antibacterial agents; even these should be used cautiously as bacteria may incorporate these agents into their genetic makeup, thus allowing resistance to develop.

Antibiotic-Resistant Bacteria

Because of our overuse and misuse of antibiotics, bacteria are becoming resistant to them. We now have penicillan-resistant gonorrhea and super-strains of staphylococcus that cannot be killed by vancomycin, the most powerful antibiotic available. There are four strains of pneumonia that are also resistant to vancomycin. Sick people are dying of bacterial infections because none of the hundreds of antibiotics is working for them. Unless serious action is taken, the world is headed for an era of drug-resistant superbugs in which children could die from bacterial infections and "we are not talking science fiction," said David Scheifele, MD, of the infectious disease division at the British Columbia Children's Hospital.

Scheifele and his colleagues found that penicillan-resistant bacteria are evident in one in eight children who have pneumococcal infections. Pneumococcal infections cause pneumonia, blood infections, and meningitis in about half a million Canadian children per year. Life-threatening forms of pneumococcal bacteria are found in about 300 children a year. Penicillin, once seen as a panacea antibiotic, is rapidly losing its ability to fight certain bacteria. Vancomycin, the antibiotic that carried the most clout, is also becoming less effective. The reality is we no longer have effective treatments for common bacteria. We must realize that we are mostly at fault for this.

Antibiotic Overuse and Misuse

Everyone has experienced the cold that never seems to end. You go to your physician, who takes a throat swab and sends it to the local lab for evaluation. Then your doctor writes you a prescription for an antibiotic, but what if it is not a bacterial infection? It could be a stubborn virus. Antibiotics do not work against viruses, only bacteria. Physicians contribute to the overuse of antibiotics by continuing to prescribe antibiotics even when they are not sure if a patient has a bacterial infection. Antibiotics should be viewed as serious medications and prescribed only for bacterial infections.

Misuse of antibiotics, which includes not completing a course of therapy, allows bacteria to mutate and become resistant to future treatment. Moreover, flushing leftover antibiotics down the drain or allowing them to go to the landfill contributes to our antibiotic-resistant bacteria problem. Worse yet is saving the antibiotic to treat undiagnosed illnesses at a later date that may not be bacterial in origin.

We add to our overexposure to antibiotics by eating animal products. Domestic animals are fed large quantities of antibiotics to keep them healthy in their unnatural environments. Over 50 percent of the antibiotics produced in North America are fed to farm-raised animals indirectly in their feed or as prescribed by veterinarians. We then ingest these antibiotics when we consume the animal product. Beef, poultry, and farm-grown fish are laden with antibiotic residues. Farmers must search for safer ways to encourage animal growth and health. In the meantime we should buy organically fed and raised animals from our local marketplace.

Good Old Soap and Water

Good hygiene, especially washing your hands often and for at least one minute, is the most effective method of controlling the spread of bacteria. There may not be an antibiotic that works for every bacterium. We must change our way of thinking and realize that we should rely on our immune system to battle bacteria the way it was designed to do.

MOTHER NATURE'S IMMUNE MODULATORS

Fish Oils Control Immune Function

Omega-3 fatty (DHA/EPA) acids, which are found in cold-water fish, mackerel, sardines, salmon, and halibut, improve T-helper-1 immune cells and reduce inflammatory interleukin-6 and interleukin-1. Several research articles have shown that with the addition of omega-3 fatty acids to the diet, the production of potentially "bad" interleukin-1 and interleukin-6 was normalized and the number of the healthy T-helper-1 cells responsible for controlling the immune system increased dramatically. Rheumatoid arthritis, allergies, and immune suppression are a few of the diseases that respond to omega-3 fatty acid supplementation.

Glutathione, an Essential Immune Nutrient

No other antioxidant is as important to overall immune health as L-glutathione. It ensures that our immune cells stay predominantly in the T-helper-1 state, making the immune system better able to fight cancer, bacterial infection, and viruses. It controls IL-6, 4, and 10, effectively reducing allergic reactions and inflammation. Reduced L-glutathione, selenium, alpha lipoic acid, whey proteins, N-acetylcysteine, and L-cysteine increase glutathione levels in the body's cells.

Spirulina Enhances the Good Guys

Spirulina is a blue-green algae that is rich in antioxidants, vitamins, minerals, and other nutrients. Immunologists at the University of California at Davis School of Medicine and Medical Center found that adding spirulina to cultured immune cells significantly increased the production of infection-fighting immune factors. Their findings are published in the Fall 2000 issue of the *Journal of Medicinal Foods*. A number of animal studies have shown spirulina to be an effective immunomodulator. While extensive human studies have not been done, the UC Davis researchers found that "nutrient-rich spirulina is a potent inducer of interferon-gamma [13.6-fold increase] and a moderate stimulator of both interleukin-4 and interleukin-1 beta [3.3-fold increase]," says Eric Gershwin, professor and chief of the Division of Rheumatology, Allergy and Clinical Immunology at UC Davis.

Sterols and Sterolins, Your Daily Immune Nutrient

Sterols and sterolins are called the forgotten nutrient because although they have been studied extensively (thousands of studies have been performed), few have heard of them. They are the missing key to immunity. Researchers found that sterols and sterolins work by activating a gene on the T-helper-1 cell, enhancing the secretion of the "good" cytokines gamma-interferon and interleukin-2. As a result, the potentially "bad" inflammatory cytokines interleukin-6, 4, and 10 are controlled. *The Journal of Immunopharmacology* found that a 20–920 percent increase in T-cell response was found in subjects taking sterols and sterolins. *The International Journal of Sports Medicine* looked at marathon runners to see if the addition of sterols and sterolins would prevent the immune suppression and inflammatory reactions characteristic in high-intensity athletes. All immune parameters improved or remained stable after a marathon run in those in the treatment group and, most important, there was a decrease in interleukin-6 and an increase in DHEA. Sterols and sterolins are safe to take every day as they selectively increase an underactive immune system and/or control an overactive one. Their use in autoimmune disease (lupus, rheumatoid arthritis, etc.) is where they really shine because we have few things that put these diseases into remission. Their profound effect on the immune system will change the way we treat disease in the future.

Vitamins: Regulators of Immunity

Vitamins B_6, C, and E increase resistance to infection and improve T-helper-1–mediated immunity and the ability of cells to digest invaders and debris. All of these nutrients also reduce the damage caused by stress.

An increase in T-cells, interleukin-2, and a reduction in inflammatory agents were found in 10 subjects who took 400 mg of vitamin E and 1000 mg of vitamin C for 28 days. Low or deficient levels of vitamin E in the body are related to certain cancers, especially those of the gastrointestinal tract and lungs. Vitamin E appears to prevent cancers of the breast and prostate by inhibiting cancer cells from multiplying. A 14-year study involving 5000 British women showed that low blood levels of vitamin E increased breast cancer risk by 500 percent. Vitamin C is essential to ensure a predominance of good T-helper-1 function and vitamin B_6 speeds up the immune system's response to invaders.

Now that you understand the intricacies of the immune system and how integrated it is with other systems in the body, the next section will provide you with the knowledge necessary to optimize your immune system by keeping your digestive and cardiovascular systems in tip-top shape.

CHAPTER 4

NUTRITION:
FOODS THAT HARM,
FOODS THAT HEAL

Nutritionists and dieticians tell us that we can get our basic requirement of vitamins and minerals from the foods we eat. This is only a true statement if we are eating a varied diet of organic fruits and vegetables (seven to ten half-cup servings), lean fish, meats or poultry, whole grains, and good fats. But what if you are eating the standard American diet (SAD), full of trans fatty acids, very few vegetables and fruits, and meats loaded with hormones and antibiotics? Most people do not eat breakfast, grab something fast for lunch, and have a typical dinner that includes a piece of meat with two vegetables. Coffee is the North American breakfast food of choice.

Adequate nutrition is just not good enough anymore. The recommended daily intake (RDI) of nutrients does not provide us with the optimal level of nutrients we require to live long and disease-free lives, but only the minimal requirement to survive. Cancer, heart disease, diabetes, low IQ, miscarriages, birth defects, and immune dysfunction result when we do not consume enough nutrients to keep the cells of our body running smoothly. Environmental toxins and the excessive stress we are exposed to have bankrupted our nutritional reserves.

Food can be used as medicine either to prevent disease or for treatment and recovery from disease. Conversely our food choices can also be detrimental, yet we resist changing our diets until a health crisis forces us to rethink our nutritional choices. The following are some points for you to think about when deciding what to eat:

- Thirty nutrients are removed during the milling process of grains.
- A 1993 *Lancet* study of 85,095 healthy people found that coronary heart disease was strongly associated with the consumption of vegetable-oil margarine.

- Processed oils contain no plant sterols and sterolins, which are essential for immunity.
- Food manufacturers are only interested in shelf life.
- We are exposed to thousands of chemicals in our home and drinking water, many known to deplete nutrients in the body.
- Cholesterol-lowering medications deplete the body of coenzyme Q10, which is important for heart function.
- Only 9 percent of North Americans get adequate vitamin C in their diet.
- Birth control pills deplete vitamin B_6 and folic acid.
- We eat 150 lbs (68 kg) of sugar per person per year (that is 20 tsps/100 mL per day).

Cambridge University found that an increase in vitamin C equivalent to consuming one extra serving of a fruit or vegetable per day was associated with a 20 percent reduction in the risk of all types of mortality. The researchers conclude that small increases in our daily intake of vitamin C could have large effects for longevity.

The consumption of refined carbohydrates in the form of white breads, white pastas, and sweets has increased by 40 percent.

Simple changes in your diet can have a dramatic difference. You don't have to make a complete change in the way you eat, but at least make a few modifications.

- Avoid all margarines and processed oils; use butter or coconut butter.
- Cut back on sugar.
- Eat organically raised fish, beef, chicken, and eggs.
- Eat a rainbow of fruits and vegetables.
- Eat only fermented dairy products, such as yogurt.
- Drink only one cup of coffee a day, preferably made from organically grown coffee beans.

Good food choices start at the grocery store. Abram Hoffer MD, Ph.D, founder of the *Journal of Orthomolecular Medicine* and a pioneer in the field of nutritional medicine, recommends avoiding the inner aisles of the grocery store, which is where the toxic, destroyed, packaged, and processed foods are found. Think about it—all the fresh, whole foods are located in the dairy, produce, meat, and poultry sections. Hopefully, your grocery store sells whole grains in bulk and at their bakery. Many stores are now offering organic meats, eggs, and vegetables. Try shopping only the circumference of the store the next time you go shopping.

ORGANIC FOOD OR FRANKENFOOD?

Each and every cell contains genes that determine the characteristics and attributes of an organism. Specific genes dictate whether your hair will be blond or chestnut, whether a flower will have thorns or not, or if a cabbage will be green or purple. Genes are the building blocks of our existence.

Biotechnology, in the form of genetically modified foods, is a rapidly growing industry that creates food by tinkering with its genetic blueprint. By establishing a process that could never have occurred in nature, they remove genes or insert them in different locations of their sequence. We are told that we need bigger yields from our farmers' fields and that fungus and pest-resistance is essential. Food manufacturers want foods that will have a longer shelf life to prevent them from spoiling.

Although we have used genetic engineering to create hybrid plants and enhance certain traits, it was accomplished through the use of the plant's own reproductive process, not by rearranging genetic code. Through the marvels of modern engineering, scientists are no longer satisfied with cross-breeding the same species. Fish genes are being implanted in tomatoes and virus genes are crossed with potatoes. Mutant varieties of food are being created without any examination of their consequences on the human body. We are the subjects of a genetic experiment and it could take decades before the ramifications are apparent. When we have created new diseases or decreased our life span, it will be too late. Scientists who oppose the use of genetic engineering in our food sources believe that rising numbers of allergies and other illnesses may in part be a result of this worldwide experiment.

We don't know the long-term implications of eating food designed not to rot, grow mold, or be palatable to bugs, so it would be best to avoid them altogether. Choose organic produce to ensure that you are not eating food grown from genetically altered seeds.

EATING TOO MUCH DEPRESSES IMMUNITY

As the saying goes, "Too much of a good thing can be bad for you." Experiments conducted by the National Institute on Aging demonstrated that when animals were fed 50 percent fewer calories per day, their thymus size was maintained, T-cell function improved, and their immune response was enhanced. This study focused on high-calorie consumption, but it did not distinguish between the *types* of calories consumed. Diets that were heavy in meat or sugar would definitely have a negative impact on immune function, whereas calories consumed through legumes, fruits, vegetables, nuts, and seeds would boost immunity. However, it is a known fact that gaining even an additional 20 lbs (9 kg) can lower your immunity. Weight maintenance is a crucial aspect of optimizing your immune system.

Harvey and Marilyn Diamond, nutritionists and the authors of

Fit for Life, point out that there may be a reason for overeating, aside from the possible psychological factors. Your body may be clogged up with waste due to a suboptimal digestive system or bad nutrition and nutrients cannot be absorbed. The body is waiting for nutrients and expecting to be fed, so it tells you that you are hungry when you should actually be satisfied.

Opting for food that is nourishing and rich in nutrients is integral to health and vitality. Once you make the switch and substitute natural, whole food for the processed junk you've been eating, you will notice that you will stop craving foods and require less food.

WHAT IS A CARBOHYDRATE?

There are two types of carbohydrates: complex (unrefined) and refined. Refined carbohydrates include baked goods, white pastas, and any sugar-laden food. Complex carbohydrates are found in fruits, vegetables, legumes, nuts, seeds, and whole, unrefined grains. Increase the number of complex carbohydrates and reduce the refined carbs you eat. I believe that if we eliminated all white pasta, white rice, white flour, and white sugar from our diet, diabetes, high blood pressure, high cholesterol, and cancer rates would drop dramatically.

Within the complex carbohydrate category there are foods that have an effect on the rate of release of insulin entering the bloodstream. Too much insulin or too fast a release of insulin has health consequences and is linked to the development of diabetes, obesity, and increased aging, to name a few effects, so choose foods from the low-glycemic list below.

High-Glycemic Foods
(Promote a dramatic rise in blood sugar and insulin)

- honey
- corn chips and granola bars
- instant cereal and quick-cooking grains
  (like instant cream of wheat or oatmeal)
- breakfast cereals, including muesli
- whole grains
- cookies
- corn and white potatoes
- bananas and fruit juices

Moderate-Glycemic Foods
(Promote a moderate rise in blood sugar and insulin)

- old-fashioned oatmeal (slow-cooking type)
- legumes, beans, and peas
- yams and sweet potatoes

Low-Glycemic Foods
(Choose more of these foods than the others)

- yogurt
- fruits: grapefruit, cherries, plums, peaches
  (should be limited to two servings per day)
- nonstarchy vegetables: broccoli, cauliflower, kale, asparagus,
  romaine lettuce

The following is a review of a clinical study presented on October 30, 2000, at the annual meeting of the North American Association for the Study of Obesity. A study, funded in part by the Atkins Center for Complementary Medicine, was conducted to evaluate the effect of a low-carbohydrate, high-protein/fat diet in achieving short-term weight loss. Researchers at the Center for Health Services Research in Primary Care, Durham, N.C., reported data from a six-month study that included 51 individuals who were overweight, but otherwise healthy. The subjects received nutritional supplements and attended bi-weekly group meetings, where they received dietary counseling on consuming a low-carbohydrate, high-protein/fat diet. After six months, subjects experienced an average weight loss of 10.3 percent and an average decrease in total cholesterol of 10.5 mg/dL.

Twenty patients chose to continue the diet after the first six months, and after 12 months, their mean weight loss was 10.9 percent and their total cholesterol decreased by 14.1 mg/dL.

"This study of overweight individuals showed that a low-carbohydrate, high-protein/fat diet can lead to significant weight loss at one year of treatment," says William S. Yancy, MD, fellow, Health Services Research, Center for Health Services Research in Primary Care, Durham, N.C.

The reason for losing weight by eating a low-carbohydrate, high-protein/fat diet was explained by the results from another clinical study, supported by a grant from The E. Donnall Thomas Resident Research Program. In this prospective study, 18 overweight and obese adults, including nine males and nine females, were instructed to follow the low-carbohydrate, high-protein/fat diet. Dietary intake was evaluated before and two weeks after starting the diet. On average, subjects consumed 1000 kcal less per day two weeks after than before starting the diet. The reduction in calories correlated highly with each subject's weight loss.

SWEET SUICIDE

A single can of soda contains 10–12 tsp (50–60 mL) of added sugars. Our average annual per capita consumption of sugar is over 150 lbs (68 kg), which is an increase of 20 percent in the last 10 years; obesity has increased over 30 percent in that same time frame.

The Sinful Side of Sugar

Sweet and addictive, sugar is undeniably a pleasurable food. Lurking in many common foods and masquerading as dozens of pseudonyms, not-so-sweet sugar has dangerous health implications. Fructose, galactose, glucose, lactose, maltose, and sucrose are the most common names for sugar, but *The Sugar Addict's Total Recovery Program* lists almost 100 different names for sugars added to our foods.

Although sugar advocates would like us to believe that sugar is a good, natural food that provides us with quick energy, high sugar consumption correlates to increased rates of diabetes, heart disease, obesity, poor immune function, hyperactivity, tooth decay, nutritional deficiencies, and *Candida albicans* yeast infections. Sugar is at the root of so many problems that it should probably be sold with a warning that says "Sugar can increase your risk of developing cancer, heart disease, varicose veins, kidney disorders, arthritis, diabetes, obesity, migraine headaches, and high blood pressure." The functioning of our immune system is also severely hampered by sugar consumption.

Soda pop outsells unsweetened juice by 10 cans to one. A single can of soda pop can contain more than 10 tsp (60 mL) of sugar. Lendon Smith, MD, and coauthors report in *Beyond Antibiotics* that 100 g of sugar or 20 teaspoons (your average daily dose) from glucose, fructose, sucrose, maple syrup, honey, or orange juice can cause a significant decrease in the ability of white blood cells to engulf and destroy bacteria. This decrease in immune function was present five hours after the sugar was consumed. With the threat of antibiotic-resistant bacteria, avoiding sugar to enhance our immune system's ability to destroy bacteria just makes sense. One hundred grams or 20 teaspoons sounds like an exorbitant amount of sugar unless you know that peanut butter, tomato soup, fruit yogurt, packaged instant oatmeal, baked beans, mustard, and relish are just a few of the many food items that contain copious amounts of sugar.

The negative effects of sugar consumption have been well documented in medical journals around the world. Sugar is the culprit in increasing our risk of certain cancers, especially breast and colon cancer. It causes heart disease, raises triglycerides and blood pressure, lowers your body's production of antibodies, causes macrophages to be inactive, increases infection rate in diabetics, and causes deficiencies in B vitamins, chromium, copper, and molybdenum. Most important, sugar reduces immunity.

Your immune cells, when under the influence of sugar, are unable to march around the body fighting invaders. A form of paralysis takes place and these cells are rendered ineffective. Sugar also increases the growth of Candida albicans, a yeast organism responsible for poor nutrient absorption, chronic fatigue, depression, weight gain, and digestive upsets.

Naturally occurring sugars are not as devastating when consumed in whole food form. For example, sugar in the form of a whole apple is better than the juice of an apple without the fibre. Similarly, a whole carrot is much better than only the juice of the carrot. The sugars in concentrated juices, maple syrup, rice syrup, barley malt, honey, and beets are only slightly better than table sugar in reducing a negative immune response and increasing cholesterol and triglycerides. Concentrated fruit juices are also high in sugar, so beware that your children are not drinking too much of them. Whole foods with their natural sugars are the best choice. Never choose aspartame or other artificial sweeteners; they are extremely toxic. Aspartame rapidly turns into dangerous formaldehyde in the body. If you have to choose between sugar-sweetened foods and aspartame, choose sugar. Even with all of sugar's foibles, it is not nearly as toxic as aspartame.

Fake Sweeteners Are Dangerous

If sugar is so bad, should we switch to sugar-free substitutes like aspartame (Nutrasweet)? No, aspartame, more sinful than sugar, is a synthetic substance made up of phenylalanine, aspartic acid, and methanol (wood alcohol). Canada's Health Protection Branch regulates methanol, a potent neurotoxin, and has banned the food supplement phenylalanine for safety reasons, yet allows aspartame to be sold freely. Opponents of aspartame say there are links between aspartame and memory problems, seizure disorders, birth defects, headaches, and brain tumors. Although no long-term studies have proven these side effects, I would recommend a safer option, especially for children.

A 1992 abstract published in *Science Health Abstracts* reported that sucralose, an artificial sweetener, shrunk the thymus glands of rats by up to 40 percent when taken in large doses. Because the thymus is so important to a healthy immune system, the Center for Science in the Public Interest requested that further studies be performed before sucralose was released in the United States. This was ignored and sucralose, sold under the name Splenda™, is available as a sweetener in North America today. Sucralose is a chlorinated sucrose derivative, with no long-term human research. Hundreds of studies have been performed using sucralose, some of which show hazards. Critics say the studies were inadequate.

ASSASSINS LURK IN PROCESSED FATS

Standard supermarket oils are damaged goods and contain no nutritional value. Supermarket oils go through a process of deodorization, rendering them odorless, colorless, and tasteless. They are then treated with sodium hydroxide and phosphoric acid—both corrosives. After being bleached, they are finally heated to frying temperature to extend their shelf-life.

Partially hydrogenated oils, shortening, and margarine are liquids fabricated to become solids with the help of hydrogenation, a process that alters the shape of oil molecules turning them into toxins resulting in trans fatty acids—a noose around our neck.

Alberto Ascherio, the lead researcher on a team from the Harvard School of Public Health and the Wageningen Centre for Food Sciences in the Netherlands, published a review in the June 1999 issue of the *New England Journal of Medicine* stating that "Coronary heart disease (CHD) kills 500,000 Americans each year. According to our estimations, if trans fats were replaced by unsaturated vegetable oils, we would expect to see at least 30,000 fewer persons die prematurely from CHD each year."

Trans fatty acids raise LDL cholesterol (the bad cholesterol) and total cholesterol. Many products that claim to be cholesterol-free are actually high in trans fatty acids, which have been associated with increasing rates of heart disease. A product may have some virtues, but if it also contains trans fatty acids, it cannot promote good health. It has been proven that trans fatty acids cause obesity, cancer, and heart disease. Food labeling regulations in Canada do not require manufacturers to disclose how the product was made unless they are making a specific health claim. But even when fat-free claims are made, the labeling criteria let one fact slip through—the trans fatty acid content. Rarely will you see this value on the label.

Fascinating Fat Facts

Frying, smoking, barbecuing, and pickling have been linked to stomach and esophagus cancer, especially deep-frying, because they increase the destructive free radical formation of fat molecules.

Research published in the *Journal of the National Cancer Society* showed that men who ate meat four or five times weekly were four times more likely to develop colon cancer than those who ate it once a month.

The June 1995 issue of *Cancer Causes and Control* published a study conducted by the University of Southern California School of Medicine that linked hot dogs with a higher incidence of leukemia in 232 children. Children 10 years and under with leukemia were compared to a control group of healthy children. Those children with the highest incidence of leukemia ate more than 12 hot dogs every month. That same issue reported studies conducted on children whose fathers ate hot dogs prior to conception and mothers who ate one hot dog weekly during pregnancy. The risk of developing brain tumors doubled. Researchers suspect that the trigger is the carcinogenic nitrosamines, metabolites of nitrates, which are used as preservatives in hot dogs and other luncheon meats.

Eliminating red meat from the diet can reduce inflammation in arthritis and MS sufferers. Red meat contains arachidonic acid, a pro-inflammatory substance.

Throw away your killer fats and oils, and any product that says hydro-genated or partially hydrogenated. Hang on to the extra-virgin olive oil. See the recipe section in this book to learn which fats to use and how to change your family recipes into healthy fat recipes.

Low Fat, Low Life Expectancy

Contrary to what popular magazines would have you believe, low-fat diets will not make you immune to disease. Low rates of breast cancer have been found in women who live in Spain, Greece, and Italy where 50 percent of their dietary intake comes from fat, specifically cold-pressed extra-virgin olive oil.

For the Inuit and other indigenous peoples, fat comprises approximately 60 percent of their traditional diet, yet they have the lowest rates of arte-riosclerosis, diabetes, and cancer. The fats they eat are rich in essential fatty acids, an important component of a healthy immune system. The diets of most affluent countries and the standard American diet (SAD) are roughly 40 percent "bad" fats that are severely deficient in essential fatty acids.

Marketing mavens have hypnotized North Americans into relying on labels that read "sugar-free," "caffeine-free," "cholesterol-free," and "no fat." If a product is sugar-free, then it probably contains aspartame; if it is fat-free, it is most likely loaded with sugar. Have you noticed that most products are sold on the basis of what they lack instead of what benefits they may have? Processing removes healthy nutrients from foods, result-ing in a chemically altered toxic soup of ingredients. I taught my children to read the labels of food before they eat them. The rule of thumb is if you can't pronounce the ingredients, don't eat it.

The Cholesterol-Free Scam

The term "cholesterol-free" is the biggest scam in the marketing industry. Most items that say cholesterol-free never had it in the first place; it is just a ploy to make you think that it is healthy.

Oxidized cholesterol that is found in packaged foods is a serious health problem. Powdered eggs and milk, cake and bread-machine bread mixes, and packaged processed meats like bologna and hot dogs are loaded with oxidized cholesterol. Cholesterol can even oxidize in the body if there is a deficiency in antioxidant nutrients. Real eggs and

Take the Trans-Fatty Acid Test

The next time you are in the supermarket, read the labels of your usual purchases. Add up all the percentages of fat. Chances are that it will not total an even 100 percent. The percentage that is missing is the trans-fatty acid content.

butter, in moderation, are not the culprits. Cholesterol gets out of hand when not enough fresh vegetables and fruits are consumed in the diet. Fiber in fresh produce is paramount in regulating cholesterol. Avoid packaged foods as much as possible—remember Abram Hoffer's advice!

THE DANGERS OF DAIRY AND EGGS

Milk has been described as the most political food and rivals cholesterol in terms of controversy over its role in the human diet. According to Robert Cohen, in his book *Milk, The Deadly Poison*, "Milk and dairy products represent the major portion of America's diet. According to the United States Department of Agriculture (USDA), in 1995, the average American ate 584 pounds of milk and dairy products, nearly 40 percent of the diet is dairy." Jane Heimlich, author of *What Your Doctor Won't Tell You*, states in the introduction to Cohen's book that "One glass of milk, even low fat milk, is awash in fat (equivalent to three slices of bacon), cholesterol, antibiotics, bacteria [see page 7 for an article on mycobacteria, Crohn's, and milk] and the most distasteful ingredient—pus.... Cows are now being injected with bovine growth hormone (rBGH) to enhance milk output. A disturbing consequence of rBGH is the increase in the insulin-like growth factor (IGF-1), a contributing factor in the growth and proliferation of cancer." Bovine growth hormone is not injected into Canadian cows as of yet. The National Dairy Council would have you believe that milk is nature's perfect food and hails it as the elixir to build muscle and strong teeth and prevent brittle bones. But the research is not there to support their claims.

In April 2000, the Harvard School of Public Health issued a press release revealing the data from an 11-year study conducted with Brigham and Women's Hospital on the link between dietary calcium and the risk of prostate cancer. The hypothesis was that calcium lowers the body's levels of vitamin D, which is known to protect against prostate cancer. Their research supported that theory. Researchers found that men who drank more than six glasses of milk per week had lower levels of the protective form of vitamin D than men who drank fewer than two glasses of milk per week. Some data indicated that calcium may have a part in causing cancer to spread from the existing tumor. More research needs to be conducted to understand the underlying biological mechanisms.

Vitamin D toxicity brought on by heavy milk consumption is another worry. Milk has been fortified with vitamin D since its deficiency was found to cause rickets. This practice has continued in spite of the knowledge that minimal sunlight exposure will give us enough vitamin D. Dairies are not closely regulated for the levels of vitamin D they add to milk, resulting in varying amounts ranging product from product. A study released by the *New England Journal of Medicine* in April 1992 revealed that of 42 milk samples, only 12 percent were within the expected range. Infant formula was tested and they discovered seven out of 10 had twice the content declared on the label; one formula had four times the amount listed.

Robert Cohen has done extensive research on the detrimental effects of drinking the engineered milk of today. Please go to www.gotmilk.com or www.notmilk.com or order his book toll-free (1-888-NOT-MILK).

Eggs should also be eaten in moderation. In a study of 16,000 Seventh-Day Adventists, women who ate eggs at least three times per week had a three times greater risk of fatal ovarian cancer than women who age eggs less than once a week. Fried eggs showed the strongest association with fatal ovarian cancer, possibly due to cholesterol oxidation and the manufacture of ovarian hormones. If you have ovarian cancer or are at risk, avoid eggs.

CAFFEINE: WHAT YOU DON'T KNOW WILL HURT YOU

Excess consumption of caffeine can lead to heart palpitations, twitchy eyelids, high blood pressure, anxiety, sleep disturbances, stress, osteoporosis, restless legs, urinary tract infections, and fibroid breast cysts, to name a few problems. Caffeine has a strong presence in North American drinking habits, and not just in your morning latte. Soda pop, tea, chocolate, over-the-counter medications such as Excedrin™ and Midol™, and even decaffeinated coffee have caffeine. Caffeine causes magnesium to be excreted, which is a serious problem because North Americans tend to have a magnesium-deficient diet.

Caffeine Countdown Per 6 oz cup (180 mL)	
Alertness pill (No-Doz, Vivarin)	100–200 mg
Drip coffee	103 mg/cup
Cappuccino	75 mg/cup
Instant coffee	57 mg/cup
Soft drinks	26–34 mg/cup
Black tea	36 mg/cup
Analgesics (Excedrin, Anacin)	35–65 mg
Iced tea, instant	30 mg/cup
Green tea	30 mg/cup
Chocolate	18 mg/cup
Decaf	2 mg/cup
Herb tea	0 mg/cup

(Reprinted with permission from *The Osteoporosis Solution* by Carl Germano and William Cabot.)

CONTAMINATED WATER

A common element of science fiction stories is that water becomes scarce and more valuable than gold. Well, the future is here. Finding pure, clean water is an arduous task and many of us have stopped drinking water from the tap. In fact, I cannot think of anyone I know who does. In Canada, the quality of our drinking water, or lack thereof, hit us full force in the spring of 2000 when residents of Walkerton, Ontario, discovered that the water they had been drinking was contaminated with E. coli, resulting in the death of seven people and the hospitalization of almost 1000 more.

Water companies have added fluoride, chlorine, and chloramine to water supplies to make it "safer" for us. Clear-cut logging methods have upset the natural soil layer, allowing microorganisms such as Giardia lamblia and Cryptosporidium oocysts to take up residence in our tap water. Plastic residues, solvents, pesticides, herbicides, and inorganic metals have also made their way into our tap water.

Distilled water is a dead liquid, devoid of oxygen, and should not be consumed. It contains less than 1 mg of oxygen per liter and can only sustain dangerous anaerobic organisms. Molecules with a positive or negative charge seek the extra charge they need. This is what causes raindrops to pull together. Deoxygenated water searches for extra charges and will take it from your body if there are none immediately available. Distillation is not an effective purification process because although it removes many of the nasties, solvents remain and can be treated only with a carbon filter.

One component of the municipal water purification process is using aluminum sulfate to remove impurities. Water's metallic taste is due to the presence of alum, a compound that can cause neurological dysfunction. A 10-year study took place in 75 villages in the south of France with roughly 3777 people who were 65 years old. They discovered that those who drank water with 100 mcg of aluminum per liter double their risk for Alzheimer's disease. In the eighth year of the study, 280 cases of senile dementia and 200 more cases of Alzheimer's disease were reported by the researchers. Most cases arose in villages with more than 100 mcg aluminum per liter of water. The link between aluminum and Alzheimer's disease has not been definitively established, but evidence certainly suggests that we should avoid consuming tap water until proven otherwise.

ENVIRONMENTAL ESTROGENS LINKED TO INCREASED RISK OF CANCER

We hear plenty about the hormone estrogen. Should women take synthetic estrogen to halt menopausal symptoms for protection against heart disease and osteoporosis? Does estrogen replacement therapy cause breast cancer? Do some men and women have an overabundance of estrogen and is that why we are seeing higher rates of prostate and breast cancer? These questions are still largely unanswered. Now another estrogen alarm bell has been raised—the concern is estrogen-like substances found in our foods and environment.

Environmental estrogens (xenoestrogens, meaning foreign) are organochlorines, chemical compounds unknown in nature that are created by the chemical industry for plastics and pesticides. These synthetic substances, found in plastics, detergents, pesticides, and feminine hygiene products, are now associated with an increased risk of breast, ovarian, uterine, and testicular cancers, reproductive problems, and endometriosis. Xenoestrogens are estrogen mimickers that have the ability to disrupt delicate hormone balances in the body. Scientists are discovering that even in tiny amounts, environmental estrogens may be dangerous, and with long-term exposure they build up, creating hormonal disruption.

While there is much debate over these claims, both camps agree that high levels of these environmental contaminants can disrupt the endocrine systems of both humans and animals and produce toxic effects on tissues, causing cancer, infertility, birth defects, and developmental problems.

Xenoestrogens Lurking in Your Cupboards

There are more than 100,000 xenoestrogens in use today with over 1000 new ones created each year. Xenoestrogens are found in organochlorines, chemicals used for PVC (polyvinyl chloride) plastics, particularly molded plastics. That means plastic containers that store yogurt, cottage cheese, juice and milk jugs, and baby bottles may all be made with organochlorines. Studies have discovered the presence of over 175 different organochlorines in human tissue and fluid, especially breast milk. These pollutants can also leach out of plastics into our food, especially if heated in a microwave. Organochlorines are used in dry cleaning, bleaching (bleached feminine hygiene products, tampons, and pads), fire prevention, and refrigeration. Pesticides and other chemical agents such as kepone, dioxin, PCB, methoxychlor, and DDT are other pollutants containing xenoestrogens.

While the body's natural elimination cycle removes excess estrogen, it does not eliminate xenoestrogens, which accumulate in fatty tissues found in the breast and prostate. Organochlorines contribute to cancer in many ways: they can cause genetic mutations and the proliferation of cancer cells, enhance the cancer-causing effects of other chemicals, or disrupt our hormonal balance. While avoiding xenoestrogens whenever possible is ideal, ensuring adequate intake of the right foods and supplements can help build your nutritional defense and help eliminate xenoestrogens.

MAD COW DISEASE AND MEAT PRODUCTS

Mad cow disease (bovine spongiform encephalopathy, or BSE) has North Americans evaluating not only the beef on their plates but the scraps left over from the slaughterhouse. Animal scrap recycling has the blessing of the Canadian Food Inspection Agency's animal health division, which allows beef scraps to be manufactured into animal feed, cosmetics, components of vaccines, and gelatin, among other things, yet in the wake of mad cow disease, these by-products may be cause for concern. Claude Lavigne Ph.D., deputy director of the Canadian Food Inspection Agency's animal health division, confirms that bovine-containing products from Europe are still being imported into Canada. Also, we are still using feeding practices, now banned in Europe, that led to mad cow disease in the first place—that is, feeding our cows the remains of ground-up cows in their feed. We upset nature's delicate balance by feeding our cattle (and other animals and farm-raised fish) the scraps of other animals and now BSE is the result. Purchase only organically fed and raised beef and other meat products and wild fish that are not fed the ruminets of cows possibly containing BSE.

HEALING FOODS

Now that you have learned about the harmful foods and substances affecting our food supply, let's explore all of the wonderful healing foods that provide solutions for optimal health.

SAFELY SWEET

Stevia, a wonderful herb (*Stevia rebaudiana*), adds a touch of sweetness without the detrimental side effects of sugar. The stevia herb in its natural form is approximately 10 to 15 times sweeter than common table sugar. Some studies report that stevia reduces plasma glucose levels in normal adults. With our increased rates of diabetes and syndrome-X, stevia consumption may have a protective effect on blood sugar.

Stevia, which is available in health food stores, has antimicrobial activity, protecting us against colds and flu while lowering blood sugar levels in diabetics. Stevia, which has no calories, is not allowed to be marketed as a sweetener in Canada and health food stores must promote it as a sweet little secret.

Stevia for Diabetics

Diabetes associations in North America have been recommending artificial sweeteners as an alternative to sugar. Stevia is a great alternative to artificial sweeteners, which have long-term negative health effects. Stevia leaves have been used as herbal teas by diabetic patients in Asian countries. In a study published in 1993, no side effects were noted in diabetics after eating stevia for years. Two other research studies published in 1981 and 1986 found that stevia extract can actually improve blood sugar levels. Brazilian researchers at the Universities of São Paolo evaluated the role of stevia in blood sugar. Sixteen healthy volunteers were given extracts of 5 g (0.17 oz) of stevia leaves every six hours for three days. A glucose tolerance test was performed before and after taking stevia and the results were compared to another group who did not receive the stevia extracts. The study participants taking stevia were found to have significantly lower blood sugar levels.

The sweet secret of stevia lies in a complex molecule called stevioside, which is a glycoside composed of glucose, sophorose, and steviol. It is this complex molecule and a number of other related compounds that account for *Stevia reubaudiana*'s extraordinary sweetness.

Whole foods markets are popping up everywhere across the nation and many stores are mandated not to order foods full of sinful ingredients like aspartame, trans fatty acids, and sugar. Support these stores and enjoy the rows of fresh organic produce and shelves of foods sweetened with stevia.

FATS ARE GOOD FOR YOU

There are fats that can kill you and most of us eat them every day, but there are also fats that can heal you and you should be including them in your diet. It is true that fats are associated with cancer, heart disease, diabetes, and arthritis, but not all fats are bad.

Can a good fat go bad? Yes, when seeds and nuts are processed into margarines, oils, and shortenings—the kind we usually find in our supermarket—every essential nutrient is destroyed or extracted. This process also changes fat molecules into disease-causing molecules, unusable by the body and toxic too.

Why Are Essential Fats So Essential?

When taken in combination with a plant-based diet, essential fatty acids (EFAs) and the sterols and sterolins they contain are effective at enhancing immunity. Research has demonstrated this fact over and over again. The two most talked about essential fatty acids are omega-3 and omega-6. Omega-3 is found predominantly in cold-water fish (sardines, herring, tuna, mackerel, and salmon) and flaxseeds, while omega-6 can be obtained from seed and herb oils (such as pumpkin seeds, walnuts, evening primrose, and borage).

The essential fatty acids are essential because they break down to make good prostaglandins, a crucial component for regulating cellular activity. Essential fatty acids protect the body by helping to fight infections, yeast, and bacteria.

Types of Fats

Saturated fats are semisolid at room temperature. Sources of saturated fats are animal fats (red meat, pork, lamb) and dairy products (milk, cheese). These fatty acids are associated with LDL, the "bad" cholesterol.

Monounsaturated fats remain liquid at room temperature; they solidify in cold temperatures. Sources of these fatty acids are olive, canola, and peanut oils. These fatty acids are associated with HDL, the "good" cholesterol.

Polyunsaturated fats, which are omega-6 fats, remain liquid at room temperature and stay in that form in colder temperatures. Sources of polyunsaturated fats are corn, safflower, sesame, soy, and sunflower oils.

Superunsaturated fats are even more liquid at room temperature and don't solidify unless frozen. Their freezing point is lower than for omega-6 oils. These fats include omega-3 essential fatty acids from flaxseed and fish. These fatty acids are associated with HDL, the "good" cholesterol, and are heart-protective.

Fats for a Healthy Future

Fats that heal are found in a variety of delicious sources. Avocados, dark green vegetables, olives, whole grains, fatty fish, unrefined cold-pressed oils, and nuts and seeds are rich in essential fatty acids and are therefore cancer protective. Flaxseed is rich in essential fatty acid, but should be combined with sunflower or sesame seeds or oil to balance the essential fats. It contains phytonutrients with a high concentration of lignans, which are cancer-fighting agents. (See page 105 for more information on lignans.)

In addition to being anticancer, lignans are antifungal, antibacterial, and antiviral. Ground flaxseed is an excellent source of fiber and contains seven more lignans than the oil. It is easy to add at least 1 tbsp (15 mL) of ground flaxseed to your diet. Coffee grinders can double as flaxseed grinders.

Nut and seed oils are also rich in the immune-enhancing sterols and sterolins. These life-enhancing substances make oils look cloudy, so manufacturers remove them (and their healing properties) and turn the oils into the odorless, colorless, tasteless variety we find in supermarkets.

To ensure you are getting enough EFAs, you should be eating 1 tbsp (15 mL) of ground flaxseeds and sunflower seeds, and 1–2 tbsp (15–30 mL) of essential fatty acid oil with three capsules of sterols and sterolins daily. Buy only organic, cold-pressed, unrefined oil. If it is clear and almost colorless, it has been refined, so leave it on the shelf. The two brands of oils that I use are Omega Nutrition and Udo's Choice Oil. Omega Nutrition also has a wonderful range of culinary oils, including pumpkin seed, pistachio nut, sesame seed, and more.

YOGURT, NATURE'S PERFECT FOOD

Poor nutritional choices and excessive use of antibiotics weaken the body's ability to attack and destroy potential disease-causing bacteria, parasites, and viruses. Probiotics, including lactobacillus acidophilus, lactobacillus bulgaricus, and bifidobacterium bifidum, are found in a healthy digestive tract and are a few of the important microorganisms that enhance immunity. Yogurt is an easy way to get those beneficial bacteria working for you.

High in potassium and rich in protein, calcium, phosphorus, vitamins B_6 and B_{12}, niacin, and folic acid, yogurt is often called nature's perfect food. It supports the immune system and kills harmful bacteria in the intestines. Even those who are lactose intolerant can usually eat yogurt without pain or discomfort as the fermentation process breaks down the lactose. Eating yogurt regularly reduces the risk of vaginal yeast infections and can ease tummy troubles such as diarrhea and food poisoning. It has been reported that children who eat yogurt show greater resistance to the flu.

The "Benefits of Yogurt," a report published in the *Journal of Immunotherapy*, found that yogurt with acidophilus eaten over several months increased gamma-interferon, the immune-enhancing protein that prevents viruses from replicating in the body. There was also a reduction in the inflammatory responses of the intestines. IgE, an effective destroyer of parasites, is enhanced when the diet includes Lactobacillus bulgaricus.

Not all yogurt is created equal. When you're in the supermarket, pass on the ones with fruit and sugar added and get the plain yogurt. Manufacturers are required to add bacterial cultures to yogurt that has gone through heat processing, but aren't required to tell you if they are alive or not. Read the label and get the yogurt that tells you exactly which bacterial cultures are included and if it contains active or living cultures. Having one cup of probiotic-rich yogurt daily will boost your immunity, but if you can't manage this or you really can't stomach the taste, you can take probiotic supplements instead, available in the health food store.

Yogurt, which is fermented, has many healing properties and the enzymes produced during the fermentation process eliminate many of the negative consequences of drinking milk before fermentation. Buy organic yogurt whenever possible.

Flaxseeds

Ground flaxseeds are another beneficial addition to the diet. Flaxseeds are rich in essential fats, antioxidants, fiber, and phytochemicals called lignans, which bind to estrogen receptors and xenoestrogens and help to inhibit the growth of estrogen-dependent cancers. Various studies have been conducted on the health benefits of flaxseeds. Recently, one study published in *Nutrition and Cancer* reported that 28 postmenopausal women who added ground flaxseed to their diets showed significant improvement in estrogen balancing. The American Medical Association reported in July 2001 that flaxseeds rich in lignans and essential fatty acids are extremely important for protecting the colon and prostate. Grind flaxseeds in a small coffee grinder but only grind what you are going to eat. If stored, ground flaxseeds will go rancid and lose many of their health-giving properties.

Soy Foods

The many plant chemicals in soy products are an important part of an immune-building diet. Saponins, one component of soy foods, prevent cancer cells from multiplying and they also lower cholesterol. Soy foods, such as soybeans, soymilk, and tofu, also contain phytoestrogens called isoflavones. The isoflavones daidzen and genistein are weak phytoestrogens that can help protect against hormone-related cancers. They prevent harmful estrogen from entering cells by taking their place. As a weaker estrogen, they reduce the symptoms of menopause, inhibit tumor growth, and reverse cancer within the cell, thus stopping prostate and breast cancer. Genistein has been shown to slow the development of cancer, particularly breast cancer. While these plant estrogens may mimic estrogen, studies show that the estrogens contained in soy are weak estrogens that are able to bind to receptors that would otherwise bind with stronger estrogens or xenoestrogens. This effect is especially important, as allowing the stronger estrogens to bind to the receptors can result in a greater likelihood of cell proliferation, cancer growth, and thyroid and adrenal disruption. Soy foods are also very rich in another phytonutrient, sterols and sterolins, known to improve immune function and lower cholesterol. For those who dislike the taste of soy products, sterols and sterolins, daidzein, and genistein are also available in a supplement form.

The strongest anticancer properties are found in fermented soy products like, tempeh, miso, fermented soy powder, and soy sauce. Soy is easy to add to the diet and delicious as well. Soy is available in many forms such as tofu, tempeh, miso, milk, cheese, pepperoni, burgers, and hot dogs. The medium and hard blocks of tofu can be diced and tossed into a stir-fry, or marinated in your favorite sauce and pan-fried. Soft tofu can be blended into delicious shakes.

Anyone who has an allergy to milk can drink soymilk. Soymilk can be enjoyed hot or cold and comes in a variety of flavors—original, vanilla, carob, cocoa, and green tea. If you like green tea ice cream, green tea soymilk is for you.

Vegetables

Cruciferous vegetables were the first food the American Cancer Society promoted as a cancer preventative. These vegetables can help lower our risk of developing many diseases and sex-hormone-dependent cancers. In particular, cruciferous vegetables, members of the Brassica family—such as cabbage, Brussels sprouts, broccoli, cauliflower, radishes, turnips, kale, kohlrabi, and collard greens—affect estrogen metabolism and lower cancer risk. During the digestion of these vegetables, an enzyme is released that forms indole-3-carbinol, or indoles for short, which are potent cancer-inhibitors. Indoles affect estrogen metabolism in three key ways. First, they reduce the amount of unhealthy estrogen while regulating the amount of healthy estrogen in the body. Second, indoles speed the removal of unhealthy estrogen from the body. And third, they can increase the activity of enzymes that detoxify the body of carcinogens. In addition, cruciferous vegetables produce di-indolylmethane (or DIM). Di-indolylmethane is approximately 10 times more effective than indoles for estrogen balancing. DIM and indoles are also available as nutritional supplements; studies have shown they can help improve overall estrogen balance.

Researchers at the Fred Hutchinson Cancer Research Center in the US noted that it only took three half-cup servings per week of broccoli, Brussels sprouts, and cauliflower to decrease the risk of prostate cancer by 41 percent. Studies have shown that cruciferous vegetables also slow colon cancer growth, reduce intestinal polyps, and eliminate excess estrogens, thereby preventing breast cancer. They also have an abundance of glutathione, that powerful detoxifier that gets rid of cancer-causing agents.

The 1927 *American Medicine Journal* wrote, "Cabbage is therapeutically effective in conditions of scurvy, diseases of the eyes, gout, rheumatism, pyorrhea, asthma, tuberculosis, cancer, and gangrene." The best way to consume cruciferous vegetables is raw, but if your digestion system is not accustomed to roughage or is just plain sensitive, steaming them will preserve more nutrients than boiling. For every one cup of raw vegetables that you eat, you will need to eat two cups of steamed vegetables. Overcooking should be avoided as the process destroys any beneficial nutrients and their immune-boosting power.

If you want to stock up on the enzymes mentioned above that deactivate cancer cells and target them for digestion and elimination from the body, you want broccoli. Broccoli contains sulphoraphane, the phytonutrient that stimulates cancer-fighting enzymes. Broccoli sprouts have 10 times the sulphoraphane than mature broccoli. In fact, sprouting cruciferous vegetables is a great way to get the biggest nutritional bang for your buck. Do not buy store-bought sprouts. They often contain molds and are suspected of being exposed to salmonella contamination. Sprouting seeds in a jar on the kitchen windowsill is much safer.

PLANT POWER

Plants contain phytonutrients, the most important weapon in your immune system's arsenal. Food is energy for your trillions of cells. Gladys Block and colleagues at the University of California at Berkeley analyzed the 170 controlled clinical trials on the protective effects of fruits and vegetables against cancer. Fruits and vegetables contain hundreds of phytonutrients, and dozens of these have been evaluated for their healing properties (see table below).

The perfect diet for a supercharged immune system is predicated on the power of plants. Fruits, legumes, grains, vegetables, nuts, seeds, and sea vegetables are foods that heal. They are best eaten fresh, whole, raw, and, if at all possible, organic. Like tomatoes, avocados, peppers, and cucumbers are classified as fruits because they have seeds in them. They also make tasty combinations with other fruits. At your next meal, try putting a banana or mango with an avocado, or peaches and nectarines with cucumber.

COMMON PHYTONUTRIENTS IN FOODS

Phytonutrient	Food	Action
allicin and allyl sulfides	garlic, onions, leeks	reduce the risk of stomach and colon cancer
anthocyanidins	red pigment in berries; grape skin, cranberries	antioxidant, anti-inflammatory
carotenoids	dark green, yellow, red, and orange vegetables and fruits	anticancer, antioxidant, and protective in heart and eye diseases
catechins	green tea, berries, tea	antiviral, anticancer, antibacterial
ellagic acid	grapes, strawberries, walnuts, raspberries, black currants, apples	anticancer, antimutagenic
indoles and indole-3-carbinol	broccoli, Brussels sprouts, cabbage, kale, watercress	anticancer, removes excess estrogens
isoflavonoids, genistein, and daidzein	soybeans	deactivates excess estrogens, anticancer, and reduces menopause symptoms
lignans	flaxseeds and whole grains	blocks excess estrogen and dihydrotestosterone (DHT), anticancer
lycopene	tomatoes, red grapefruit, watermelon	prevents prostate cancer
phthalides	carrots, celery, parsley, coriander, fennel	anticancer
polyphenols	green tea	protects gastrointestinal tract, anticancer
sterols and sterolins	all fruits, vegetables, nuts, seeds, soy products, and shellfish	anticancer, immune modulating
sulforaphane	broccoli, cabbage, cauliflower	anticancer
triterpenoids	soybeans, citrus	anticancer

Avocado

Avocados have been given a bad rap. Physicians have been warning heart patients and those on weight-reduction diets to avoid the avocado. Superhero of the immune system, the avocado is rich in the powerful detoxifier glutathione.

Glutathione-rich avocados actually help cleanse the body of dangerous oxidized fats. Avocado has been wrongly dismissed as a healing food due to its fat content, but it contains monounsaturated fats, the ones we recommend to help the body deal with oxidation and free radicals. Potassium and chromium are also found in avocados. Potassium is used to treat high blood pressure, water balance in the body, and kidney, heart, and adrenal function. Chromium works to help control blood sugar levels by helping insulin work more efficiently. It is used for the treatment of hypoglycemia, diabetes, and high cholesterol, and to normalize triglyceride levels and to increase fat loss.

Fiber

A good bowel movement at least once a day is essential for a healthy immune system, and fiber is the means to do it. Not only does fiber comb out the debris in the intestinal tract, it eliminates toxins and regulates cholesterol levels. In his lectures, Udo Erasmus, author of *Fats That Heal, Fats That Kill*, recommends that you should have at least one large bowel movement a day, or two to three smaller ones (about 12 in/30 cm of waste should be excreted in total). The feces should be soft, easy to pass, and float—if it sinks in the toilet bowl, you are not getting enough fiber in your diet.

For a healthy bowel you need to eat at least 20 g of fiber per day. There are two types of fiber, soluble and insoluble. Soluble fiber is the pectin in apples, the gooey stuff in cooked cereal, and the slippery substance surrounding soaked flaxseed. It absorbs water and swells to ten times its weight, forming a gel in the intestinal tract. This bulkiness slows down food and lends to that full feeling, which is very beneficial if you are trying to lose weight. Insoluble fiber is also called roughage and does not get broken down during the digestive process. Found in whole-grain cereals and breads, vegetables, and fruit, it sweeps out the intestinal tract and is eliminated with the other waste.

Brazil nuts in the shell are an excellent source of fiber, selenium, sterols, and sterolins—all important to keep the immune system healthy. I also like to grind flaxseeds fresh every morning and add it to my cereal or cook it into a delicious pudding.

Fruits

Dark-colored fruits are bursting with immune-boosting anticancer ingredients. The highest levels of antioxidants and phytonutrients are held within the dark pigments of cranberries, strawberries, bilberries, blueberries, and raspberries. Blueberries and cranberries contain powerful antioxidants and free radical scavengers called anthocyanins. They suppress urinary tract infections by preventing bacteria from adhering to the wall of the bladder. Vitamin C-rich berries are a tasty and healthy addition to your diet.

Over a dozen recognized antioxidants are found in grapes and a cancer-preventing phytonutrient called reservatol. Grapes also contain selenium, the powerful flavonoid quercetin, and ellagic acid. Green grapes are not as rich in antioxidants as red and purple grapes. Research conducted on grapes is showing that they may enhance natural killer cell activity and put small tumors into remission. They fight allergies, unclog arteries, reduce cholesterol, and suppress oxidation. Proanthocyanidin oligomers (PCO) are an extract from grape seed and have exhibited immune-enhancing functions against cancer. (A reminder about genetically engineered food—biotech grapes do not have seeds in them, so they cannot naturally reproduce or provide us with PCO.) If you want to take PCO supplements, you need at least 100 mg per day, 500 mg if you are combating allergies.

Ellagic acid is found in grapes, black currents, raspberries, strawberries, and walnuts. It is a polyphenol with powerful anticancer and antimutagenic properties. Scientists believe it is those properties in strawberries that provide effective protection against prostate cancer. Remember to buy organic, as berries are often heavily sprayed with pesticides and fungicides.

A healthy immune system is found in those people who eat plenty of fresh, phytonutrient-rich fruit. Enjoy the benefits of watermelon, berries, grapes with seeds, limes, lemons, oranges, and grapefruit. Citrus fruits are loaded with flavonoids, carotenoids, and vitamin C. Grapefruit is also packed with lycopene and glutathione, the master nutrient of the immune system. Choose fruits, preferably organic, to optimize your immune system.

Garlic

For over 5000 years, garlic has been the treatment of choice for everything from foot fungus to cholesterol. Over 2500 scientific studies have been published praising its virtues and deservedly so, for it is an amazing healing herb. Current research focuses on garlic's antifungal, antiviral, anti-inflammatory, anticancer, and antibacterial properties used in the treatment of asthma, colds and flu, diabetes, ear infections, and heart disease.

Garlic is comprised of over 200 compounds, including sulfur and trace minerals. Although most information about garlic emphasizes the benefits of the compound allicin, like most food, garlic's power lies in the synergy of many compounds, not just one. Sulfur, another compound found in garlic, is an effective free radical scavenger and a "super" antioxidant. The immune system is able to fight infected and cancerous cells because sulfur enhances the function of natural killer cells. Selenium is also present in garlic and is one of the recommended 10 immune system nutrients. In addition to its ability to protect against stomach cancer, it also helps detoxify an immune system burdened with heavy metal toxins, especially mercury.

Greens

It may seem impossible to consume seven to 10 half-cup servings of fruits and vegetables, but try to eat as many as you can and drink the rest as freshly squeezed juice or green drinks (see the following). Juicing several fruits or vegetables will provide your body with plenty of phytonutrients, especially sterols and sterolins. You don't want to lose the benefit of the fiber for the sake of the juice, so be sure to put the fiber left over from juicing back into the drink or add it to quick bread or muffin recipes.

Drink immediately after juicing as many phytonutrients will be destroyed if exposed to air for too long. Drink the juice in small amounts so you can "chew" it for a few seconds (with your mouth closed) before you swallow. The chewing encourages salivary enzymes to begin digestion. Fresh-squeezed juice is good for you, but you may consume too much sugar in juices, so limit yourself to one juice daily.

One easy way to get a good dose of phytonutrients and fiber is in green drinks. They are considered a superfood because they can contain alfalfa, wheat grass, barley, brown rice germ, green tea, grape seeds, ginkgo biloba, bee pollen, sprouted grains and soy, milk thistle, spirulina, chlorella, dulse, probiotics, Siberian ginseng, bilberry, licorice root, and phosphatidyl choline. Superfood drinks will contain any combination of these ingredients to give you a convenient drink to supplement your diet.

They are excellent for people on the run and teenagers. You can drink them straight up, mixed with organic fruit juice, or in a power shake. Toss them into your emergency kit, hiking pack, or travel bag for a quick pick-me-up when you need a boost. I recommend Green Alive, Udo's Beyond Greens, and greens+.

Mushrooms

A growing field of scientific study is concentrating on the immune-enhancing properties of mushrooms. Mushrooms have had a solid reputation in Asia for hundreds of years, and it has only been in the last 20 years that

North American research is catching on to their antiviral and antitumor action. Shiitake mushrooms are probably the best known and are considered to be antitumor and helpful in controlling hypertension. They enhance the production and use of vitamin D and increase macrophage activity in the immune system. Shiitake can suppress the further cell division of viruses and can reverse the suppression of T-cells. In clinical studies, reishi mushrooms have shrunk and eliminated tumors and increased gamma-interferon and T-cell activity. Reishi also suppresses histamine release, making it an excellent food for asthmatics. Maitake mushrooms are known as the "King of the Mushrooms" because they can grow to 20 in (50 cm) in diameter and weigh up to 100 lbs (45 kg), but also because they exhibit the greatest efficacy of all the mushrooms in preventing tumor growth. Supplementation with mushrooms has been helpful for boosting the immune system of women with breast cancer, especially during chemotherapy.

Mushrooms are easy to include in salads, soups, and stews. Finding these exotic mushrooms fresh is a bit of a rarity in North America, but in the dried form they taste just as good. Reconstitute them by soaking them in water, but when you're done, don't throw out the water; you can use it for soups and stews. When you are eating mushrooms, try to make sure that they are accompanied with food that is rich in vitamin C. Studies show that vitamin C enhances their immune-boosting power. If you really don't like the flavor of mushrooms, you can take a food supplement containing their marvelous extracts.

Tomatoes

Tomatoes are rich in lycopene, a type of carotene that provides protection against cancer. Lycopene is a red pigment that is also found in watermelon, rosehip, and pink grapefruit, but no food is a better source than tomatoes. One cup of tomato juice contains 25 mg of lycopene, compared to a slice of watermelon, which has only 14.7 mg. A raw medium tomato has less lycopene (3.7 mg) than processed tomatoes such as in juice, sauce (28.1 mg in a half-cup), or paste (13.8 mg in 2 tbsps/30 mL). Tomatoes also contain iron and are good sources of lignans and vitamins A and C. They neutralize uric acid (a by-product of high protein diets) and cleanse the body of toxins.

A study investigating lycopene was conducted by a professor of medicine and oncology at the Karmanos Cancer Institute in Detroit. Dr. Kucuk and his colleagues observed 30 men who were scheduled for the surgical removal of their prostate. In each case the prostate cancer was localized. During the three weeks before surgery, participants either received a placebo without intervention or 15 mg of lycopene as a pure tomato extract twice daily. After the prostates were removed, the glands were examined for any differences between the study group and the control group. It was discovered that the group receiving lycopene had smaller tumors, and that they were more commonly confined to the prostate. They also found lower levels prostate specific antigen serum, used to detect prostate cancer. As well, the tumors demonstrated signs of regression and a decrease in malignancy.

As an oil-soluble phytonutrient, lycopene is absorbed better if eaten with oil. Drizzle a little flaxseed or olive oil on your tomato salad or add it to your spaghetti sauce and you will absorb up to 70 percent of the lycopene present.

PROTEIN POWER

Our bodies require 20 essential amino acids to facilitate the production of protein for cellular repair and the manufacture of CP-450, a protective enzyme that acts as a free radical scavenger and decreases the risk of breast cancer. Of those 20 amino acids, 12 can be made within the body and the remaining eight we must get from our food. Sources come from protein such as legumes, fresh fish, free-range poultry, eggs, nuts, seeds, soy, and dairy products. A depressed immune system can be a result of protein deficiency. Osteoporosis, weak nails and thin hair, wrinkled skin, lack of muscle tone, breast cancer, and poor repair are all associated with inadequate protein consumption.

Some people have greater protein requirements than others. If you are very active, exercise strenuously, or do heavy labor, or you are pregnant you will need more protein than a couch potato. The average person should make protein 15–20 percent of their diet (see chart below). When choosing your protein sources, opt for free-range poultry and eggs and wild fish over farm-grown, to avoid contamination from antibiotics and growth hormones. Purchase nuts in the shell and buy organic legumes when you can. If you need to keep your glucose levels stable, split up your protein requirements into three or four small portions and eat them spaced throughout the day. Women rarely get enough protein in their diet and as a result I formulated a protein drink especially for them called Sisu Women's Whey. It contains whey and fermented soy and is sweetened with Inulin and stevia.

Exercise Category	Recommended Protein Intake (gm/lb)
Sedentary	0.36
Moderate	0.36–0.5
Endurance	0.5–0.8
Strength	0.6–0.8
Teenage	0.6–0.9

(From Chapter 16 of *The Complete Idiot's Guide to Total Nutrition for Canadians* by Leslie Beck (Toronto: Prentice Hall Canada, 2000.)

WATER, THE LIFE SAVER

After oxygen, water is the next most essential nutrient we consume. We could last months without food, but without water we would die in about a week. Seventy-five percent of our body is water.

Dr. Fereydoon Batmanghelidj, author of *Our Body's Many Cries for Water*, says that most of us suffer from severe chronic dehydration, which is responsible for many of our illnesses. By drinking more water, we can cure ourselves of angina, rheumatoid arthritis, asthma, colitis, constipation, edema, gout, headaches (including migraines), hypertension, ulcers, obesity, fatigue, osteoporosis, and neck, muscle, and back pain. And your bouts of forgetfulness? Brain tissue is 85–90 percent water, and research documents that brain cells begin to shrink after prolonged dehydration. Water prevents aging. As you get older, your sense of thirst decreases, conspiring even further to prevent you from drinking what you need.

If you doubt the curative benefits of water, consider this: 7–11 qt (6.5–10.5 L) of water are required for the digestion of a meal (3 pt/1.5 L for saliva, 2 qt/2 L for gastric juices, bile and other secretions); the kidneys need 1 qt (1 L) of water for every 1.5 oz (45 mL) of waste removed; 1 pt (470 mL) of water is required for one day of exhaling (more if the climate is arid); and the skin sweats up to 1 qt (1 L) of water an hour in dry conditions. Dr. Batmanghelidj's theory does not seem so extreme now.

Most of us have heard that we should drink at least six glasses of water daily. Thirst is a bad indicator; if we feel thirsty, then we have already been dehydrated for far too long. According to Dr. Batmanghelidj, you should use your weight to find out how much water to drink.

Determine your weight in pounds and divide by two. That is the number of ounces of pure, filtered water you should drink every day. For example, if you weigh 175 lbs, you need to consume 87.5 oz or roughly 11 glasses. That is a lot of water to drink in one day, so you need to drink water whether you are thirsty or not. Drink two glasses before breakfast and keep large water bottles everywhere to remind you to take a sip—in the office, in the car, in your gym locker, even on the end table beside your bed or favorite reading chair. Hot weather warrants doubling or tripling your intake.

Coffee, tea, soft drinks, and juice do not count. (The only exception is herbal tea.) For every cup of non-water that you drink, add another 8–10 oz (250–300 mL) of water. Substances in these beverages, especially caffeine, are diuretics, which force you to lose more water than you consume.

Tap and distilled water should not be consumed. A reverse-osmosis (RO) water system, combined with a carbon filter, is the best type of water filtration system for your home. In an RO system, a synthetic membrane filters out contaminants as the water passes through.

GREEN TEA:
MUCH MORE THAN A COFFEE SUBSTITUTE

Herbal teas are a good substitute for caffeine and come in a variety of flavors such as peppermint, licorice, chamomile, and dandelion. Studies indicate that green tea is a powerful antioxidant and anticarcinogen. Green tea contains epigallocatechin gallate (catechins for short), a substance that inhibits tumor growth and lowers cholesterol. As part of a larger compound in green tea, it is more powerful than vitamin E in the fight against free radicals and supports immune system function. High consumption of green tea (up to 10 cups a day) is thought to contribute to a lower incidence rate of breast and lung cancer. Drink a cup or two before meals to cleanse your palate and prepare your liver for digestion.

Research is also being conducted into green tea's fat-burning properties. A small study revealed that participants who took three green tea capsules daily increased their fat burning without accelerating their heart rate.

In 1999, several studies were published in Sweden, Taiwan, and the United States describing green tea's efficacy in inhibiting COX-2–related arthritis. Not only is green tea as good as COX-2 anti-inflammatories, the Napralert Database identified 51 other anti-inflammatory compounds present in green tea. The USDA Phytochemical Database also identified 15 antiulcer compounds in green tea, supporting evidence that long-term use can also inhibit ulcers caused by prolonged NSAIDs use. Advertisements for Celebrex or Vioxx may celebrate their ability to relieve pain, but little is said about their likelihood of inducing ulcers. Green tea is a safe and natural alternative.

You now have a good understanding of the foods and beverages that have powerful healing properties and the ones you should avoid, but we all know that as hard as we try, our schedules and lifestyles may prevent us from eating perfectly every day. The next chapter will teach you about the food supplements, vitamins, minerals, plant nutrients, amino acids, and neutraceuticals that can act as an insurance policy for health or powerful treatments if you are already affected by disease.

NUTRITIONAL SUPPLEMENTS

Food supplements are exactly that—supplements to the foods you eat. Vitamins, minerals, amino acids, coenzymes, essential fats, and the phytonutrients and extracts from foods and herbs are all called food supplements. All are based on the premise that if we can correct the underlying nutrient deficiencies caused by our inadequate diet, health can be achieved. Hundreds of thousands of research papers have been published in well-respected journals worldwide touting the health benefits of nutrients. The evidence is irrefutable—we need nutrients.

You learned in the last chapter that whole foods contain powerful healing substances, but it is difficult to consume all of those nutrients every day in the correct dosages to achieve and maintain optimal health and longevity. Supplementing a good diet with nutrients is like putting money into your savings account to ensure that you never become bankrupt. Whether you are a seemingly healthy person or someone suffering from illness, nutrients can make a difference. In the condition section I will recommend the specific dosage of each nutrient for each disease.

VITAMINS

In order for a substance to be classified as a vitamin, the body must not manufacture all that it requires and it must be obtained from the foods we eat and be essential to life. Deficiencies can cause illness and death. Fourteen essential vitamins and several vitamin-like substances have been identified. Vitamin-like substances, like coenzyme Q10, are initially manufactured by the body, but production declines as we age. Vitamins are classified as fat soluble or water soluble, meaning they require either fat or water to be absorbed and transported. Fat-soluble vitamins, including A, D, E, and K, are stored in the liver and fat tissues of the body. Vitamins B and C are water soluble and any excess is excreted in the urine and sweat. Water-soluble vitamins should be taken every day to ensure adequate levels.

Enzymes and coenzymes act as catalysts to ensure absorption and assimilation of each vitamin. For example, enzymes must break down vitamin B_6 to its assimilated form, pyridoxal-5-phosphate, before it can be absorbed. If you are deficient in the enzyme required, absorption would be difficult. As well, vitamins often need cofactors in the form of minerals or plant nutrients, such as a bioflavonoid, to better absorb vitamin C and conversely, certain minerals can inhibit or interfere with the absorption of vitamins (iron reduces the absorption of vitamin E).

I mentioned in Chapter 4 that the recommended dietary allowances (RDA) or the more recent recommended dietary intake (RDI) do not provide for optimal health. They were designed only to prevent deficiency diseases like scurvy and rickets.

Synthetic Versus Natural

Products backed by published clinical trials should always be chosen over those with no human research whenever possible. Companies that spend time and money in proving the effectiveness of their products should be supported. Natural vitamins and minerals are found in the whole foods you eat. They come bound to carbohydrates, proteins, lipids, and fats. Ninety-nine percent of the vitamins and minerals we buy today are synthesized, meaning they are produced in the laboratory. They are chemically identical to the nutrients found in food with the exception of vitamin E, which should be taken only in the natural form. By taking your vitamins and minerals with meals, you can ensure better absorption.

Fillers, binders, and flowing agents are used in the manufacture of nutrients. Fillers are used to fill up a capsule (some nutrients take up such a small amount of space that a filler has to be used), binders are used to make tablets stick together, and flowing agents are used to keep the machinery from sticking during the tableting or encapsulation process. Look for nutrients that state on the label "No magnesium stearate, no ascorbyl palmitate" (these are often used as flowing agents) and look for allergen-free fillers.

Vitamin A

Two types of vitamin A are available: preformed vitamin A, or retinols, and precursor vitamin A (known as beta-carotene) sourced from plants. Beta-carotene is converted into vitamin A in the body. Stored in the liver and fat soluble, it prevents night blindness, infections, and hyperkeratosis (hardened red bumps on the back of the arm located at the base of follicles). Beta-carotene is one of the top 10 nutrients because it acts on the immune system by increasing levels of T-helper cells and maintaining the health of the mucosal membrane in the gastrointestinal and respiratory tracts (thus keeping out invaders). It improves thyroid function, normalizes blood glucose and insulin, and treats acne, asthma, and bronchial infections. It promotes cell division, white cell activity, and increases the response of antibodies. Vitamin A helps to increase the good immune factors that turn off the inflammatory and pain-causing immune factor, interleukin-1. Vitamin A is an antioxidant that fights cancer and heart disease. It also increases interferon's influence as an antiviral and enhances activity in the thymus. Adequate dietary protein, zinc, and B vitamins enhance its absorption.

Beta-carotene sources include dark green, red, and deep yellow-orange vegetables. Vitamin A sources include egg yolks, liver, kidney, full-fat milk and cheese, butter, cod liver oil, and halibut oil. Toxicity has occurred when high doses of over 50,000 IU were taken over a long term, but this is rare. When vitamin A is taken in recommended doses toxicity is not a problem. Too many carrots or dark vegetables can cause a harmless orange color to appear on the palms of the hands, soles of the feet, and the end of the nose. This is often seen in babies who love carrots and eat them every day.

Vitamin B$_1$

According to a U.S. Department of Agriculture study, 45 percent of Americans consume less than the recommended dietary allowances of vitamin B$_1$, known as thiamine.

In the late 1800s, deficiencies of vitamin B$_1$ brought on by eating polished instead of whole-grain rice led to beriberi, a disease that resulted in wasting muscles, mental confusion, edema, heart problems, and difficulty in walking. Experiments conducted to understand this phenomenon led to the discovery of this first B vitamin. Vitamin B$_1$ is necessary for healthy mental function and protects us against the aging effects of stress. It mimics acetylcholine and takes part in the production of energy production in the brain. For this reason it is usually recommended for treatment of Alzheimer's, fatigue, depression, tingling sensations in the legs, and mood disorders. It is beneficial to the cardiovascular system as it builds blood and strengthens the heart. A 200 mg dose of thiamine was given to patients with congestive heart failure, and after six weeks 22 percent showed improvement in breathing, walking, and a reduction in edema. It also helps the digestive system to regulate appetite, produce stomach acid, and break down carbohydrates. It is a great mosquito repellent as well because mosquitoes hate the skin of someone taking thiamine, so they won't bite.

Brewer's yeast and organ meats are the richest sources of vitamin B$_1$. Soybeans, brown rice, sunflower seeds, peanuts, and whole wheat are just some of the other foods that are rich in vitamin B$_1$. It is highly sensitive and its efficacy is reduced when a person is exposed to sulfites, alcohol, and the tannins in coffee and tea. Reduce or eliminate as many of these as possible from your diet.

What Is a Free Radical?

Little was known about free radicals as recently as 40 years ago. Today free radicals are considered the main component in aging and disease progression. Many diseases, such as rheumatoid arthritis and cancer, are the result of free radical damage to the body. Free radicals are a natural by-product of everyday reactions that produce energy for the body. Digesting and metabolizing foods causes the largest production of free radicals in the body. The energy is produced by reactions between many substances and oxygen. Without energy production, our body cannot survive. Think of the serious impairment to life that chronic fatigue syndrome causes with its malfunctioning energy production. Molecules including oxygen, fatty acids, amino acids, and DNA are the basic components used to build and repair the body. Molecules are held together by electrons; stable molecules have electrons that are paired. When a molecule does not have a pair, it becomes unstable and reactive. A free radical is the unstable molecule that is highly reactive and searching for a pair to make it stable. It will do anything to find a partner, including stealing and damaging other molecules to get what it needs. If a stable molecule loses an electron, it then becomes a free radical, which then steals an electron from another molecule and so on. Stealing an electron from another molecule creates a chain reaction, resulting in the release of thousands of free radicals, which cause damage and destruction until the reaction is squelched. Think of a tiny spot of rust on the fender of your car. If this tiny spot is left unattended, it will eventually become a big rusty hole. Fortunately, free radical damage can be easily kept in check by using potent antioxidants, including vitamin E, vitamin C, selenium, and vitamin A.

Exposure to toxins such as tobacco smoke, prescription drugs, environmental pollutants, radiation, and even exercise that lasts 30 minutes or more can increase free radical reactions in the body. Our immune system normally produces exorbitant amounts of free radicals to destroy invading bacteria and viruses. Free radical production is a process developed by our bodies to eliminate potential dangerous substances, but if left unchecked, free radical damage can do more harm than good. This is where the exciting field of nutrition plays a role. Destruction of healthy cells can be avoided by simply improving diet and adding nutritional supplements, especially antioxidants and nature's powerful protectors, phytochemicals.

Vitamin B$_2$

Vitamin B$_2$ (riboflavin), when taken in a B-complex, turns urine a fluorescent yellow-green color. Vitamin B$_2$ is essential for energy production and metabolism. Glutathione, B$_6$, C, E, and niacin enhance its actions. Research has shown that it protects against free radical damage and esophageal cancers. It is crucial for metabolizing all nutrients and for forming antibodies and red cells. It has been used to prevent migraines and sickle cell anemia. Carpal tunnel syndrome has been relieved with 100–500 mg of riboflavin taken with equal amounts of vitamin B$_6$. Rosacea symptoms have improved over several months with 50 mg per day of riboflavin.

Deficiency in vitamin B$_2$ can result in eye problems such as cataracts, weak visual acuity, and sensitivity to light, and anemia similar to that of iron-deficiency anemia. Signs of deficiency include cracks at the edges of the mouth, chapped lips, swollen inflamed tongue, bloodshot eyes, sensitivity to light, and crusty skin. Birth control pills inhibit the absorption of riboflavin, so women taking them should also take 100 mg of vitamin B$_2$ per day to protect against this effect.

Sources of vitamin B$_2$ include green leafy vegetables, soybeans, whole grains, almonds, raw mushrooms, organ meats, dairy products, and eggs.

Vitamin B$_3$

One of the B-complex family, vitamin B$_3$ (niacin, nicotinic acid, niacinamide) is an important component of nicotinamide adenine dinucleotide (NAD) and nicotinamide adenine dinucleotide phosphate (NADP), enzymes involved in over 200 reactions in the body. Niacin is beneficial in lowering blood cholesterol levels and triglycerides (see page 27 in Chapter 2). It helps the digestive system by maintaining hydrochloric acid in the stomach and bile secretion, and is used to stop both diarrhea and gingivitis and the resulting tooth loss. Niacin is excellent for cardiovascular health. When a daily dose of 2000 mg of niacin was given to patients who had previously had heart attacks, the recurrence rate was cut by 30 percent. Niacin also takes part in the production of adrenal and sex hormones, and helps the nervous system. In addition, niacin plays a role in energy production, antioxidant mechanisms, and detoxification. It is also being investigated for possible anticancer properties.

Niacinamide has shown some effect in reducing the need for insulin in diabetics. There have been favorable reports of its efficacy in rheumatoid arthritis and osteoarthritis. It has also been used to treat anxiety and to help people withdraw from benzodiazepines

Another powerful antioxidant version of B$_3$ called NADH is being explored for its ability to give healthy people a noticeable boost in energy and for its therapeutic properties for those suffering from Alzheimer's disease, chronic fatigue syndrome, and Parkinson's disease.

When you supplement with niacin, there is a harmless flushing effect of the skin that can take up to half an hour to go away. If you find the skin flushing uncomfortable, use non-flushing niacin, inositol hexanicotinate. Do not use sustained-release niacin as studies have shown it to be toxic to the liver.

Vitamin B_3 is available in avocados, whole grains, legumes, eggs, milk, fish, organ meats, peanuts, peanut butter, and poultry.

Vitamin B$_5$

Pantothen means "everywhere" and because of its wide availability in foods, it is rare to have deficiencies in vitamin B_5, or pantothenic acid. Organ meats, fish, poultry, milk, whole grains, legumes, mushrooms, nuts, eggs, sweet potatoes, broccoli, cauliflower, oranges, and strawberries are all sources of vitamin B_5. It is required for its supportive role in energy conversion of fats, carbohydrates, and protein; for optimizing adrenal function; and for manufacturing red blood cells.

It is an important vitamin because it supports the adrenal glands, is a constituent of coenzyme A, and produces cortisol and steroid hormones. It also plays a role in controlling blood sugar metabolism. Vitamin B_5 has been used to reduce the symptoms of discoid lupus. High doses of vitamin B_5 were shown to improve the symptoms of rheumatoid arthritis and osteoarthritis. Vitamin B_5 supplementation is used to alleviate symptoms of allergies, digestive disorders, and stress. Pantethine, the more active form of vitamin B_5, has been shown to reduce cholesterol and triglycerides up to 30 percent. It is also used to control cellulite (with great results) and "burning feet" syndrome.

Vitamin B$_6$

Vitamin B_6 (pyridoxine and pyridoxal-5-phosphate), one of the top 10 nutrients for supporting immune function, is also needed to make antibodies and slow tumor growth. Unfortunately, vitamin B_6 is a common deficiency. It is a crucial component in cell replication and is therefore extremely important during pregnancy and controlling homocysteine (see Chapter 2). Vitamin B_6 lends itself to proper functioning of enzymes, red blood cell and antibody formation, mucous membranes, and the skin—all areas where cells multiply quickly.

Because of its part in the manufacture of neurotransmitters and hormones, vitamin B_6 is required for optimal brain and nervous system function. It is vital for the utilization of many nutrients, including B_{12}, magnesium, and niacin. Vitamin B_6 also prevents the thymus from shrinking and may decrease insulin requirements. It is also recommended for asthma, cardiovascular disease, carpal tunnel syndrome, PMS, autism, nausea during pregnancy, and osteoporosis. A daily dose of 100 mg may prevent the recurrence of oxalate kidney stones.

Vitamin B_6 should be taken in conjunction with the other B vitamins in a complex. This is the way they are found in nature and each has a synergistic effect on the other. Those who have liver problems or lack the enzyme to break down vitamin B_6 should use pyridoxal-5-phosphate (P-5-P), the active form of vitamin B_6. Magnesium is a cofactor required for vitamin B_6 absorption. If using a nutritional supplement of B_6, look for one with added magnesium.

Deficiencies in vitamin B_6 can be recognized by symptoms of depression, learning disabilities, acne, arthritis, weakness, anemia, and seborrheic dermatitis. There may also be glucose intolerance or convulsions (particularly in infants).

Vitamin B_6 is found in cantaloupe, bananas, cabbage, green leafy vegetables, Brussels sprouts, organ meats, eggs, whole grains, soybeans, and saltwater fish.

Vitamin B_{12}

Vitamin B_{12} works with other B vitamins to support DNA synthesis and the formation of red blood cells. It also maintains the structure of the myelin sheath, the covering around nerve cells that ensures speedy communication of the neurotransmitters. Vitamin B_{12} supplementation is indicated for people with Alzheimer's, diabetic neuropathy, depression and other emotional problems, asthma, multiple sclerosis and other motor neuron difficulties, shingles, and HIV/AIDS. Those with multiple sclerosis should take 1000 mcg per day to slow the destruction of the myelin sheath. Vitamin B_{12} 1000 mcg injections also reduce shingles outbreaks and the painful neuropathy associated with them. Anemia is the first symptom of B_{12} deficiency. Pernicious anemia, common in the elderly, is caused by inadequate B_{12} intake or gastric absorption problems.

Vegans and some vegetarians are at risk for vitamin B_{12} (cobalamin) deficiency because the better sources of B_{12} are in meat products (especially kidney and liver), fish, eggs, and cheese. Sublingual vitamin B_{12} or B_{12} injections are advised for those avoiding meat-based diets.

Folic Acid

Without folic acid (folate, folacin), DNA synthesis could not occur and cells would not divide. It is the most essential nutrient an expectant mother can take before and during pregnancy to optimize the formation of her fetus's nervous system. Deficiencies during gestation have been linked to a range of birth defects, including spina bifida and a higher incidence of miscarriages, preeclampsia and placental problems. In adults, deficiencies increase homocysteine levels and can contribute to atherosclerosis.

Folic acid is necessary to improve appetite, produce sufficient stomach acid, form red blood cells, metabolize protein, and prevent anemia. It also elevates serotonin levels in the brain.

Folic acid can be found in asparagus, citrus fruit, lentils, legumes, whole grains, salmon, organ meats, dairy, beets, but especially green leafy vegetables (folic = foliage). The typical Western diet, however, emphasizes meat (low folic acid content) over vegetables (high folic acid content), so deficiencies are quite common as a result. Supplementation can alleviate that problem and there is a form of folic acid called folinic acid that is more efficient at raising the nutrient's levels in the body.

Choline

Choline, which is essential in manufacturing the neurotransmitter acetylcholine and other components of our cell membranes, transforms into phosphatidyl choline and sphingomyelin. It is also necessary for nerve function, metabolism of fats, and liver and gallbladder modulation. Choline is present in meat, milk, and whole grains, but is also present in the form of lecithin in egg yolks, legumes, and grains.

Acetylcholine is required for many processes in the brain, including memory. Deficiencies of choline can lead to heart, kidney, and liver troubles, high blood pressure, growth problems, Alzheimer's disease, and bipolar depression.

Vitamin C

The late Linus Pauling spent half of his life heralding the benefits of vitamin C. Pauling died at the age of 93 due to prostate cancer, but assured us that his life was extended by several decades due to his consumption of vitamin C. Thousands of research papers and almost as many books have been written about this essential nutrient. Emanuel Cheraskin titled his book *Vitamin C: Who Needs It?*, and then provided over 50 double-blind studies to prove that we all need vitamin C. In Jack Challem's book, *Syndrome X*, he states that "study after study shows that low levels of vitamin C are intertwined with and contribute to diabetic complications, heart disease, kidney disease and eye disorders. It lowers glucose and it normalizes insulin's response to glucose."

Research has now confirmed that vitamin C is antiviral, antibacterial, and anticancer. It is known that a prostaglandin (PGE1), which plays a major role in regulation of T-cell function, is enhanced by vitamin C. Vitamin C also enhances complement and C1 esterase, without which the entire enzymatic

Vitamin C to Bowel Tolerance

How much is too much vitamin C? Robert Cathcart, MD, says that we each have our own ascorbate limit, which is determined by stress, nutritional status, and current state of health. To determine your own personal vitamin C requirements, start taking gram doses of vitamin C until your bowels become loose. At this point, reduce the dosage until bowel movements are normal. This is your personal vitamin C requirement. Depending on your current health and lifestyle choices, this level may fluctuate from day to day or week to week. The RDA is 60 mg per day. Most people require much more.

cascade of complement would not occur and non-self cells would not be destroyed. Taking as little as 1000 mg of vitamin C per day increased T-cell activity and 500 mg per day increased glutathione levels by 50 percent. Glutathione, as you will see later, is extremely important to immune function because it eliminates toxic substances from the body, enhances cellular oxygen, and activates enzymatic reactions.

Vitamin C Facts:
- The National Institute of Aging states that only 9 percent of North Americans are in an optimal vitamin C state.
- Each cigarette smoked eliminates 25 mg of vitamin C from the body.
- 10 g doses of vitamin C daily may make birth control pills ineffective.
- 1000 mg per day increases sperm motility and fertility.

In order to get the minimum requirement of vitamin C, we would have to eat five vine-ripened fruits and vegetables each day. Foods high in vitamin C include Brussels sprouts, cabbage, cauliflower, collard, mustard greens, broccoli, black currants, kale, parsley, chili peppers, citrus fruits, and sweet red and green peppers.

Vitamin D

Vitamin D, another fat-soluble vitamin, is also called the sunshine vitamin because 15 to 20 minutes of sunlight a day on bare skin can give us our daily dose. Those living in the northern hemisphere often have deficiencies of this vitamin because poor climates with extended cloud cover do not allow for adequate sun exposure. Most dairy products are now fortified with vitamin D to prevent rickets and vitamin D deficiency diseases. See page 68 for health problems associated with excessive milk consumption and vitamin D toxicity. Vitamin D is considered a hormone as well as a vitamin. As we age, our bodies are less efficient at manufacturing vitamin D. A deficiency in vitamin

D leads to decreases in calcium absorption in the intestine and increases its excretion via the kidneys, promoting osteoporosis. Many disorders are promoted by vitamin D deficiency, and the resulting decrease in calcium; these include osteoarthritis, muscle cramps, and twitching. It is essential for the manufacture of thyroid hormone and many with hypothyroid are often vitamin D deficient. Psoriasis can also be improved as vitamin D halts the proliferation of skin cells (this is thought to be why those with psoriasis have an improvement when they are exposed to the sun).

These foods are good sources of vitamin D: fatty fish (including cod, tuna, and halibut), egg yolks, cod liver oil, blue-green algae, and fortified milk products.

Vitamin E

Known as an antiaging vitamin, vitamin E is also a powerful antioxidant that prevents damage to cells, especially nerve cells, and protects against the effects of stress. It lowers cholesterol, strengthens capillaries, prevents clotting, and improves blood flow. Also a top 10 nutrient and crucial to healthy immune function, vitamin E protects the thymus and white blood cells from oxidative stress and viral illnesses such as AIDS and hepatitis. It improves cell-mediated immunity, enhances digestion in cells (phagocytosis), and increases resistance to infection. Vitamins C and E work cooperatively to increase the number of T-cells, tumor necrosis factors, and good immune factor IL-2, and reduce inflammation. Vitamin E appears to prevent cancers of the breast and prostate from developing by inhibiting cancer cells from multiplying. A 14-year study involving 5000 British women showed that low blood levels of vitamin E increased breast cancer risk by 500 percent. Due to vitamin E's free radical scavenging abilities, your risk of cancer can be cut by 50 percent with a daily dosage of 400 IU. Large-scale studies are now showing that vitamin E supplementation can lower our risk of colon cancer.

It also decreases the negative effects of stress. Stressors cause the release of our stress hormone, cortisol, which then causes the inflammatory immune factor interleukin-6 to be released. Vitamin E increases the good immune factors that keep interleukin-1 and interleukin-6 under control. Vitamin E's healing abilities affect a vast range of conditions such as cancer, diabetes, dementia and Alzheimer's, cataracts and macular degeneration, leg cramps and pain, skin disorders, arthritis, allergies, PMS, and cardiovascular disease.

Vitamin E can be found in food sources such as eggs, organ meats, pressed vegetable oils, and dark green vegetables. It is also found in almonds, but you would need 9 lb (4 kg) of these nuts to get enough vitamin E to boost immunity! There are natural and synthetic forms of supplements available, but the natural is far superior and the best vitamin E supplements will also contain mixed tocopherols including beta, delta, and gamma-tocopherol. Look for d-alpha-tocopherol or d-alpha-tocopheryl acetate or d-alpha-tocopheryl succinate, which are the natural forms. Do not use the forms with the prefix dl-. You can also buy vitamin E in a water-soluble form called micelized vitamin E. Caution: Because vitamin E has blood-thinning action, do not take it with Warfarin (Coumadin), a blood thinner.

Vitamin K

Our liver uses vitamin K, called the "Koagulation" vitamin, to make protein factors that are essential to form blood clots. Vitamin K is manufactured in the body by bacteria that live in our intestines. Deficiency is rare. Babies are given injections of vitamin K at birth to prevent bleeding until their gut bacteria can produce vitamin K. However, some experts on vitamin K and blood clotting believe that babies should not be injected and instead kept safe from bumps and bangs and protected in a bassinet for the first few weeks of life. Vitamin K regulates clotting in the blood, making it beneficial for excessive menstrual bleeding. It is necessary for activating bone protein to increase bone mineral density to offset osteoporosis. A more recent application of vitamin K has been as a supplement during cancer treatment. There is an unusual property in vitamin K that allows it to enhance anticoagulant therapy, which prevents tumors from metastasizing, even during chemotherapy.

Sources include green vegetables, green tea leaves and extracts, liver, and dairy products. Too much vitamin K can cause excessive sweating and flushing.

VITAMIN-LIKE NUTRIENTS

Alpha Lipoic Acid

Alpha lipoic acid's principal role is to convert glucose to energy. More potent than vitamins C and E, it is also able to recycle these vitamins in the body as well. ALA (lipoic acid, thioctic acid) is soluble in both water and fat, so it is able to protect our cells (both inside and out) against damage from toxins. The German government has approved alpha lipoic acid for the treatment of diabetic neuropathy. In one study the regeneration of nerve tissue was observed. It also inhibits the ability of viruses to replicate.

Diabetics or pre-diabetics take note: alpha lipoic acid in a dose of 600 mg per day can lower glucose levels, improve insulin sensitivity, and improve the body's ability to burn glucose.

Coenzyme Q10

CoQ10, noted as "the spark of life," plays an essential role in producing energy in the cells. A powerful antioxidant with antiviral, antibacterial, and antitumor properties, it is most noted for its heart-protective effects and now researchers have realized it is also a potent immune nutrient. CoQ10 is currently being studied for its effectiveness in reducing the rate of degenerative illnesses such as amyotrophic lateral sclerosis, Parkinson's disease, and Huntington's disease. Promising research has also shown that doses of CoQ10 over 300 mg inhibit the growth of breast tumors.

CoQ10 is depleted as we age. At the age of 50 we produce half the amount of CoQ10 as we did when were 20. Although CoQ10 is available from foods such as peanuts, organ meats, and fatty fish, it is difficult to obtain enough of it from diet alone. You would have to eat pounds of those foods every day, but CoQ10 is available as a supplement; it should be taken when you are eating healthy fats or oils, to enhance absorption.

MACRO MINERALS

Minerals act as coenzymes, work synergistically with vitamins, control many biochemical actions, and provide normal cell function and healthy bones and blood. Without enough of a certain mineral, some vitamins cannot be assimilated. Minerals are grouped as either macro or trace minerals. Macro minerals include calcium, magnesium, phosphorus, potassium, and sodium. Trace minerals, needed in minute or trace quantities, include boron, chromium, copper, iodine, iron, manganese, molybdenum, selenium, and zinc.

Calcium

Two percent of our total body weight is made up of calcium. It is needed to build bones and teeth, control muscle function, transmit nerve impulses, keep the heart beating, and promote blood clotting and wound healing. It is helpful for arthritis, rheumatism, menstrual cramps and menopause, osteoporosis, and hypertension and preeclampsia in pregnant women.

Numbness, difficulty in sleeping, nervousness or heart palpitations, tooth decay, and muscle cramps can all signal a deficiency in calcium. Contrary to what most people think, milk is not the perfect source of calcium. Sea vegetables, kale, mixed greens (such as collard leaves and dandelion and turnip greens), Brazil nuts, almonds, sunflower seeds, and tofu have as much or more calcium than milk. Given the controversy over the increasing dangers of milk products, the Physicians for Responsible Medicine do not recommend giving milk to children, so it is important to know that you have alternatives (read more about milk in Chapter 4).

Calcium absorption is reduced by eating a diet that is too high in meat or drinking carbonated soft drinks. The tannins in tea, saturated fats, bran, and dietary fiber all inhibit the uptake of calcium.

Magnesium

Magnesium is essential for proper immune function, is anti-inflammatory, treats fibromyalgia, protects against diabetes and loss of bone, lowers high blood pressure, and prevents dental cavities. It is considered an antiaging nutrient that also promotes a healthy nervous system and reduces stress.

If your heart is jumping out of your chest, or if you have a twitchy eyelid, leg cramps, or restless legs, you are probably magnesium deficient. Deficiency often develops due to unhealthy diet choices and excessive caffeine consumption (caffeine causes a more rapid depletion of the mineral). Magnesium, the fourth most abundant mineral in the body, is essential for over 300 enzymatic and metabolic reactions and is essential to a peak operating immune system. Diets that focus on plant foods contain more magnesium: tofu, whole grains, green leafy vegetables, nuts and seeds, and legumes. Meat, fish, and dairy products are low in magnesium.

Phosphorus

Because it is involved in most reactions in the body and is required for the metabolism of nutrients, phosphorus is vital to our health. Good dietary sources include meat (especially poultry and glandular meats), fish, nuts and seeds, eggs, yellow cheese, and whole grains. Phosphorus participates in the growth and repair of cells, the building of teeth and bones, and the production and release of energy. It also improves kidney, heart, nerve, and muscle function.

Phosphorus is beneficial for alleviating stress and arthritis, promoting growth in children, and maintaining healthy gums. Symptoms of its deficiency can be observed through fatigue, weight loss or gain, loss of appetite, nervous disorders or irregular heartbeat, rickets, and pyorrhea.

Potassium and Sodium

Potassium and sodium work together to balance cellular fluid levels, and regulate blood pressure and muscle contraction. Potassium supports adrenal and kidney function, heartbeat, and calms the nerves. It participates in glucose-to-glycogen conversion, hormone secretion, and keeps the pH balance from becoming too acidic or alkaline. Potassium also prevents acne and enhances growth.

The ideal ratio of potassium to sodium in our diet is 5:1. The average North American consumes so much salt that the ratio is 1:2. Too much or too little potassium is equally bad—the key is balance. The richest sources of potassium are dried apricots, potatoes, tomatoes, avocados, and bananas, but other plant foods and fish have significant amounts as well.

A lack of potassium results in increasing constipation, acne, dry skin, edema, thirst, nervousness, and weakened reflexes. A lack of sodium results in a loss of appetite and weight, increased gas, muscle wasting, and vomiting.

TRACE MINERALS

Although they are required in smaller amounts, trace minerals are very important for good health. How much we get from our food, however, depends entirely on the condition of the soil it was grown in, as the plants' uptake can be poor if the soil is depleted or if pesticides are used. Choose certified organic products to get the highest trace mineral content from foods.

Boron

Good dietary sources of boron are fruits and vegetables. Boron is required for vitamin D activity to stimulate the absorption and use of calcium. It is also recommended for preventing osteoporosis and arthritis. A lack of boron in postmenopausal women forces calcium and magnesium to be excreted and lowers estrogen and testosterone concentrations in serum.

Chromium

Whole grain foods and meats are staples for chromium in the diet. Chromium is highly significant in glucose tolerance factor (GTF), the compound that is key to maintaining insulin stability, stimulates the synthesis of fatty acids and cholesterol, activates digestive enzymes, and protects RNA and DNA. Because of its influence on insulin (and its suppression of sugar cravings), chromium is prescribed for diabetes, hypoglycemia, and weight loss. It also works to lower triglyceride and blood cholesterol levels. Deficiency of chromium leads to glucose intolerance and atherosclerosis.

Copper

Shellfish and legumes are the richest dietary sources of copper, but it is also found in avocados, raisins, and dark green leafy vegetables in lesser amounts. Copper is essential for several enzyme actions, so its deficiency can be apparent in many areas of the body: weakened blood vessels, abnormal bones and joints, elevated LDL cholesterol and lowered HDL cholesterol, and impaired brain and immune function. Copper supplementation is recommended for heart disease, sciatica, and osteoarthritis and rheumatoid arthritis. It is also more effective than iron in treating anemia. It may be inhibited or depleted by high doses of vitamin C, zinc, iron, and other minerals.

Iodine

The major source of iodine is seafood, specifically seaweeds such as kelp, nori, and dulse. Iodine is critical to the production of thyroid hormone, it regulates estrogen in breast tissue, and also protects against harmful electromagnetic radiation. Fibrocystic breast disease, miscarriage, stunted growth, increased risk for infant mortality, mental disabilities, thyroid problems, and goiter are just some of the possible outcomes of iodine deficiency. Since iodine was added to table salt, the deficiency rate has plummeted. Iodine deficiency can result from overeating foods that block iodine absorption (called goitrogens), such as turnips, mustard, cabbage, soybeans, pine nuts, and peanuts.

Iron

There are two types of iron: heme and nonheme. Heme iron is available in meat products and is more easily absorbed. Nonheme is found in plant foods and is not as well absorbed. As the carrier of oxygen in the blood and carbon dioxide to the lungs, iron is essential to our existence. Iron is also important in the enzymatic reactions that, among other things, synthesize DNA and produce and metabolize energy. It also helps us resist disease and tolerate stress.

Iron deficiency is very common. Children under two, the elderly, and females, especially pregnant women and menstruating women, are at risk for deficiency. Craving ice chips or dirt are signs of iron deficiency. Floradix is a wonderful nonheme iron supplement that normalizes iron levels without constipation.

Manganese

Manganese is crucial to the enzymes that control blood sugar, thyroid hormone activity, and the metabolism of energy. It is required for the nervous and immune systems, and prevents cells from suffering free radical damage and the resulting inflammation. Manganese is used in treatments for allergies, fatigue, asthma, diabetes, and epilepsy, as well as sprains, strains, and inflammation. A lack of manganese can lead to bone loss, lowered HDL cholesterol, and problems with the skin, hair, and nails. Diabetics require manganese to fully utilize insulin. Plant foods such as whole grains, nuts, green leafy vegetables, and dried fruits are excellent sources of manganese.

Molybdenum

Molybdenum is a required coenzyme for the enzymes that are involved in detoxification of alcohol and sulfites, and controls uric acid formation. People with esophageal cancer tend to have low levels of molybdenum, so it is speculated that its detoxification qualities include cancer-causing agents. Deficiencies can bring on cavities and sulfite sensitivities that express symptoms such as headaches, nausea, disorientation, and a racing pulse. Molybdenum also mobilizes iron and nitrogen metabolism. Whole grains, dark green leafy vegetables, and legumes are the best sources of molybdenum.

Selenium

Insufficient selenium makes us highly susceptible to cancer, viruses, and free radical damage. Selenium is one of the most potent free radical scavengers, which we call antioxidants. Areas of the world that have low selenium levels have correspondingly high levels of cancer and viruses. For example, Harold Foster, of the University of Victoria, found that breast cancer rates were strongly correlated to soil selenium levels. As well, Zaire, which has extremely low soil selenium levels, has unusually high rates of HIV infection. Also interesting is a study published in the *Journal of the American College of Nutrition* that showed dormant coxsackie virus B3 became active and extremely virulent in selenium-deficient mice. The researchers noted that the public health implications of this are significant with the increase in RNA viruses such as AIDS, polio, and influenza. Optimal selenium levels may have profound protective effects against the activation of viruses.

Selenium is essential to the production of a powerful enzyme called glutathione peroxidase, which is important in detoxifying the body from environmental toxins. Selenium deficiency causes poor resistance to viruses and bacteria, and reduces T-cell activity and antibody production. Imagine an immune system that is unable to mobilize its T-cells and natural killer cells to destroy pathogenic bacteria and viruses. This is exactly what occurs in a selenium-deficient immune system.

Another study involving rheumatoid arthritis (RA) patients showed that selenium supplementation is important in reducing the production of inflammatory prostaglandins, leukotrienes, and free radicals, which are thought to cause most of the damage seen in RA conditions.

Brazil nuts, still in the shell, are an excellent food source of selenium. One or two Brazil nuts a day provide adequate selenium. You will notice throughout the book that certain foods will be recommended over and over for their powerful healing benefits. Brazil nuts are also rich in phytosterols, which are another important nutrient for the immune system. Selenium should be supplemented in doses of 100–200 mcg daily to enhance immune function and obtain a disease-protecting effect.

Zinc

We mentioned in Chapter 3 that the thymus gland is like the orchestra director or commanding officer of a very large army. Without a healthy thymus, we just can't have an immune system that accomplishes the job. Zinc is the most important mineral to the thymus gland, so important that even if you have a small or malfunctioning thymus, zinc supplements can reverse and rejuvenate this gland. Causes of zinc deficiency include the following:

- vegetarian diets (phytates in plant foods inhibit zinc and other minerals)
- low red meat consumption
- nonconsumption of seafood
- diets, especially high-carbohydrate diets
- copper toxicity
- low stomach acid
- digestive disorders
- aging, especially if you are over 45

In a review article by Ananda Prasad, he stated that there are over 300 enzyme systems in the body that require zinc. A deficiency can result in poor growth (as seen in children), small testes, anorexia, slow wound healing, delayed puberty, and skin problems. Especially important to the scope of this book is the effect that inadequate zinc has on our immune system. Zinc is required for cell-mediated immunity and proper cell division as well as for DNA synthesis. Prasad also found that when 30 mg of zinc was provided daily to zinc-deficient elderly subjects, levels of interleukin-2 and thymulin, an important hormone secreted by the thymus, were increased. Remember—interleukin-2 authorizes killer T-cells to attack.

Zinc's antiviral activity was examined in a double-blind, placebo-controlled trial with 37 cold-infected subjects. Zinc lozenges containing 23 mg of zinc were taken at two-hour intervals. After seven days, over 85 percent of the participants were symptom-free compared to half of the placebo group. Zinc lozenges are now commonly prescribed for the cold virus, but remember, even too much of a good thing can be bad. One study of 11 subjects who took 300 mg (150 mg twice a day) of zinc daily for six weeks found that the immune system was suppressed.

EXTRA SPECIAL NUTRIENTS

Beta Glucan

Japanese and Chinese medicine has been using beta glucan from mushrooms since the beginning of time. Derived from baker's yeast, mushrooms, and oats, beta-1,3/1,6 glucan stimulates macrophage cells, a role that is vital to a healthy immune system. It is a powerful antioxidant and an effective medication for lowering blood cholesterol. Beta-1,3 glucan has also been used for viral infections such as HIV, Epstein-Barr, and herpes, and in candidiasis. Research is currently underway to confirm its effectiveness in cancer treatment and in lowering cholesterol and triglyceride.

Chondroitin

Chondroitin sulfate, which is used for treating pain in over 100 arthritic conditions, is a component of cartilage. It acts as a lubricant for joints and prevents cartilage deterioration. It is nature's shock absorber for joints and gives the joint spaces access to nutrients. Experiments comparing chondroitin sulfate to NSAIDs reported chondroitin to be more effective at stopping edema and inflammation. It is often supplemented with glucosamine sulfate (see page 104).

Colostrum

Colostrum is the yellow fluid produced by a mother's mammary glands to nourish her baby for the first 24 to 72 hours after giving birth. It contains carotenoids such as lycopene and beta-carotene, essential fatty acids, immunoglobulins IgA, IgD, IgE, IgG, and IgM (as well as antibodies from diseases that mom was previously exposed to), growth factors, lactoferrin (a potent, natural antibacterial, antiviral, and anti-inflammatory), vitamins, minerals, enzymes, amino acids, and more. Colostrum is designed to protect the baby during the initial weeks of life and stimulate the development of the infant's immune system.

In order to make colostrum available to everyone, cows were chosen as a good source because they make gallons of colostrum in the first hours after the birth of a calf. Bovine colostrum has been used successfully to alleviate diarrhea in AIDS patients and to prevent the onset of illness from shigella infection. Colostrum has been used to help the immune system fight viruses and bacteria, and promote wound healing. It is also an effective treatment for diarrhea, leaky gut, and overall bowel health, and reduces inflammatory cytokines, including interleukin-6.

DIM (Di-indolylmethane)

Di-indolylmethane (DIM) is one of several powerful phytonutrients found in cruciferous vegetables, including cabbage, broccoli, and Brussels sprouts. It is a powerful estrogen regulator and enhances the production of 2-hydroxyestradiol and 2-hydroxyestrone, the "good" forms of estrogen. DIM also lowers 16-hydroxyestrone, a carcinogenic form of estrogen.

Research studies have shown that high levels of 16-hydroxyestrone are seen in women with breast cancer and low levels of the 2-hydroxyestrogens have been linked to breast, uterine, and cervical cancer, and lupus. Long-term exposure to xenoestrogens found in our environment or estrogens in hormone replacement therapy are associated with many health risks. A healthy ratio of 2-hydroxyestrone to 16-hydroxyestrone is essential to reducing the risk of certain cancers and improving apoptosis (cell death) in cancer treatment.

DIM is beneficial for both men and women. Not only does it reduce the risk of estrogen-related breast cancer for women, who may or may not be taking any type of hormone replacement, but it can also regulate rising estrogen levels in men during andropause (the male menopause), which can lead to prostate gland enlargement. DIM is 10 times more potent than its precursor indole-3-carbinol and is more effective as a dietary supplement.

5-Hydroxytryptophan

5-hydroxytryptophan (5-HTP) enhances the body's production of sero-tonin and works as a natural antidepressant. Supplementation with 5-HTP has proven as equally effective as Prozac and other selective serotonin reuptake inhibitors (SSRIs) and tricyclic antidepressants, but without the side effects. It calms the nerves and appetite while enhancing mood and restful sleep. 5-HTP relieves chronic pain and modulates smooth muscle function in the cardiovascular and digestive systems. It is used predominantly in cases of insomnia and depression and to suppress appetite.

Flavonoids

Flavonoids are the most prevalent phytonutrient family in the plant kingdom. Discovered by Albert Szent-Gyorgi in 1936, they include anthocyanidin, astragelin, catechin, hesperidin, isoflavones, kampherol, luteolin, naringin, pycnogenol, and quercetin. Quercetin is commonly recommended as a potent antiallergy nutrient capable of inhibiting inflammation of the airways and the release of histamine. Flavonoids are antibacterial, anticancer, antiestrogenic, and anti-inflammatory. They also prevent allergies, stimulate weight loss, promote circulation, reduce the risk of osteoporosis, and more.

Glucosamine Sulfate

Commonly regarded as the "arthritis cure," glucosamine sulfate allows cartilage, invertebral discs, and ligaments to regenerate. It also acts as a shock absorber and anti-inflammatory. More than a dozen human trials have demonstrated that glucosamine sulfate improves arthritis symptoms by 50–80 percent; is equal to or more effective in controlling pain and inflammation than non-steroidal anti-inflammatory drugs (NSAIDs); and can regenerate joint tissue. Chondroitin and glucosamine sulfate are generally taken together. Plant sterols and sterolins can turn off the damaging inflammatory process, allowing glucosamine to repair the joint.

IP-6 (Inositol Hexaphosphate)

Phytic acid, also known as IP-6, is found in the cells of all mammals, including humans. It exists in the seeds of grains and legumes, but is removed during milling and processing. IP-6 is required to control cell division and is located predominantly in the brain and skeletal and heart muscle. IP-6 acts as an antioxidant, binding with excess iron during energy production in cells to prevent free radicals from forming. Its antioxidant action can prevent tissue inflammation and damage from asbestos. In addition to its anticancer and antitoxin activity, it is useful for kidney stones, heart and liver diseases, sickle cell anemia, fat metabolism, diabetes, cholesterol, psychiatric diseases, and preventing birth defects. In laboratory animals IP-6 has been shown to enhance natural killer cell activity. No human research at this time has shown that IP-6 can fight cancer.

Lignans

Lignans are one of today's superfoods. Plant lignans are found naturally in foods high in dietary fiber, such as flaxseeds. Plant lignans are converted in the colon by bacterial fermentation into human lignans. Lignans are structurally similar to estrogens and work as weak estrogens or antiestrogens, removing excess estrogens that may be harmful. They balance estrogen metabolism in women and men. Lignans have also been found to be antibacterial, antifungal, and antiviral. Researchers are investigating the effects of lignans on humans. In 1990 the National Cancer Institute in the United States launched a program to learn more about plant chemicals and disease prevention. Flaxseed was one of the six food groups targeted for study. Flaxseed is the richest source of plant lignans. Flaxseed fiber consumption results in an average of 100–800 percent greater lignan production. Defatted flaxseed has up to 30 percent more lignans than whole or ground flaxseeds.

MSM (Methylsulfonylmethane)

MSM is a form of sulfur that was first detected in humans in the 1960s. Until recently, research into MSM has been shadowed by its cousin, dimethylsulfoxide (DMSO), a naturally occurring sulfur compound. DMSO, a potent antioxidant, is also approved by the FDA for the treatment of interstitial cystitis.

MSM, according to the authors of *MSM: The Natural Solution for Pain*, relieves pain and reduces inflammation, scar tissue formation, muscle spasms, and more. A six-week study, published in *The Journal of Anti-aging Medicine*, was conducted with eight patients receiving 250 mg of MSM twice a day and six receiving a placebo. Those who were treated with MSM had better than 80 percent reduction in pain. Veterinarians commonly use MSM to treat joint and muscle injuries in animals. Gram quantities are recommended.

Multimune

Decades of research have shown that the following 10 key nutrients are important for immune health. They include: vitamins A, B_6, C, and E; the minerals magnesium, selenium, and zinc; coenzyme Q10, reduced L-glutathione, and alpha lipoic acid. Most people do not want to take 10 separate nutrients every day, so I formulated this product to provide all 10.

Multimune contains vitamin A (1600 IU); vitamin C mineral ascorbates, magnesium ascorbate, calcium ascorbate (1000 mg); vitamin E, d-alpha tocopherol (100 IU); vitamin B_6 in the form pyridoxal-5-phosphate (45 mg); magnesium glycinate, citrate (120 mg); zinc citrate (15 mg); selenomethionine (100 mcg); coenzyme Q10 (30 mg); reduced L-glutathione (45 mg); and alpha lipoic acid (30 mg).

Multimune contains 99.9 percent pure raw materials; no fillers, binders, or flowing agents (ascorbyl palmitate or magnesium stearate) are used in the manufacturing process to ensure a super-clean, hypoallergenic, highly absorbable antioxidant supplement.

NAC (N-Acetylcysteine)

N-acetylcysteine is a combination of the amino acid cysteine and a protein known to enhance intracellular glutathione. NAC is utilized as an antidote for acetaminophen poisoning in hospitals as it supports liver function to metabolize the acetaminophen and restore glutathione levels that were depleted by acetaminophen. NAC promotes thinning of mucous and as a result is quite beneficial in treating chronic bronchitis. It is also touted as the hangover cure for its ability to detoxify the liver and prevent nausea and vomiting caused by chemotherapy.

In cancer studies, NAC enhanced the effect of macrophages and leukocytes. Further studies reveal it to be cancer-preventative as it disables the method that cancer cells use to attach to DNA.

PC SPES

PC SPES, which means prostate cancer hope (*spes* is Latin for hope), is a combination of seven Chinese herbs with the addition of saw palmetto.

The Chinese herbs include Scutellaria baicalensis, Rabdosia rubescens, Dendrantherma morifolium, Glycyrrhiza glabra (licorice), Panax pseudo-ginseng or Notoginseng, Ganoderma lucidum, and Isatis indigotica. Although these herbs have been evaluated and used clinically to provide anti-inflammatory, antioxidant, or estrogen-like activity, it is the specific combination of these herbs and their synergy that provides a powerful anticarcinogenic effect.

PC SPES's estrogen-like action decreases testosterone and the prostate-specific antigen levels. As well, PC SPES enhances the body's immunity by promoting macrophage and T4 cell activity. It also slows the growth of malignant cells and stimulates programmed cell death. When used as a complement to radiation therapy, PC SPES can increase the efficacy of radiation by 10 percent.

A joint study, published in January 2001 by the Dana-Farber Cancer Institute and Harvard Medical School, concluded that PC SPES worked well for those men with androgen-independent prostate cancer. Of 23 subjects, 12 demonstrated a reduction in prostate-specific antigen (PSA) of more than 50 percent.

Probiotics

Several hundred bacteria inhabit the human body, including beneficial bacteria that reside in the small and large intestines and vagina. Probiotics, meaning "for life," include Bifidobacterium bifidum, Lactobacillus acidophilus (the most prolific), Lactobacillus bulgaricus, and Enterococcus faecium, which is known to colonize the colon. Many health benefits are obtained from a diet rich in friendly bacteria, which enhance our immune system, improve digestion, treat *Candida albicans* yeast infections, and improve our bad bacteria-fighting ability.

PS (Phosphatidylserine)

Phosphatidylserine (PS), a phospholipid, is a component of cell membranes throughout the body. It is highly concentrated in the brain and aids the conduction of neurotransmitters (chemical messengers), including serotonin and dopamine. PS has been heavily researched in Europe and is used to treat cognitive decline in the elderly and those with Alzheimer's disease. PS improves memory, mood, and the ability to learn new words and ideas.

Reduced L-Glutathione

Glutathione, made up of the amino acids cysteine, glycine, and glutamine, is the most potent detoxifier. A cell contains two forms of glutathione—

oxidized (GSSH) and reduced (GSH)—and if it is a healthy cell, it will have more reduced glutathione than oxidized. Reduced glutathione, also known as active, is able to donate electrons. When vitamin C or E has been used, the cell can regenerate the oxidized vitamins with the help of reduced glutathione. If the ratio of GSSH to GSH is out of balance, then the cell will have no spare electrons to regenerate the used vitamins and the cells will eventually become sick.

No other antioxidant is as important to overall immune health as reduced L-glutathione. It ensures that our immune cells stay predominantly in the T-helper-1 state, making the immune system better able to fight cancer, bacterial infection, and viruses. It controls IL-4, 6, and 10 effectively, reducing allergic reactions and inflammation. Reduced L-glutathione, selenium, alpha lipoic acid, whey proteins, N-acetylcysteine, and vitamin C increase intracellular glutathione levels.

SAM-e (S-adenosylmethionine)

SAM-e is a major component of all body tissues and is manufactured using a combination of methionine and adenosine triphosphate (ATP). SAM-e turns harmful homocysteine into helpful methionine. Homocysteine is one of the culprits that can lead to arthritis, heart disease, cancer, and depression. SAM-e heals cartilage and eases inflammation of arthritis, migraine headaches, and possibly fibromyalgia. It is crucial for producing melatonin, the hormone that regulates our waking and sleeping patterns and alleviates depression. SAM-e enhances cognitive abilities and aids in liver detoxification. In one study, more than 1000 participants with depression were given SAM-e. The SAM-e group showed greater improvement than depressive patients who took antidepressant medication.

Sterols and Sterolins

Next to carotenoids, sterols and sterolins (phytosterols) are the most researched plant nutrient. Over 4000 published studies to date have examined phytosterols and 120 studies are double-blind, placebo-controlled human trials. Phytosterols include beta-sitosterol and its glucoside beta-sitosterolin, campesterol, brassicasterol, stigmasterol, ergosterols, and avenasterol. Among the various sterols, beta-sitosterol and beta-sitosterolin (called sterols and sterolins for short) have the most exciting disease prevention and treatment applications. They were isolated in 1922 with the earliest research evaluating their anticancer effects.

The sterol superstars are found abundantly in all plant materials and also in shellfish. Raw, unprocessed nuts and seeds and their oils are the richest sources of sterols. Unfortunately, standard food-processing methods destroy the sterols and sterolins contained in foods, stripping the finished product of any health-giving properties. Freezing fruits and vegetables destroys the sterolins, and boiling vegetables causes the sterols and sterolins to be released into the cooking water.

We call sterols the forgotten nutrient because although thousands of research studies have been performed on this nutrient, it has not been given the recognition it deserves. Rheumatoid arthritis, cervical cancer, diabetes, immune function, prostate problems, HIV, herpes, hepatitis C, allergies, stress-induced immune suppression, chronic fatigue, tuberculosis, breast cancer, and high cholesterol are only some of the diseases where sterols and sterolins have been shown to be extremely effective. A proprietary blend of plant sterols and sterolins called Moducare has been extensively researched. The following provides an overview.

Sterols, Allergies, and Asthma:
Our immune system causes allergic symptoms in its bid to rid the body of what it sees as invaders. This is not a normal response and occurs only in those who have an overly sensitive immune system. In an allergy-prone person, when the immune system encounters an allergen such as pollen, the T-helper-2 cell releases an immune factor called interleukin-4. IL-4 promotes IgE to attach onto mast cells which then secrete histamine, which is responsible for the watery eyes, itchy skin, and other symptoms. In asthmatics the situation is even worse because not only does the immune system release IL-4 but also interleukin-6. In asthmatics IL-6 causes lung tissue damage that, if not controlled, can lead to reliance on steroid medications and puffers. The key to halting allergies in their tracks is stopping IL-4 from being released in the first place and controlling IL-6. Sterols and sterolins halt the release of IL-4, so histamine is not released and allergies are controlled. As well, sterols and sterolins normalize the release of IL-6 and protect lung tissue from further destruction.

A 12-week study of 24 rhinitis patients was completed in spring 2001 under the direction of P. Bouic, L. Rabie, and M. MacDonough. Patients were given three capsules daily of Moducare. The study results showed a significant decrease in circulating IgE levels, an increase in the good T-helper-1 cells, and an increase in the ratio of Th-1 to Th-2. As well, patients reported fewer sleep disturbances and a reduction in itching, postnasal drip, mucous output, sneezing, fatigue, and 50 percent less conjunctivitis (inflammation of the inner mucous membrane of the eyelids).

Sterols and Cervical Cancer:
Over 65,000 cases of cervical cancer are diagnosed each year in North America. Over 10,000 women will die from this silent killer. The fear of cervical cancer sends most women to their doctor for an annual PAP smear, which will hopefully detect precancerous or cancerous cells. One cause of cervical cancer or precancerous cervical lesions is the human papilloma virus, HPV (the same virus that causes warts on our skin). A pilot study using plant sterols and sterolins for stage three CIN III

(a classification for cervical cancer) cervical lesions involved 13 women, who were divided into two groups. Seven were given plant sterols and sterolins and six were given a placebo (a fake pill). The results of the study showed that three patients in the treatment group receiving plant sterols and sterolins had no sign of CIN III cervical lesions. The lesions were gone and the other four women had no progression of disease. All six in the placebo group had no improvement in the disease. In fact, three patients in the placebo group showed signs of disease progression in the form of tissue infiltration, which required hysterectomy or other surgery.

Sterols and Sterolins and Chemotherapy: Plant sterols and sterolins have also been shown to halt the negative effects of chemotherapy. When cancer patients took plant sterols and sterolins six weeks before chemotherapy, they did not become nauseous, lose their hair, or get mouth sores or skin lesions. We know that phytosterols increase natural killer cell activity and the release of the body's own cancer-fighting immune factor, gamma-interferon. Many studies are currently underway in the United States to evaluate the tumor-fighting ability of phytosterols.

Sterols and Hepatitis C: Over 4 million North Americans are infected with hepatitis C. Liver specialists are overwhelmed as they struggle to deal with the increase in the incidence of this disease. It is the leading cause of liver transplants in North America. Over 85 percent of patients develop chronic hepatitis as the virus slowly and insidiously destroys the liver, and 5 percent of patients develop liver cancer. Plant sterols and sterolins have been shown to halt the destruction of liver cells by normalizing inter-leukin-6 levels and controlling inflammation in the liver, while stimulating the good immune factors interleukin-2 and gamma-interferon, which destroy the virus. Physicians using sterols and sterolins to treat hepatitis C have already seen liver enzymes and viral load normalize within 90 days of the treatment.

Sterols are Great Stress Busters: Chronic stress is so negative that it can promote and exacerbate most diseases. Numerous studies have linked our ability to deal with stress to our susceptibility to the common cold and more serious diseases such as cancer. Adults who have recently lost a loved one or been divorced or separated tend to have the highest cancer rates. Unrelieved stress gradually weakens and suppresses our immune system, causing disease. Marathon running causes consistent stress to the immune system and adrenal glands. In one research study (a double-blind trial) marathon runners in the treatment group were given plant sterols and sterolins prior to participation in the run with the hopes of alleviating post-marathon sickness caused by declines in both red and white blood cell counts. Results of the study showed that marathon runners who received

STEROL CONTENT OF COMMON FOODS

	Betasitosterol W/betasitosterolin mg/100 mg edible portion	Campesterol	Stigmasterol
VEGETABLES			
Asparagus	14	3	5
Barley	98	33	101
Beet root	13	—	6
Brussels sprouts	17	6	1
Cabbage	7	2	2
Carrot	7	1	3
Cauliflower	12	3	2
Cucumber	14	—	—
Ginger root	10	1	4
Squash, white	89	2	—
Lettuce, romaine	21	2	11
Melon	16	—	—
Okra	15	3	6
Onion	15	12	1
Peas	108	—	—
Pepper, red	7	3	2
Potato, sweet	8	3	1
Potato, white	40	—	—
Pumpkin	12	—	—
Radish greens	22	6	—
Soybean	30	9	11
Taro	11	3	6
Turnip greens	9	2	—
Yams	7	2	2
FRUITS			
Apple	11	1	—
Apricot	16	1	—
Banana	11	2	3
Cherry	12	—	—
Fig	27	1	2
Grapefruit	13	2	2
Lemon	8	—	—
Orange, navel	17	4	2
Peach	6	1	1

STEROL CONTENT OF COMMON FOODS

	Betasitosterol W/betasitosterolin mg/100 mg edible portion	(continued) Campesterol	Stigmasterol
FRUITS			
Pear	7	—	—
Pomegranate	16	tr	tr
Strawberry	10	tr	tr
SEEDS AND NUTS			
Almond	122	5	3
Cashew	130	13	tr
Chestnut	18	2	2
Coconut meat	27	3	7
Pecan	88	4	2
Pine nut	84	14	tr
Pistachio	90	6	2
Sesame seed	443	91	78
Sunflower seed	349	61	75
Walnut	87	6	—
VEGETABLE OILS			
Flaxseed	46	9	29
Olive (France)	91	1	3
Olive (Italy)	84	1	3
Sunflower	60	8	8
Wheat germ	67	tr	22
Soybean	53	20	20
Cocoa butter	59	26	9
Safflower	52	9	13
LEGUMES/BEANS			
Azuki	37	1	36
Broad	95	8	9
Kidney	91	3	31
Mung	13	2	8
Peanuts	142	24	23
GRAINS			
Buckwheat	164	20	8
Corn	120	32	21
Rice bran	735	257	289

STEROL CONTENT OF COMMON FOODS

	Betasitosterol W/betasitosterolin mg/100 mg edible portion	(continued) Campesterol	Stigmasterol
GRAINS			
Whole wheat	40	27	—
SPICES, DRY			
Clove	242	—	14
Fenugreek	100	18	7
Ginger	56	10	18
Oregano	177	12	15
Paprika	119	29	18
Thyme	152	3	8
SEAFOODS	TOTAL STEROLS		
Haddock	97		
Pollock	80		
Salmon	99		
Shrimp	209		
Lobster	171		
Crab	244		
Oyster	362		
Clam	518		
Scallop	681		

In order to consume 100 mg of plant sterols per day, you would have to eat about 16–25 oz (500–700 g) of fresh fruits and vegetables, 7 oz (200 g) of whole wheat flour without additives, or 8 oz (250 g) of potatoes (not boiled). If you want to achieve maximum immunity, you would have to double this daily requirement.

the sterols and sterolins had no decline in immune function and no increase in the inflammatory immune factor, interleukin-6. As well, cortisol levels remained stable in the sterols and sterolins group, indicating a reduction in adrenal stress to the run. They also had an increase in DHEA levels. The runners in the placebo group showed immune suppression, a drop in DHEA, and an increase in cortisol. You don't have to be a marathon runner to experience stress and its negative effects. Stressful situations promote the release of cortisol, our stress hormone, which in turn causes the secretion of the negative immune factor interleukin-6. Abnormal levels of IL-6 are associated with osteoporosis, autoimmune disease, asthma, inflammatory diseases (including arthritis), and more. We know that phytosterols are effective in reducing IL-6, cortisol, and other negative immune factors. They also improve DHEA, a hormone known to help fight the effects of stress.

Sterols, Heart Disease, and DHEA: A team of Canadian researchers discovered that an error in the regulation of certain immune cells that fight bacterial infections may be implicated in heart attacks and strokes. Josef Penninger, an immunologist at the Amgen Institute and the Ontario Cancer Institute at Princess Margaret Hospital in Toronto, found that the bacteria chlamydia can cause the body's immune system to target the heart, causing inflammation and plaque buildup in the arteries, which leads to heart disease and heart attacks. In a study published in the *International Journal of Immunopharmacology*, plant sterols and sterolins have been shown to improve the ability of the immune system to fight bacterial infections. Sterols and sterolins, not antibiotics, may be the way to treat bacterial-induced heart disease.

Physicians know that people with low levels of the hormone DHEA have higher rates of arteriosclerosis (hardening of the arteries). In a study published in the *International Journal of Sports Medicine*, researchers reported that participants taking plant sterols and sterolins had an increase in DHEA and a decrease in cortisol levels. Scientists believe that, like cholesterol, plant sterols and sterolins may be used by the body to make DHEA, thereby protecting us from hardening of the arteries.

Sterols and Prostate Problems: Urologists in Germany have been using plant sterols and sterolins for over two decades to treat enlarged prostates. In one double-blind, placebo-controlled study, 200 patients of an average age of 65 with Benign Prostatic Hypertrophy were given sterols and sterolins for six months. The treatment group showed a rapid reduction of the symptoms mentioned above and an increase in peak urinary flow and a decrease in inflammation. Researchers also found that when they compared the effectiveness of sterols and sterolins to the drug Proscar, the sterols and sterolins were better. Another German study involving 177 patients found that improvements in symptoms occurred within 30 days. The PSA (prostate-specific antigen test) scores were also normal when patients took sterols and sterolins. As well, it was found that sterols and sterolins halt the conversion of testosterone to dihydrotestosterone (DHT). DHT is thought to be involved in stimulating new cells to be deposited in the prostate, causing swelling and decreasing urine flow.

Wobenzym

Wobenzym is a protein-digesting supplement that has been used in Germany for over 50 years for the treatment of inflammatory disorders, bowel disease, cancer, and pain. It consists of the bioflavonoid rutin and the enzymes amylase, papain, bromelain, pancreatin, trypsin, chymotrypsin, and lipase. It can be taken as a suppository, in tablet form, or by injection. Cancer cells are covered in a very thick coating that prevents them from being detected by the immune system. Wobenzym digests the protein coating so that the immune system can recognize and attack the cancer. Research has also shown that wobenzym reduces inflammation and pain. A study in Austria comparing the effectiveness of diuretics and wobenzym for the treatment of edema and pain in mastectomy patients found that wobenzym was more effective.

HORMONE SUPPLEMENTS

DHEA (Dehydroepiandrosterone)

Important for regulating immune function, dehydroepiandrosterone (DHEA) is also called the "mother" hormone because it is able to convert into several other steroid hormones. It has acquired widespread popularity as an antiaging nutrient. Along with its ability to control age-related disorders, it helps repair and maintain tissues, control allergic reactions, and balance the activity of the immune system. It controls the inflammatory immune factors IL-1 and IL-6 and cortisol while enhancing gamma-interferon and interleukin-2, our cancer- and virus-fighting cytokines. DHEA acts as an anti-inflammatory and stimulates natural killer cell activity. When we are experiencing stress, our adrenal glands secrete cortisol, the stress hormone, causing a drop in DHEA. Conversely, when DHEA is increased, cortisol and inflammatory immune factors are controlled.

Diabetics and those with atherosclerosis are often low in DHEA. Research has demonstrated that the number of antibodies attacking the "self" cells is reduced with DHEA, thereby controlling autoimmune disorders such as rheumatoid arthritis and lupus. A report published in *Science News* stated that DHEA was added to prasterone (a drug for lupus) after it was found to elicit fewer symptomatic flare-ups in women with lupus. If you live in Canada, where DHEA is not available for sale, take Moducare, which is a precursor to DHEA (meaning your body makes DHEA from it). Have your doctor check your DHEAS level to see if it is in the normal range.

Melatonin

Produced in the pineal gland, melatonin has been referred to as the sleep hormone and antiaging nutrient, but it is also a potent antioxidant. Melatonin regulates our internal clock, which is known as our circadian rhythm. Melatonin is secreted in the dark in greater quantities up until about 3 a.m., at which point it begins to abate and slowly raises the body temperature by morning. Drugs commonly prescribed as sleep aids suppress stages 3 and 4 of the sleep pattern, which prevents the most beneficial, restful portion of sleep. Those who sleep with a light on can interfere with the secretion of melatonin. In an experiment conducted with elderly volunteers, melatonin increased the efficiency of their sleep, helped them fall asleep more quickly, and reduced occurrences of awakening in the night. Studies have found melatonin to be helpful for jet lag, insomnia, preventing cluster headaches, and possibly Alzheimer's by interfering with the formation of a plaque that can kill brain cells. It is also cancer-protective and an immune system booster. Research in the Netherlands suggests that melatonin may protect against estrogen-dominant cancers.

Melatonin may interfere with some antidepressants, including Prozac, so consult your physician before taking it.

BOTANICAL MEDICINES (HERBS)

Herbs have been a part of nature's apothecary since the beginning of time. Many of the common drugs sold today were originally derived from plants, including digitalis from foxglove and aspirin from willow bark. Around the globe researchers are evaluating the healing properties of herbs. Many believe that a cancer cure may one day be found in the jungles of the world. Herbal medicines are available in many forms: tincture, tonic, dried, fresh, or in capsules. There are hundreds of herbal medicines. I will highlight the most scientifically studied and common remedies in the following sections.

Aloe Vera

Aloe vera contains polysaccharides, amino acids, vitamins, minerals, sterols and sterolins, and aloin. A wonderful healing and soothing herb for the stomach, aloe vera also acts as a laxative. It has wonderful emollient action and heals sunburn and skin abrasions. Cancer patients can take aloe vera during chemotherapy to soothe an upset gastrointestinal tract.

Astragalus

Two thousand species of astragalus (*A. membranaceus*) have been identified. It has been used in China as a herb to strengthen the life force or *qi* of a person. Astragalus contains flavonoids, polysaccharides, selenium, and amino acids. Research at MD Anderson University Cancer Center found that astragalus improved immune function, restoring T-cell counts to normal in cancer patients. Astragalus is an effective diuretic and its heart-protective effects are well known. In one study, Chinese researchers found that it protected against viral myocarditis caused by coxsackie B virus. Heart attack patients taking astragalus showed improvements in

EKG results and angina. There have also been anecdotal reports of its positive effects in fibromyalgia and chronic fatigue syndrome. Alzheimer's sufferers should also take astragalus to improve memory.

Bilberry

Bilberry (*Vaccinium myrtillus*) is a wonderful herb that improves night vision, prevents circulatory disorders by strengthening capillaries and improving circulation, and treats kidney and urinary tract disorders, diarrhea, gout, and inflammation. Anthocyanidins are the active ingredient in bilberry. One study showed that 50 people who took bilberry had no worsening in cataracts. Europeans have used bilberry as an effective remedy for varicose veins and atherosclerosis.

Black Cohosh

Black cohosh (*Cimicifuga racemosa*) is used to treat problems associated with menopause and menstruation. It contains potent phytoestrogens that bind to estrogen receptor sites and mimic the effects of estrogen. Night sweats and hot flashes are effectively controlled in most women by taking black cohosh. Painful periods, cramps, and endometriosis are lessened by this herb's estrogen-balancing effects.

Boswellia

Boswellia, an extract from the Boswellia serrata tree, has been extensively studied in humans and found to have several powerful antiarthritic effects. It inhibits inflammatory factors; acts as an analgesic; and may also improve circulation to damaged joints and inflamed tissue. In one study 70 percent of rheumatoid arthritis patients had a reduction in pain and stiffness. To prove these potent effects, researchers gave 17 of the patients who had been receiving Boswellia in the study a placebo pill instead and their symptoms returned. A standardized dose of 200 mg twice a day was given to research subjects. Boswellia has also been found to be just as effective as NSAIDs in reducing pain and inflammation. It has also been studied in ankylosing spondylitis in dosages of 600 mg per day with excellent results. Boswellia is a powerful anti-inflammatory, halting 5-lipoxygenase, IL-6, IL-1, and autoantibody production.

Chaste Tree Berry

Chaste tree berry (*Vitex agnus castus*), commonly known as the hormone regulator Vitex, has been used in Europe for over 40 years as a remedy for female menstrual cycle disorders, low sexual drive, and infertility. Studies have shown that an extract of this herb can lower levels of the hormone prolactin. This is important because high levels of prolactin can decrease progesterone levels. Without progesterone, estrogen can build up in the system, increasing cancer risk. Low levels of progesterone can be addressed through supplementation with this herb, resulting in protection against estrogen imbalance. Chaste tree berry also stimulates the production of lutenizing hormone, thereby increasing progesterone. PMS symptoms, menstrual cramps, heavy periods, endometriosis, uterine fibroids, hot flashes, night sweats, and acne have been controlled with Vitex.

Cranberry

Cranberry fights urinary tract infections by inhibiting bacteria from adhering to the bladder wall, especially those caused by E. coli. Cranberry is rich in vitamin C and anthocyanidins, enhancing immune function. Do not drink sweetened cranberry juice. You can buy unsweetened at the health food store and mix it with unsweetened apple juice or water for a refreshing drink.

Devil's Claw

My very first article almost 20 years ago was on the powerful antiarthritic effects of devil's claw (Harpagophytum procumbens) root from Africa. Since then many new studies have confirmed devil's claw as a potent anti-inflammatory. A study of 50 patients suffering from arthritis showed that arthritis symptoms and the severity of pain were markedly decreased by using devil's claw. Controlled clinical research in Europe compared the efficacy of a standard antiarthritic drug, phenylbutazone, with that of devil's claw. The results revealed devil's claw to be more effective in reducing pain and inflammation without unpleasant side effects associated with the drug; 1.5–3 g of standardized devil's claw should be taken daily. A more recent study comparing devil's claw with diacerhein (a European analgesic) and their effect on osteoporosis revealed that devil's claw was as effective as diacerhein in reducing pain and was better tolerated.

Dong Quai

Dong quai (Angelica polymorphia, A. sinensis, A. acutiloba) has been used to normalize menstruation, enhance sexual desire, and stop fibrocystic breasts in women. Chinese medical texts have recommended it for inflammation, liver disorders, high blood pressure, digestive upsets, ulcers, and constipation. Dong quai is an all-round tonic for the body, eliminating fatigue and sluggishness.

Echinacea

Echinacea (*Echinacea purpurea*, *E. agustifolia*, and *E. pallida*) is an immune enhancer that stimulates macrophage function. Three double-blind, placebo-controlled trials have shown that when echinacea is taken as prescribed, it shortens the duration of colds and flu. People with auto-immune disorders such as lupus, rheumatoid arthritis, HIV, or TB should not take echinacea. (See page 38 in Chapter 3 for further information.)

Evening Primrose Oil

Omega-6 fatty acids can be converted in the body to gamma linolenic acid (GLA) with the cofactors zinc and vitamin B_6. GLA inhibits the production of the inflammation-causing prostaglandins and leukotrienes, which are overactive in autoimmune disorders. In one study, patients taking GLA from evening primrose oil were able to decrease their dosage of NSAID medication significantly and felt much better as compared to those in the placebo group. GLA has also been used in very high doses to eliminate the symptoms of multiple sclerosis. Several randomized double-blind, placebo-controlled trials involving rheumatoid arthritis patients found that there was a significant reduction in both tender and swollen joints, and the need for pain medication was reduced along with inflammation upon supple-mentation with GLA. By down-regulating overzealous inflammatory processes, GLA is an effective treatment for autoimmune disease.

Garlic

See Chapter 4, page 80.

Ginkgo Biloba

An antioxidant belonging to the flavonoid family, ginkgo biloba neutralizes free radicals, but is renowned for its effects on memory and its ability to improve circulation. It is very helpful in reducing the symptoms of asthma, including wheezing, coughing, and shortness of breath, and reduces the frequency of attacks. Ginkgo has been suggested for those with Raynaud's disease, tinnitus, Parkinson's, and multiple sclerosis.

Ginseng (Panax, American, and Asian)

Ginseng is often referred to as the panacea herb, meaning it has many treatment applications. There are several types of ginseng: Panax quin-quefolius and Panax ginseng (Asian), and Siberian ginseng. The active ingredients include ginsenosides, triterpenes, saponins, and glycosides, which enhance the immune system and protect the cardiovascular system. Ginseng acts as an adaptogen, regulating many systems in the body while supporting the adrenal glands. It improves learning and memory, reduces the effects of aging, regulates digestion, and has been known to increase sex drive and energy. A large Korean study found that people who took ginseng had a lower incidence of cancer compared to those who took no ginseng.

Goldenseal

Goldenseal (*Hydrastis canadensis*) is revered as a potent immune booster, and virus and tumor fighter. It is often called the "poor man's ginseng" because it too is an overall tonic for many body systems. It contains two main active ingredients—hydrastine and berberine—both recognized drugs in several countries. Berberine has been studied for its antibiotic action and effectiveness in treating canker sores and ulcers. It also acts as a digestive aid and stimulates bile secretion. Crohn's disease and diverticulitis may also benefit from this potent herb. Goldenseal is an excellent gargle for sore throats, cankers, and gum disease.

Grape Seed Extract

Grape seeds are rich in PCOs (procyanidolic oligomers), potent antioxidant phytochemicals. They protect us from free radicals and blood vessel damage seen in those with atherosclerosis. Research has shown that grape seed extract is effective in controlling histamine release, thereby blocking allergic reactions. It has been used for varicose veins, clogged arteries, and to improve circulation. It is thought to stop the release of the "bad" prostaglandins responsible for the pain of arthritis and other inflammatory disorders. Diabetics can take it to protect against retinopathies.

Guggul

Native to India and commonly used in Ayurvedic medicine to lower cholesterol, gugulipid is the standardized extract of the mukul myrrh tree (*Commiphora mukul*). Several clinical studies have confirmed that guggisterones, the active ingredient, have the ability to lower triglyceride levels and LDL cholesterol by inhibiting the liver's production of cholesterol and increasing its metabolism of LDL cholesterol. Gugulipids also raise HDL, the "good" cholesterol. Gugulipids have been shown to be free of side effects and have a similar action to cholesterol- and triglyceride-lowering medications. Michael Murray, ND, in his book *Heart Disease and High Blood Pressure*, reports that "typically total cholesterol levels will drop from 14 percent to 27 percent in a 4 to 12 week period, while LDL cholesterol and triglyceride levels will drop from 25 to 35 percent and 22 to 30 percent respectively. HDL cholesterol levels will increase by 16 to 20 percent."

Those who are trying to lose weight will definitely want to take guggul as a food supplement. It stimulates the thyroid gland and increases metabolism, thereby promoting weight loss.

Hawthorn

Many double-blind, placebo-controlled studies have shown that hawthorn (*Crataegus species*) is an effective heart tonic. In Germany hawthorn is prescribed for slow heartbeat, angina, and mild heart failure. Dramatic improvements were seen in a study of 30 heart patients with congestive heart failure; 15 took hawthorn and the others took a placebo. A statistically significant improvement was seen in the treatment group after eight weeks of hawthorn extract. Look for standardized hawthorn containing 15 mg of procyanidin per 80 mg capsule.

Licorice

Licorice (*Glycyrrhiza glabra*) is a sweet root with marvelous virus-fighting capabilities. In Great Britain scientists are evaluating licorice's action on hepatitis C. It has commonly been used to treat indigestion, heartburn, peptic ulcers, and inflammation of the intestines. Cold sores and active shingles outbreaks benefit from topical licorice creams and ointments. Licorice stimulates the production of cortisone, which is important to immune function. It also enhances interferon production. High doses of licorice can increase blood pressure. Look for deglycyrrhizinated licorice, which does not raise blood pressure.

Milk Thistle

Widely known for its detoxifying properties, milk thistle (*Silybum marianum*) promotes bile flow, liver cell reproduction, and overall liver function, and is a tonic for the other organs involved in detoxification—the gallbladder, spleen, kidneys, and stomach. Milk thistle can break down poisons such as alcohol, carbon monoxide, and nicotine that enter the bloodstream. It is also an effective antidote for those who eat the poisonous death-cap mushroom and stops the mushroom toxins from destroying the liver. It is usually suggested for treating hepatitis, cirrhosis, and jaundice. Milk thistle works by preventing hepatotoxic materials from entering the cell and by stimulating the regeneration of the liver. It also stops the circulation of toxins in the intestines and liver and raises glutathione levels to stimulate antioxidant activity. Hepatitis patients who are given milk thistle recover more quickly than those who are given a placebo. It is also thought that milk thistle may halt the development of gallstones. Look for Nature's Way milk thistle standardized to 80 percent silymarin. Most of the human research has been done using their product.

Pygeum

Pygeum (*Pygeum africanum*) is used to treat prostatitis, benign prostatic hypertrophy (BPH), incontinence, and urinary tract disorders. Phytosterols are the main active ingredient in pygeum with anti-inflammatory, diuretic, and antiedema actions. In a study of 18 patients with BPH or chronic prostatitis, pygeum improved all urinary symptoms within 60 days. In another placebo-controlled clinical trial of 120 patients with BPH, the pygeum group experienced a significant reduction in the number of daily trips to the toilet and more complete emptying of the bladder. In another international, multicentered, double-blind, controlled study that lasted 60 days, 236 patients with benign prostatic hypertrophy showed an improvement in all urinary symptoms. Dosages of 150 mg of standardized pygeum per day are required.

St. John's Wort

In Germany, doctors prescribe St. John's wort (*Hypericum perforatum*) 20 times more often than the leading prescription antidepressant. St. John's wort is as effective as Prozac and other antidepressants, but without side effects. More than 20 studies have proven that St. John's wort is an effective treatment for depression. In addition to depression, it is indicated for anxiety, insomnia, and seasonal affective disorder. Researchers trying to determine St. John's wort's effectiveness have proposed a couple of hypotheses: first, it seems to slow the rate of serotonin reabsorption by the brain, which is beneficial because depression is linked to low levels of serotonin; second, it decreases levels of IL-6, which is also important because depression is associated with excess adrenal activity. While self-medication is safe in cases of mild symptoms, treatment for serious depression should be monitored by a health care professional.

Saw Palmetto

Extracts of saw palmetto (*Serenoa repens*) are being used throughout the world to treat benign prostatic hypertrophy. Numerous double-blind, placebo-controlled clinical trials have demonstrated that saw palmetto improves urinary flow, alleviates nocturnal voiding, and reduces the number of times one needs to urinate during the day. Saw palmetto extract has been compared to Proscar, a common drug prescribed to BPH patients in North America. Results showed that saw palmetto was equivalent or better in its action without the side effects associated with Proscar (which causes impotence), and it was less expensive.

Saw palmetto works by blocking the conversion of testosterone to dihydrotestosterone (DHT) by inhibiting 5-alpha reductase and preventing the binding of DHT. The action of this increases the elimination of DHT. It also reduces the inflammation associated with BPH and reduces the effects of estrogen and progesterone on the prostate.

French researchers discovered that saw palmetto berries are rich in essential fatty acids as well as sterols and sterolins. Moducare, a proprietary blend of sterols and sterolins, contains a higher percentage of sterols and sterolins than saw palmetto (see sterols and sterolins and the prostate in this chapter).

Tea Tree

Tea tree (*Melaleuca alternifolia*) oil has been found effective against viruses, fungi, and bacteria. One study performed in 1995 found tea tree oil stopped Staphylococcus aureus found in hospitals. Other studies have confirmed tea tree oil's ability to eliminate nail fungal infections, vaginal yeast infections caused by candida, and control acne. Tea tree cream is soothing to herpes and shingles eruptions. It is a safer and more effective alternative to toxic head lice preparations. Head lice are killed quickly.

Turmeric

Esteemed by Ayurvedic practitioners for centuries, turmeric (*Curcuma longa*) contains anti-inflammatory curcuminoids. These reduce pain by blocking the enzymes that cause inflammation. Several double-blind studies have shown dramatic improvements in symptoms experienced by rheumatoid arthritis sufferers. Turmeric is also an antioxidant and improves the liver's flow of bile to gently regulate hormone function. Use standardized extracts containing 500 mg of curcumin.

White Willow

White willow (*Salix alba*) bark is nature's aspirin. It is an ancient remedy used to treat fevers and arthritic complaints. Salicin is its active ingredient. Many human studies have evaluated willow bark's ability to temporarily relieve pain and reduce inflammation and fever. Standardized willow bark is available and dosages range from 200–1000 mg.

CHAPTER 6

STRESS, EXERCISE, AND DISEASE

STRESS: MORE THAN DANGEROUS

- Over 40 percent of adults suffer adverse health effects due to stress.
- Stress is now linked to heart disease, cancer, gum disease, immune dysfunction, and more.
- Over US$12 billion is spent annually in North America on stress-management programs, products, and services.

The old adage "One man's stress is another man's pleasure" is truly a profound statement when it comes to our health and longevity. Excessive or chronic stress, either physical or mental, has a detrimental effect on the optimal functioning of the immune system, our antiaging hormones, and promotes disease. Stress is like the card that finally tips the balance and collapses the house of cards, bringing everything crashing down. An immune system that is in top operating order will be only minimally affected by small stressors, yet that same system can be toppled by a continual stream of small stressors or by one big stressor, such as the death of a loved one.

According to many researchers, stress and its negative effects on the body have surpassed the cold virus as the most common health problem in North America. Living with continual stress or just feeling as if you can't get out from under stress is enough to cause disease. The effort to succeed, to compete, to have more, and do more have all contributed to many of our health problems. Too much stress, combined with inadequate nutrition, is the cause of most of our health complaints.

Although we may not be aware of them, there are many stressors that affect us daily: noise, crowded cities, our polluted environment, a lack of exposure to the sun, driving, crime, racism, pathogens, a lack of joy in our lives, abuse, school, work, negative emotions, over-exercising, chronic allergies, lack of sleep, trauma, angry emotions, intense heat or cold, depression, loneliness, and much more. When these stressors accumulate, they wreak havoc with our immune system and disrupt our delicate hormone balance.

Scientists now confirm that our response to stressors has a profound effect on our bodies' ability to protect us from everyday infections and the rate at which we age. In *The Stress of Life*, Dr. Hans Selye wrote, "If a microbe is in or around us all the time and yet causes no disease until we are exposed to stress, what is the cause of the illness, the microbe or the stress?" A serious illness is often preceded by a major life stressor such as a death, the loss of a job, the illness of a loved one, even moving or the birth of a baby. A lower immune resistance caused by excessive stress, inadequate nutrition, and toxins in the environment is the pendulum that swings toward illness and increased mortality.

The body has developed mechanisms to protect it from the damaging effects of stress. The fight-or-flight response is one way the body deals with extreme situations of stress. Upon realizing we are in danger, the brain sounds an alarm, telling our adrenal glands to secrete adrenaline and cortisol, which mobilize the body to fight or run. This response is supposed to be a short-lived reaction, yet today most of us are in and out of this state continually due to the stressors mentioned above. As a result, our immune system becomes imbalanced and produces too many inflammatory cytokines, and our adrenal glands become exhausted, weakening several body systems, especially the cardiovascular and endocrine systems. (See "The Immune System and Stress" in Chapter 3, page 45.)

The link between stress and several diseases has been thoroughly evaluated by universities around the world. The following sections are highlights from that research. I have not mentioned heart disease and stress because we are all very familiar with this connection. (For more information on heart disease and stress, see pages 20 and 21 in Chapter 2.)

Aging

Stress has been found to accelerate brain aging and can result in the loss of neuronal function and death of some brain cells. Elevated cortisol levels caused by stress can compromise the function of neurons responsible for learning and memory.

Autoimmune Diseases

People with multiple sclerosis, rheumatoid arthritis, and other autoimmune disorders have suggested to their doctors that there is a connection between the flare-ups of their disease and the stressors they are exposed to. Several studies have now shown that there is a strong correlation between stressful experiences and disease progression. A study at the University of California at San Francisco evaluated 48 multiple sclerosis patients aged 23 to 69 over a period of between 12 and 68 weeks. The patients rated the amount of psychological stress and stressful events that occurred during the study. The patients also had MRI scans once a month to show disease activity in the brain. The researchers found that major stressful events, as well as small daily hassles, were related to the development of new brain lesions. The researchers stated that "while brain lesions are not necessarily a sign of increased impairment, they do point to an increase in disease activity and it is the clearest demonstration yet that what patients are experiencing is in fact occurring."

As well, research reported back in 1993 that cortisol deficiencies were thought to be the problem in those with rheumatoid arthritis. When some research shows that too much cortisol causes flare-ups, how can another study show that a deficiency can cause the same action? Researchers believe that long-term excessive stress causes a continual secretion of cortisol, which eventually exhausts the adrenal glands, resulting in too little cortisol being available when it is needed. Cortisol is a hormone needed for many actions in the body. It becomes a problem only when there is an excess or a deficiency—balance is important when it comes to cortisol. The cortisol secretion rate is higher in overweight people. Losing 10 lbs (4.5 kg) can reduce the dangerous effects of a high cortisol level. (See page 45 in Chapter 3 for more information on cortisol.)

Cancer and Stress

Stanford University doctors found that among women with metastatic (cancer that had spread) breast cancer, those with high daytime levels of the stress hormone cortisol died on average one year sooner than those with normal levels of the hormone (*Journal of the National Cancer Institute,* July 2000). We know that cortisol suppresses the action of our natural killer cells, which fight cancer. One research study reported that just the stress of being told you have cancer and having to undergo many unpleasant treatments causes NK cell function to decline dramatically. DHEA enhances natural killer cell activity and cortisol lowers DHEA, so a double-jeopardy occurs. Low DHEA causes suppression of our NK cells, and high cortisol also suppresses our NK cells. We know that DHEA declines dramatically after age 50 and there is a dramatic increase in cancers among people around that age.

Gum Disease Linked to Financial Stress

Mental Health Weekly (July 26, 1999) reported that high levels of financial stress, combined with poor coping abilities, double the risk of developing gum disease. A study released by the American Academy of Periodontology found that long-term financial stress could lead to altered habits, such as teeth grinding or reduced oral hygiene, as well as salivary changes and weakening of the body's immune system. This study shows we should brush and floss and balance our checkbook to maintain healthy teeth and gums.

Osteoporosis

Scientists have shown that there is an intimate connection between the immune system and osteoporosis. Who would have ever thought that osteoporosis could be caused by a dysfunctional immune system? Research showing that our immune system may cause osteoporosis is so new that even your doctor may not be aware of this important interplay. Calcium and vitamin D supplements alone won't halt osteoporosis if your immune system is not in balance. The immune system is made up of many different types of cells that release cytokines. These cells and their cytokines destroy invaders, fight cancer cells, and regulate other systems in the body, including the body's bone maintenance system. Certain cytokines have a direct effect on bone density by causing bone loss.

When we are under stress, especially unrelenting stress, our T-helper-2 cells secrete plenty of interleukin-1, interleukin-6, and interleukin-8, which deplete calcium from our bones, causing bone loss. Stressful events cause an increase in cortisol, and cortisol's job is to get calcium from bone to make it available to the body during the stressful event. The occasional stressful situation is not a problem, but for many people who are under constant stress from financial pressures, too many activities to complete in a day, inadequate nutrient consumption from our food, and other stressful situations, bone loss can be the result. Each of us handles stress differently and stress does not mean just having a fight with your

Risk Factors for Osteoporosis

- Are you Caucasian or Asian, small-boned or thin?
- Is there a family history of osteoporosis?
- Are you peri- or postmenopausal?
- Have you taken prednisone, thyroid, or heparin drugs for extended periods?
- Are you a Type A personality?
- Are you under a lot of stress?
- Do you eat white sugar, white flour, or refined or processed foods?
- Do you drink coffee or caffeinated beverages every day?
- Do you smoke?
- Do you have poor digestion?
- Do you exercise less than twice a week or more than six times per week?
- Do you have a high-protein diet?

Answering yes to many of these questions puts you at higher risk for osteoporosis.

spouse or disliking your job; you can release cortisol from feeling cold. Stressors are different for each of us, yet one thing is clear—stress *does* contribute to bone loss.

Our bones are not static; they are constantly being broken down and restored. We can take all the calcium citrate, vitamin D, boron, and estrogen in the world, but if we do not deal with our stress we are missing the key to osteoporosis prevention. Some people are taking Fosamax, hormone-replacement therapy, and thousands of milligrams of calcium, yet still have bone loss—now we know why. Plant sterols and sterolins are the missing key—they stop bone loss! Make plant sterols and sterolins the basis of your bone-building program. Then add vitamin D, calcium citrate, soy isoflavones, and other bone-building nutrients along with weight-bearing exercise and watch your bone density improve.

Prostate Disease

North Carolina State University scientists have shown the link between stress and increased inflammation of the prostate gland in rats. The researchers believe that the hormone prolactin, released by the body during stress, causes increased inflammation in the prostate. The National Institute of Health is now evaluating the first major study on men with chronic prostatitis, and stress will be one of the factors evaluated. Stress causes an increase in inflammatory factors, so if you are troubled by prostatitis or an enlarged prostate, learn how to reduce the stressors in your life.

Skin Diseases

Arash Kimyai-Asadi and Adil Usman reviewed the literature pertaining to the role of psychological stress and the exacerbation of psoriasis, urticaria (hives), eczematous dermatitis, and herpes virus infections. They found that there is evidence linking stress to the onset or worsening of skin diseases.

Women's Health Issues

Disease frequency statistics tell us that women often have higher risk factors for contracting many common illnesses. This is true for autoimmune conditions such as lupus, multiple sclerosis, and rheumatoid arthritis, as well as depression, breast cancer, osteoporosis, fibromyalgia, and chronic fatigue syndrome. Even heart disease, which used to be predominantly a male disease, now affects women almost as often as men. Stress and our reaction to stressors, combined with poor nutrition, may be the reason we see increased rates of common diseases in women.

Along with equality, women have inherited the demands of too many tasks. It is not uncommon to find women looking after their home and children, doing overtime at work, looking after the family finances, volunteering in the community or at school, helping friends, and keeping their husbands happy. Women have increased their activities to the point where many are chronically stressed and have serious immune system dysfunction. I have talked to women who are very ill with an autoimmune disease or fibromyalgia, yet they are *still* looking after everyone else at the expense of their health. Getting to the root of

> ### "Middle" Management
> New Age Tip of the Day reported that when it comes to "middle" management, some downtime may be the key to downsizing. Studies show that chronic stress may lead to more body fat around the middle due to elevated levels of cortisol. If dieting and exercise have not whittled down your ab flab, try adding a relaxation component to your routine, such as yoga, meditation, or another stress-reducing activity.

the problem—immune dysfunction caused by poor nutrition and too much stress—is the key. Stop! Slow down, take time for yourself, and remember to eat meals. You may not feel the effects of stress immediately, but over time the deterioration in your health will become evident. Ensure good nutrition, take sterols and sterolins, include a high-potency B-complex along with a multivitamin, and learn some relaxation techniques. Buy yourself the Nike T-shirt that says "Just Say No" and read it the next time someone asks you to do another task. Your health demands it.

Virus Fighting and Stress

A research study of 82 homosexual men who were HIV positive without symptoms of AIDS was performed at the University of North Carolina School of Medicine. These men were followed every six months for over seven years. Results of the study showed that disease progression to AIDS was more rapid in the presence of severe life stressors and elevated cortisol levels. Professor Patrick Bouic in his research at the University of Stellenbosch, Cape Town, South Africa, also found that high cortisol/low DHEA causes stress-induced immune suppression and an inability to fight colds and flu. Stress lowers our immune system's ability to fight viral and bacterial infections. Antioxidant nutrients, including alpha lipoic acid, coenzyme Q10, essential fatty acids, magnesium, reduced L-glutathione, selenium, vitamins A, B_3, B_6, C, and E, zinc, and an excellent diet of organic fruits and vegetables should be adopted to supply the required nutrients to provide a powerful defense against the negative effects of stress. Practice some of the stress-busting tips for optimal immunity and maximum longevity. The mind and body are one unit, interrelated and highly complex. It may take a while for scientists to truly understand the

Stress-Busting Tips

- Breathing is a powerful de-stressing tool. Several times per day, breathe in through your nose and fill your lungs with air until your abdomen rises. Then slowly exhale from your mouth until your lungs are empty. Repeat this five times.
- Get eight hours of sleep every night and try to sleep until 7:30 in the morning.
- Just say no when you have too much to humanly accomplish in one day.
- Share the household workload with family.
- Eat seven to ten half-cup servings of fruits and vegetables every day.
- Smile. Purge negative emotions such as anger and hatred.
- Get help in dealing with grief. The loss of a loved one, a divorce, or the loss of a job all produce grief. Immune suppression is the result when grief is not dealt with.
- Carpe diem—seize the day—and live it to the fullest. Don't worry so much about tomorrow.
- Believe in yourself. Negative self-talk and continually doubting your abilities hampers your body's ability to heal.
- Notice the beauty around you. Smell the flowers, watch the sunset, and listen to the wind.
- Love your family and friends and be forgiving.
- Be good to yourself. Most of us are our own worst enemies. We focus on our weaknesses and minimize our strengths. Wake up each day and tell yourself you are a good and useful person.
- Do the things you have always wanted to do. Learn to water ski, sing in a choir, write a book, tell stories to your grandchildren, walk, garden— whatever makes you happy.
- Seek your spiritual side. This does not have to be religious, although those with strong religious beliefs generally live at peace and feel protected. Most of us believe in something greater than ourselves, a spiritual power that offers solace and helps us find the quiet place within.

intricacies of how stress affects immunity and the aging process. Today we know that having a positive attitude, a loving family, friends, and effective stress-coping strategies enhance our immune system and give us a few extra years. Do not wait another day to implement some positive changes in your life.

Stress Test to Determine Immune Status

Check off the symptoms that apply to you. Then add up your score.

❑	Unusual tiredness and/or dizziness	3
❑	Unexplained irregular heartbeat and/or shortness of breath	3
❑	Cigarettes, alcohol, caffeine, or prescription medication	3
❑	Sugar or aspartame consumption	3
❑	Headaches and/or muscle tension or joint pain	3
❑	Lack of desire for sex	3
❑	Nausea or irritable bowel/digestive problems	3
❑	Overexercise (more than four times per week) or no exercise at all	3
❑	Not taking vitamin and mineral supplements	2
❑	Poor nutrition	2
❑	Feelings of anxiety or depression	2
❑	Feelings of guilt	2
❑	Inability to cope or escape stressful circumstances	2
❑	Lack of confidence and self-criticism	2
❑	Feelings of inadequacy	2
❑	Fear of getting a disease such as cancer	2
❑	Use of antibacterial soaps	1
❑	No desire to socialize with friends	1
❑	Suppressed anger	1
❑	Inability to relax	1
❑	Fidgeting or restlessness	1
❑	Excessive appetite/loss of appetite	1
❑	Loneliness	1
❑	Insomnia or difficulty falling asleep	1

How did you score?

Over 12: You are putting yourself at risk for immune system overload. Immediately adopt the recommendations on page 130 and focus on stress reduction.

Between 6–12: You are still coping with the stressors in your life, but you need to slow down, say no once in a while, and register in a yoga class.

Between 1–5: You are in the peak range for stress management and if you keep this pace, you will reach the finish line healthy.

The next section will look at how exercise can help boost the immune system and give you a healthier lifestyle.

EVERYDAY ACTIVITIES BURN FAT

Millions of North Americans are obese and less than 25 percent of us exercise regularly. Obesity means carrying too much body fat; for women that means 30 percent or more and for men 25 percent or more body fat. Almost half a million deaths a year in North America are associated with obesity. Over US$30 billion is spent annually in North America for weight-reducing products and programs, yet rates of obesity are still rising. Heart disease, Type II diabetes, arthritis, and immune impairment are the result of no exercise and excess body fat.

Our bodies are designed to move. Early humans had to work hard just to gather food and maintain shelter. Today, with the advent of computers and remote controls, most of us probably can't remember the last time we went for a walk. Exercise means physical activity. Walking, gardening, dancing—even cleaning our homes, if we do it vigorously enough—can help burn excess fat and keep our immune and cardiovascular systems in peak performance.

These are the calories expended by a 125 lb (57 kg) woman doing 10 minutes of the following activities:

Activity	Calories Expended
Making beds	32
Weeding	49
House painting	29
Dancing	35
Swimming (crawl)	40
Tennis	56
Walking (briskly)	52
Walking (leisurely stroll)	29
Running	90
Cycling	42
Cross-country skiing	98
Downhill skiing	80
Shoveling snow	65

(*Sources:* John Foreyt, Baylor College of Medicine's Behavioral Medicine Research Center; Kelly D. Brownell, Ph.D., Yale University; and Thomas A. Wadden, Ph.D., University of Pennsylvania School of Medicine.)

EXERCISE FOR PREVENTION AND TREATMENT OF AILMENTS

You are never too old or too unfit to start an exercise program; in fact, it's all the more reason to begin. Study after study has come to the same conclusion—

inactivity promotes illness, and the right exercise for a condition can work wonders in reversing or delaying that illness. Activity encourages the flow of nutrients and oxygen and enhances mood. An article published in *Diabetes Care* by Japanese scientists confirmed that exercise, and not its accompanying weight loss, lowers triglyceride levels, improves insulin sensitivity, and stabilizes glucose tolerance in Type II diabetics.

Diseases related to excess weight:

- Type II diabetes, decreased glucose tolerance, and insulin resistance
- High blood pressure and increased risk of stroke
- Osteoarthritis (even an extra 10 lb/4.5 kg presents 40 lb/18 kg of pressure on our hips, knees, and ankles)
- Breathing difficulties and pulmonary disease
- Gout
- Endometrial cancer
- High cholesterol and lipoprotein
- Renal disease

Have no fear—weight loss can reverse these conditions.

Fitness trainers are worth every penny. They develop a program specifically for you with your health concerns in mind. Most important, they set a schedule motivating you to meet them at the gym. Their encouragement and support make working out more fun. Your local community center most likely has a fitness/workout room and many of them have trained staff to help you set up a safe program and show you how the equipment works. Fitness clubs have personal trainers. Ask the trainer what type of certification he or she has obtained and ask for references.

Aerobics without weight training will just not burn fat. You need to build muscle to burn fat. A combination of weight and cardiovascular training is the key to fat burning. *The American Journal of Cardiology* published the results of a study in which researchers compared aerobic workouts to aerobics with weight training. One group performed 75 minutes of aerobic exercise twice a week, while the second group did 35 minutes of weight training and 40 minutes of aerobic exercise twice a week. Results were spectacular in the group who combined aerobic activity with weight training—they had up to 43 percent increase in overall strength and 109 percent increase in endurance. The aerobics group had an 11 percent increase in endurance and no increase in strength. Most of us don't enjoy huffing on the treadmill or StairMaster for 75 minutes anyway. Weight training is more fun and offers more variety.

EXERCISE AND IMMUNITY

You don't have to run on the treadmill every day for hours. Research shows that excessive exercise may be detrimental to our health and increase the aging process. To encourage your immune system to thrive, participate in moderate exercise. Researchers in Toronto studied the effects of exercise on immunity in healthy young males. Each group was asked to do aerobic activity for 40 minutes per day. One group exercised five days of the week, while the other group exercised three days per week. Blood tests revealed that those who exercised five days a week had lowered antibody production, whereas those who exercised only three days a week demonstrated overall enhancement of their immune system. This does not mean that you can reduce your activity, but it does show that everything in life is about balance.

We know that low to moderate exercise is beneficial to our health and enhances immunity. Walking is the most potent immune-enhancing activity, providing movement while clearing the mind. Boost the intensity and duration of that same exercise and you will find that too much of a good thing can be bad. Overexercising causes stress on the immune system, resulting in higher than average colds, flu, and poor exercise recovery rates. Marathon runners and bodybuilders are especially prone to these negative side effects of strenuous, relentless exercise. Researchers are discovering that the function of T-cells and natural killer cells is suppressed due to overexercise. Suppression of the immune system can result, providing a susceptibility to microorganisms and viruses.

Prominent immunologists and sports physiologists have been looking into the reasons why marathon runners are prone to colds and influenza during the period immediately following a marathon race. Excessive physical stress causes tissue damage, which promotes an increase in the secretion of cortisol and pro-inflammatory factors, especially interleukin-6.

Have you ever noticed that many marathon runners or those who take part in excessively demanding repetitive sports look aged? Without a good, solid diet and nutrient program, they are actually speeding up the aging process—muscles start to waste and the skin wrinkles and sags. The body will find the nutrients it needs even if it has to steal them from muscles, bones, and connective tissues. Make sure you get the maximum nutrition for the amount of physical exercise you do.

Even if you are starting a moderately physically demanding exercise program, take precautions to ensure that your immune system has the tools it needs to protect your body. Antioxidants are essential for athletes to curb any free radicals produced during a workout. Plant nutrients are also recognized as important protectors in cases of intense activity and can prevent cellular damage caused by stress. Nutrition is the basis for health. If you go to gym or jog the neighborhood in a poorly fed body, you will damage not only your muscles but your immune system as well. Fitness starts with good, wholesome food. You must provide the proper nutrients to protect your muscles and immunity.

Sports nutrition science has become very sophisticated over the years. Researchers are emphasizing the importance of solid nutrition and sports performance enhancers.

SEX REVS UP IMMUNITY

Sex twice a week may prevent the common cold, say researchers at Wilkes University. After studying the sex habits of undergraduate students, researchers concluded that students who had sex once or twice a week had one-third more immunoglobulin A (IgA) in their saliva. Elevated levels of IgA protect us from colds, flu, and other infections. Surprisingly, more sex is not better. Researchers found that those students who had sex more than three times per week had lower IgA levels than those who rarely had sex or had no sex at all. Moderation seems to be the key.

STEROLS, STEROLINS, AND MARATHON RUNNERS

Marathon runners are a well-documented group of athletes who experience exercise-induced immune suppression. Many researchers have indicated that there are increases in immune cells while others have shown a reduction in the ability of those cells to function appropriately after high-intensity workouts. The type of immune suppression that occurs after a marathon race may be attributed to the lack of regulatory factors released by T-helper cells, especially gamma-interferon, a powerful antiviral agent. As well, increased levels of interleukin-6 are found in the blood and urine of athletes following strenuous workouts. Interleukin-6 is associated with high cortisol levels, low DHEA levels, and reduced activity of natural killer cells. During this temporary immune suppression period, microorganisms, especially viruses, have time to evade immune detection and become established, giving rise to infections in athletes.

Patrick Bouic and his research team have shown that plant sterols and sterolins are potent immune modulators (they balance the immune system) and can reverse abnormalities of the immune system. The aim of their marathon runner study was to determine whether sterols and sterolins could inhibit the radical physiological changes seen in the blood of athletes and also whether these plant fats could decrease the, muscle pain, and inflammation associated with the excessive exercise of marathon running (which is also similar to that seen in those with excessive stress in their lives).

STEROLS AND STEROLINS: PRECURSORS TO DHEA

Post-marathon results showed that those runners who received sterols and sterolins had a significant reduction in interleukin-6 compared to the placebo group. A profound effect was observed in the balance between cortisol and DHEA levels in the sterol- and sterolin-treated group. Cortisol is an immune-suppressing hormone, and in the placebo group cortisol increased as expected, yet it dropped in the treated group. This cortisol decrease was accompanied by an increase in DHEA that was statistically significant. DHEA, the immune-regulating hormone, is important in protecting us from viral and bacterial infections, as well as inhibiting new tumors from forming. DHEA protects against the lethal coxsackie B enterovirus or herpes Type 2 and Enterococcus faecalis infection. DHEA levels decline with age and it is proposed as one factor in immune dysregulation, such as raised interleukin-6 and the development of degenerative diseases, including arthritis.

A balance between the two types of T-helper cells is required for optimal immune health, and DHEA greatly enhances the action of Th-1 cells and the regulatory factors they release, including interleukin-2. By enhancing T-helper cells in turn, we increase the activity of our cytotoxic T-cells and the number of T-helper cells called to battle while decreasing interleukin-4, which causes inflammation and tissue destruction. Sterols and sterolins are precursors to pregnenolone and then to DHEA.

Dysfunction in the regulation of the immune system, caused by an overdominance of Th-2 and underactivity of Th-1, will result in low DHEA levels. This is especially true in those who use corticosteroid drugs for joint, cartilage, or muscle injuries, are under continuous stress, or who have an autoimmune disorder such as lupus or rheumatoid arthritis. Low DHEA levels are also seen in those with chronic fatigue syndrome as well as in those with poor recovery times after a workout. DHEA is a super immune hormone and in order to stay young and healthy, we must ensure adequate DHEA levels as we age.

The effects of intense exercise (a stressor) on the immune system have been debated for many years. Most of the negative effects of overexercising can be summed up to excess cortisol production (the stress hormone) and an imbalance in the ratio of Th-1 helper cells to Th-2 cells and a reduction in the antiaging super immune hormone DHEA. Sterols and sterolins improve these parameters quickly within several weeks.

14 FITNESS TIPS

Now that you know the possible dangers of overexercising without adequate nutrition, here are 14 quick strategies for losing weight, gaining muscle, and reversing disease.

- Ideally, you should do some kind of activity every day of the week, or at least three days a week or every other day. Studies in Finland demonstrated that exercising just over half an hour four times a week or 45 minutes three times a week reduces the risk of heart attack by 50 percent and stroke by 40 percent. Make sure that you alternate your higher-intensity workouts with lower-intensity ones to give your body time to recover and keep your immune system in balance. If you dance for two hours on Monday, walk on Tuesday.

- Take the stairs instead of the elevator, and walk to the corner store instead of driving your car. Every little bit of exercise helps.
- How hard you exercise during your workout is another component of success. Measured as a function of heart rate, intensity ranges between 55 and 85 percent of your maximum heart rate. Beginners will be around 55 percent; more active people will be closer to 80 and 85 percent. Whether you are a beginner or an athlete, you should be able to talk while you are exercising. If you can talk easily as if nothing is going on, then you are right—nothing is going on, so pump it up a little. If you are out of breath or wheezing, then slow down, you have pushed yourself too far too soon.
- If you are a beginner or haven't exercised since your last day of high school physical education class, don't worry if you can't start with 20-minute workouts. Even if all you can do is five minutes, just do it—and do it every day; or do it once in the morning and again in the afternoon or evening. Time yourself and add a minute every third workout. You will improve over the next few weeks.
- Variety, as they say, is the spice of life. To prevent boredom or possible injury from overuse of the same muscle groups, incorporate new types of exercise into your workouts. On your off-workout days, try other activities because they are fun, not because you can burn a certain number of calories. Exercise should not feel like one more chore on your "to do" list.
- Reduce your intake of margarines, bad oils, and processed meats. Add essential fatty acids (the fat-burning fats), and eat grapefruits (they contain naringin, a fat burner).
- Eat breakfast every day. Get a good protein drink mix. (I use Women's Whey with berries and yogurt.) Eat something with fiber; it will fill you up. (See recipe section for ideas.)
- Use a smaller plate to serve your meals, or fill up your plate as you normally would and then put back half.
- Snack all day. Four or five high-protein (one hard-boiled egg is loaded with pure protein; eat only one per day), low-carbohydrate snacks throughout the day will keep hunger pains at bay. Eat foods low on the glycemic index (see chart on page 63).
- Take 5-HTP, which will curb appetite and increase serotonin levels.
- If you are tired and stressed, your cortisol levels will remain high throughout the day. Researchers have discovered that high cortisol causes us to carry that spare tire around the middle. If you are exercising and eating correctly and you still can't budge the bulge, ask yourself why you are stressed and/or tired (see page 45 about waking times and high cortisol).

- Take these fat-burning nutrients: chromium (200 mcg per day), Citrus aurantium standardized to 6 percent synephrine (150 mg twice per day, half an hour before meals), *Garcinia cambogia* (1000 mg per day in a divided dose; sold under the name Citrimax), and carnitine (1 g per day). Drink lots of green tea, which is rich in fat-burning catechins.
- Avoid white foods (bread, pasta, rice, white potatoes), aspartame, and nondairy creamers. These foods are devoid of nutrition, make us fat, and increase our risk of diabetes.
- According to Brad King, author of *Fat Wars*, we need to do more than 20 minutes of cardio along with weight-bearing exercise to burn fat, and one of the best ways to keep your fat-burning engine revved is to do the cardio/aerobic activity after you have done your weight-bearing activity. I always dreaded doing the cardio portion of my fitness program. Getting on the bike or treadmill for 30 minutes or more at the beginning of my workout was hard and I couldn't wait to do my weight routine. When I read that it was not only okay but also actually a better way to burn fat to do the weight routine first, I was thrilled. I start with some stretching exercises, then do a variety of weight-bearing exercises. By then, lots of endorphins are running through me, so riding the bike is no longer a chore. I can actually ride for 30 minutes or more without tiring.

Adopt as many of the above recommendations as you can and watch your weight drop, your health improve, and your energy levels soar.

CHAPTER 7

A TO Z LIST
OF DISEASES

Now that you have a thorough understanding of your digestive, cardio-vascular, and immune system and how important nutrition, exercise, stress reduction, and nutritional supplements are to your health, the following section puts all of the information you have learned into prac-tice. If you have not read the earlier chapters and want to go directly to the appropriate disease, you can flip back to the appropriate chapter as recommended in the Prescription for Health when needed. It is impor-tant to understand that good food is our best medicine and nutritional supplements should augment a great diet, not replace it.

Each condition has an overview of the disease, symptoms, causes, the prescription for health (including herbs and nutrients) researched for that particular condition, health tips, other recommendations, and health facts. Nutritional deficiencies caused by poor food choices are the underlying cause of many diseases. The use of nutrition as medicine is now scientifically vali-dated. Diseases caused by inadequate diet, environmental toxins, and too much stress respond dramatically to nutrients in the appropriate doses, stress reduction, and dietary modifications.

The Prescription for Health recommendations are based on research published in scientific journals worldwide. Wherever possible, recommen-dations are gleaned from human studies or the clinical observations of ortho-molecular researchers and doctors. Some conditions list many nutrients that work for the specific disease. Several of the recommended nutrients will be available in a combination formula in your health food store so it will not be necessary to take them all separately, reducing the number of pills you have to take. If you are currently on prescription medication, consult your medical doctor or pharmacist to determine if there are any drug–nutrient interactions. As mentioned throughout the book, many prescription drugs cause a depletion of essential nutrients and many vitamins and minerals enhance the action of certain prescription medications, so it is important to discuss this with your pharmacist and doctor. Also, if you are pregnant or have a serious illness, or autoimmune disease, consult a physician or naturopath before administering these remedies. Enlist the help of your physician or seek out an alternative health care practitioner who understands nutrition as medicine. The best scenario is one in which the doctor and patient work as a team to ensure the best possible treatment to eliminate disease.

Several conditions have hereditary factors or a genetic predisposition as a contributing cause to an illness. It is important to understand that while people are born with genes inherited from their ancestors and that certain genes show vulnerability for specific diseases, this does not mean you are destined to contract the disease just because you have a genetic susceptibility. According to Chris M. Reading, MD and Ross Meillon, authors of *Your Family Tree Connection,* we can alter our genetic predisposition by changing the patterns that promote disease. For example, if you have a family history of colon cancer, you can reduce your genetic susceptibility by eating a high-fiber diet, taking antioxidant supplements, and avoiding alcohol, caffeine, and stress, which are all known triggers for promoting this type of cancer.

Certain health recommendations are important in treating each condition. Instead of listing them under each disease condition, they are explained below.

ALLERGY DETECTION AND ELIMINATION

Start a diet diary and write down everything you eat for one week and see if there is any correlation to your symptoms. Ask for a referral to an allergy specialist and get tested for possible triggers. Some allergies may be detected only with the help of an ELISA/ACT test. I recommend ELISA/ACT Biotechnologies Inc. at 1-800-553-5472 for the ELISA/ACT (enzyme-linked immunosorbent assay) allergy test to rule out delayed-onset allergies. Once you know what you are allergic to, avoid those allergens.

DIETARY RECOMMENDATIONS FOR EVERYONE

- See "How Nutrients Are Absorbed" in Chapter 1 for complete information on dietary requirements.
- Aid digestion by taking digestive plant enzymes with every meal. If gas, bloating, and bowel movements don't improve, you may not be producing enough stomach acid to break down your food properly. Hydrochloric acid supplements with meals may alleviate this condition.
- Eat seven to ten half-cup servings of organic fruits and vegetables every day. If you haven't been eating raw vegetables regularly, start

by steaming your vegetables and don't forget the digestive enzymes. Avoid white pasta, white rice, or white flour and opt for natural whole grains instead. Eat one half cup of plain yogurt with active cultures every day unless you are lactose intolerant.

- Drink eight to ten glasses of pure, filtered water every day, but do not drink during meals or else you will dilute your digestive enzymes. For every cup of caffeinated liquid that you drink, add another glass of water.
- To spark your digestive juices, add fresh-squeezed lemon juice to a cup of water or herbal tea upon waking or 15 minutes before your meal.
- Reduce the amount of sugar you eat every day. We eat on average 150 lbs (68 kg) of sugar per person per year. One teaspoon (5 mL) of white sugar causes our virus- and cancer-fighting cells to become inactive for hours. Aspartame and sucralose are not much better. Instead, use stevia, a wonderful sweet herb that is a thousand times sweeter than sugar and safe for diabetics.
- If you are not hungry when you rise in the morning or have gas, bloating, or heartburn, you may have low stomach acid. If you suspect you have low stomach acid, take one capsule (600 mg) of hydrochloric acid before a large meal. If symptoms worsen, stop—you do not have low stomach acidity. If you feel the same or better, increase your dosage by one capsule at your next meal. Keep increasing dosage up to a maximum of seven capsules or until you feel warmth in your stomach. When you feel the warmth, cut back your dosage. For some people two capsules may be adequate; for others it may take a maximum of seven. Use fewer capsules for smaller meals. Read Chapter 1 to learn more about digestive problems.
- Stop smoking—*now*. If you don't smoke but are exposed to secondhand smoke, remove yourself from the situation or ask people to butt out. Secondhand smoke has 4000 chemicals in it, including known carcinogens. Smoke that wafts from the lit end does not go through a filter and is more poisonous than what is inhaled by the smoker. Children raised in smoking environments are more prone to lung disorders such as asthma and bronchitis.
- Get regular exercise. Moderate exercise improves your circulation and overall health. Work up to 20 to 30 minutes of walking, at least five times a week. Learn more about exercise in "Exercise for Prevention and Treatment of Ailments" in Chapter 6.
- Keep a positive frame of mind. Attitude and emotional outlook play a powerful role in sickness and health. Adopt the strategies mentioned in the "Stress-Busting Tips" in Chapter 6.

NUTRIENT CAUTIONS

Vitamins and minerals are safe when taken in the recommended dosages. The following cautions show what may happen when high doses of certain nutrients are taken over the long term.

- Supplement with iron only if a blood test shows you are iron deficient. If you are supplementing with iron, monitor your intake carefully. Iron deficiencies can cause fatigue and impair the immune system, but excess iron promotes heart disease and hinders our immune system, among other illnesses. Iron can cause the depletion of zinc as well.
- Vitamin A should not be taken in high doses long term. A safe and acceptable dosage of vitamin A is 5000 IU per day. Dosages higher than this should not be continued over the long term. For example, vitamin A in a dose of 100,000 IU may be recommended for infections for several days and then discontinued. Pregnant women should avoid taking vitamin A above the recommended dose.
- Zinc in dosages of 300 mg per day can impair immune function, causing immune suppression.
- Dosages of above 200 mcg per day of selenium should not be consumed without your doctor's advice because toxicity may occur over time.
- Niacin may cause the skin to turn red, flush, and be warm to the touch (known as the histamine flush). This is not harmful and will naturally subside within a couple of hours. Niacin in the time-release form is not recommended as it has been shown to cause liver toxicity. Those taking high doses of niacin should have their liver enzymes monitored by a physician. Alternatively, inositol hexanicotinate (nonflushing niacin) does not have the toxicity problems associated with pure niacin and can be taken in large doses without side effects.
- When taking gram quantities of omega-3 fatty acids, vitamin E should be supplemented to protect against free radicals.
- Vitamin B_6 in doses of 200 mg daily over the long term can cause neurological symptoms. Pyridoxal-5-phosphate, the active form of vitamin B_6, should be taken to avoid this problem. Magnesium and P-5-P should be taken together as they work synergistically.

TROUBLESHOOTING

On the next page is a list of common symptoms that may be associated with a more serious illness that is present in the body or that may result if those symptoms are not assessed and dealt with. The following symptoms should be reported to your health-care provider. Symptoms are your body's way of telling you that something needs attention. Early detection improves healing and recovery.

SYMPTOM	POSSIBLE ASSOCIATION(S)
Blood (from vagina, anus, or penis, or in urine, stools, mucous, or vomit)	Hemorrhoids, polyps, ulcer, infections, bowel tumor, renal, uterine, or bladder cancer
Coughing (persistent), shortness of breath	Pneumonia, emphysema, lung problems, cancer, food allergy, whooping cough, allergies, asthma
Fatigue (persistent)	Addison's disease, chronic fatigue syndrome, weak immune system, restless leg syndrome, candidiasis, cancer, congestive heart failure
Fever (recurring or lasting longer than two days)	Mononucleosis, chronic infection, bronchitis, colds or flu, rheumatic problems, diabetes; a recurring or long-lasting fever should be discussed with your physician
Indigestion, gas, bloating, nausea	HCl deficiency; lack of digestive enzymes; problems with liver, adrenals, gallbladder, or pancreas; heart disease; stress; ulcers; poor nutrition; food allergy; bowel disease
Itching	Allergy, candidiasis, eczema, psoriasis, fungal infection, hives, herpes virus, shingles, restless leg syndrome, parasites, liver dysfunction
Pain (abdominal)	Premenstrual syndrome, food poisoning, food allergy, colitis, diverticulitis, hiatal hernia, irritable bowel syndrome, Crohn's disease, fibroids, endometriosis, constipation, infection
Pain (headache)	Constipation, eyestrain, sinusitis, stress, allergy, asthma, drug reaction, glaucoma, high blood pressure, nutritional deficiencies, brain tumor, depression, Wegener's granulomatosis, infection
Pain (joints, muscle, or tendons)	Carpal tunnel syndrome, arthritis, chronic fatigue syndrome, fibromyalgia, osteoporosis, gout, leg cramps, infection
Swelling	Heart or kidney problems, drug reaction, food allergy, arthritis
Thirst (excessive)	Fever, infection, diabetes
Urination (frequent or painful)	Cancer, diabetes, urinary tract infection, interstitial cystitis
Weight gain (rapid)	Thyroid problems, constipation
Weight loss (unexplained)	Parasitic infection, thyroid problem, malabsorption syndrome, hepatitis, HIV, cancer, diabetes, mononucleosis

ACNE

Acne vulgaris appears predominantly among teenagers while women between the ages of 20 and 40 cope with acne conglobata, yet acne is a condition that has affected most of us at some time in our life.

Acne is caused by an increase in the production of androgens (male hormones) stimulating the oil glands beneath the skin to enlarge and increase production of sebum and keratin. Although they are male hormones, they exist in smaller quantities in women as well. Sebum moves along hair follicles to surface on the skin and as it does, cells on the follicle are shed. The cells, keratin, and sebum adhere and plug the pore.

When the plug surfaces on the skin, it oxidizes and creates a blackhead; when the pore is blocked, bacteria grows, releasing enzymes to break down the sebum, turning it into pus. An inflammation occurs, causing whiteheads. In severe cases, pimples develop as cysts and they are more difficult to heal if a whitehead doesn't form to release the pus.

Symptoms

Red cyst-like lumps, or pimples with white or blackheads can appear on the face, neck, back, and chest. The skin may have an oily sheen to it. Attempts to hurry healing by squeezing or erupting the pimple can lead to scarring.

Causes

Deficiencies in essential fatty acids can cause an overproduction of sebum, resulting in acne. Research has shown that when the Inuit changed to Western diets, they developed acne. Far less acne is seen those eating traditional diets versus the Western diet. Eating too many of the wrong fats has also been shown to cause excess sebum production. People with specific food allergies will be susceptible to flare-ups brought on by eating the offending foods.

Hormonal imbalances or excess progesterone from oral contraceptives or postovulation in women can increase acne. Young men often experience acne when testosterone levels surge. Stressful events have also been shown to worsen or aggravate acne. Acne can also be a reaction to some prescription medications. Acne, especially around the chin, is a common symptom of taking too much DHEA in supplement form. Fortunately, the acne disappears when DHEA is reduced.

The skin is the final means for detoxification. Acne arises when the body has no other way to rid itself of excess toxins. If the liver is sluggish, it can't break down the androgen hormones causing acne. A sluggish liver also burdens the immune system. If the digestive system is not functioning efficiently, waste is left to decompose, forming toxins in the intestines instead of being eliminated at a proper pace. If toxins are left in the blood, they will be excreted through the skin. Acne, a recurring bacterial infection, can be associated with immune deficiency diseases (such as chronic fatigue syndrome; see Health Fact on page 147).

Prescription for Health

NUTRIENT	DOSAGE	ACTION
Vitamin A	50,000 IU (water-soluble Micel A) daily for three weeks. Dosages of 100,000 IU per day have been used with excellent results within several weeks. High doses of vitamin A should not be taken over the long term without medical supervision. Reduce to 5000 IU per day for maintenance after treatment period ends.	Reduces sebum production, promotes smooth, clear skin
Folic acid, vitamin B$_3$, B$_6$ B-complex	Folic acid 1 mg per day
Vitamin B$_6$ (P-5-P) 50 mg per day
Vitamin B$_3$ 100 mg in a high-potency B-complex per day	Facilitates breakdown of excess hormones
Vitamin D	400 IU per day	Promotes healing of skin
Vitamin E	400 IU twice daily	Acts as an antioxidant and encourages tissue repair
Zinc	60 mg daily. In one study 135 mg of vinc daily was as effective as tetracycline 750 mg daily without side effects.	Is essential for healthy immune function
Chromium picolinate	400 mcg daily	Improves glucose tolerance and essential fatty acid metabolism
Selenium	100 mcg daily	Enhances glutathione and fights bacteria
Artichoke	160–320 mg three times daily with meals, assuming standardized to contain 13–18 percent caffeolquinic acids calculated as chlorogenic acid	Increases bile formation and flow to digest and absorb fats
Omega-3 fatty acid	1–2 Tbsp (15–30 mL) of flaxseed oil daily	Reduces overproduction of sebum
Reduced L-glutathione	45 mg daily	Antibacterial, enhances immune function
Lactobacillus acidophilus	1 tsp (5 mL) twice daily	Improves intestinal flora (especially important if you have taken antibiotics for condition)
Moducare sterols and sterolins	One capsule of Moducare three times daily	Increases antibacterial activity and reduces inflammation

NUTRIENT	DOSAGE	ACTION
Garlic	Eat foods containing garlic	Acts as a natural antibacterial
Vitamin C	1000 mg three times daily	Repairs skin tissue and reduces inflammation
Digestive enzymes	One or two capsules with meals	Aids digestion
Milk thistle	Choose standardized extracts; use as directed	Detoxifies the liver
Chaste tree berry (Vitex)	40 drops of tincture daily	Normalizes hormones
Dandelion root	Dandelion tea as a beverage	Detoxifies the liver
Gugulipid	Standardized (*Commiphora mukul*) 500 mg three times daily	Metabolizes fats

Health Tips to Enhance Healing

- If you suspect you have low stomach acid that is hindering your digestion, see the introduction on low stomach acid, page 141.
- One study published in *Archives of Dermatology* found that 1 oz (28 g) of All-Bran cereal per day rapidly cleared acne. Researchers felt it was due to correcting constipation.
- Take digestive enzymes before a meal. Do not drink while eating or the enzymes will be diluted. Start your day with a glass of purified water with 1 tsp (5 mL) of organic apple cider vinegar or fresh-squeezed lemon juice.
- Avoid foods high in sugars, trans fatty acids, dairy, processed and refined foods, hydrogenated oils, and fried food. Follow a diet of natural whole foods that include fresh fruits and vegetables, vegetable protein as found in legumes and seeds, and grains and essential oils to ease the burden on your digestive system.
- Drink plenty of pure, filtered water, at least 8 to 10 glasses daily (see Chapter 4).
- Eat foods that encourage healthy liver function such as artichokes, rhubarb, Chinese white radish, black radish, soy, apples, and rolled oats.

Avoid:
- foods with iodized salt (aggravates acne)
- inorganic iron (inactivates vitamin E)
- foods you are allergic or sensitive to
- vitamin B_{12} (can produce or aggravate acne)
- soft drinks (they contain brominated vegetable oils, which can aggravate acne)

Other Recommendations

- Take regular saunas. The skin is the largest detoxification organ and saunas can improve elimination through the skin. Saunas are found at your local swimming pool.
- Tea tree oil topical ointments fight bacteria on the skin and reduce redness of blemishes.
- Wash your pillowcases regularly in detergents free of colors or fragrances, and rinse twice.
- Avoid using cosmetics or heavy moisturizers. Wash your face with natural soaps or cleansers, avoiding ones with perfumes and scents. Dr. Hauschka and Weleda cleansing lotions and moisturizers are excellent for acne and sensitive skin. Keep your hair clean as well.
- Exercise regularly to stimulate the circulation, the release of toxins, and proper functioning of the organs.
- Read Chapter 1 for more information on ensuring proper absorption and elimination of foods.

Health Fact

Chronic fatigue syndrome is a mixture of viral, bacterial, or parasitic infections that take advantage of a temporary breakdown in the immune system. Acne, because it is a recurring bacterial infection of the oil glands, is often associated with chronic fatigue syndrome. Repairing immune function to better fight infections can often eliminate these conditions.

ADDISON'S DISEASE

Addison's disease is a rare disorder caused by chronic and insufficient functioning of the outer layer of the adrenal gland. The adrenal glands lie on top of each kidney. They produce three types of hormones: the glucocorticoid hormones, including cortisol; mineralocorticoid hormone aldosterone; and the androgen and estrogen hormones. The glucocorticoid hormones maintain glucose regulation, regulate the immune system, and help us respond to stress. Aldosterone regulates sodium and potassium balance. With Addison's disease, the outer cortex of the adrenal glands is damaged and cortisol and aldosterone are secreted in insufficient amounts.

Symptoms

Symptoms include chronic candidiasis and gastrointestinal disturbances, including malabsorption, often beginning in infancy, although Addison's disease may not be diagnosed until symptoms become debilitating.

Aldosterone deficiency elevates the secretion of sodium and lowers potassium. This imbalance in sodium and potassium leads to low blood pressure and an increase in water excretion that could result in severe dehydration.

Addison's disease is quite often associated with diabetes, thyroid disease, ovarian failure, and pernicious anemia. Hypothyroidism may appear. Other signs are skin darkening, food cravings, blood sugar disorders, severe weakness, dizziness, weight loss, headaches, problems with memory, and darkening of the skin and mucous membranes. Diagnosis of Addison's is frequently overlooked or delayed if skin darkening is not apparent.

Causes

Addison's is predominantly caused by the immune system destroying the adrenal cortex. Addison's can also be caused by chronic infections like tuberculosis, AIDS, prolonged use of steroid medication that suppresses adrenocorticotrophic hormone, tumor growth, viral infections, and pituitary disease.

Prescription for Health

NUTRIENT	DOSAGE	ACTION
Moducare sterols and sterolins	Two capsules three times daily for one week; one capsule three times daily thereafter	Stops autoantibody production and modulates cortisol, enhances DHEA
High-potency B-complex	Two or three capsules daily	Reduces stress and is necessary for healthy adrenal glands
Vitamin C	1000 mg daily	Antioxidant; enhances immune function
Pantothenic acid	1000 mg daily in divided doses. In lupus research, up to 6 g was used with success to control autoimmunity.	Required by adrenal glands hormone activity
Astragulus	Two 500 mg capsules or 5 mL of tincture daily	Improves adrenal function and reduces stress
Licorice DGL (Enzymatic Therapy)	Chew two tablets 20 minutes before each meal.	Supports the adrenal glands, stimulates aldosterone and cortisol
Multimune containing A, C, E, P5P, selenium, zinc, magnesium, lipoic acid, reduced L-glutathione, and coenzyme Q10	Three capsules daily taken with food	Supports healthy immune function, controls inflammatory response
Raw adrenal gland	Choose product from New Zealand (free from mad cow disease).	Rebuilds adrenals

Health Tips to Enhance Healing

- Avoid the substances that antagonize the adrenal glands: alcohol, animal products, caffeine, bad fats such as fried foods, processed food, soft drinks, sugar, tobacco, and white flour products.
- Eat plenty of fresh fruit and vegetables, nuts and seeds, healthy oils, legumes, and whole grains. Have salmon, tuna, and deep-water ocean fish at meals three times a week at least.
- Drink Women's Whey or Proteins+ protein powder every day to ensure adequate amino acid complex. Amino acids are required for proper functioning of adrenal hormones.
- Protecting the glands is of the utmost importance to prevent them from becoming completely exhausted. Practice stress-reduction techniques regularly (see page 130), do not drive yourself too hard, and rest.

Other Recommendations

- See more on autoimmune disease in Chapter 3.
- See Candidiasis.
- See Malabsorption Syndrome.

Health Fact

Test Your Adrenal Function: You can test your adrenal function by comparing two blood pressure readings. Take your blood pressure after resting for five minutes. Stand up and immediately take another reading. If your standing reading is lower than your resting reading, suspect insufficient adrenal gland function.

ALLERGIES

For most individuals, allergies are a seasonal or situational problem causing unbearable symptoms. Your friend's cat or the pollens of spring may be the reason for your itchy eyes, runny nose, sneezing, wheezing, and more. Yet for many people, allergy symptoms never seem to abate. They are a constant problem. Common environmental exposures and foods trigger their allergies and promote asthmatic attacks. But why is it that only some are affected by allergies and others are not?

There are two types of allergic response: the first is a classic allergic response where the allergen (e.g., pollen, shellfish, pet dander) triggers an increase in immunoglobulin E (IgE); the reaction is immediate. This response is easily determined with a blood test, which will show a high count of IgE antibodies. The IgE antibodies meet an invader and then trigger a release of chemicals (including histamine) from mast cells that can kill or immobilize it. Allergies that are mediated by IgE are called atopic. Allergens can initiate different symptoms depending on which area of the body they settle in. An upper respiratory tract irritation will exhibit sneezing and a runny nose, while the same allergen in the lower respiratory tract will produce wheezing or coughing.

The second type of allergic response is cell-mediated or delayed-onset response. They are more difficult to diagnose as the symptoms may not occur immediately. Delayed-onset allergies are cell-mediated, showing an increase in IgG antibodies. The symptoms tend to be in the gastrointestinal tract in the form of gastric upsets, diarrhea, irritable bowel, hyperactivity (in children), and brain fog-type symptoms.

Many illnesses, including autoimmune disorders, arthritis, attention deficit hyperactivity disorder, and inflammatory diseases are associated with or arise from years of untreated or hidden allergies.

Symptoms

Allergies can elicit a cornucopia of symptoms that are so wide and varied that it can be difficult to detect an allergy over some other condition. Common reactions are sneezing, watery eyes, runny nose, itching, dermatitis, earache, congested nasal passages, headaches, hives, bloating, blurred vision, cramps, frequent urination, stomach distress, diarrhea, gas, edema, fatigue, depression, brain fog, lack of concentration, poor memory, anxiety, feeling faint, hyperactivity, insomnia, irritability, arthritic pain, and muscle pain.

Additional symptoms include:
- dark circles under the eyes
- red-rimmed or swollen, watery eyes
- red, burning ears
- runny nose
- constant nose rubbing (some allergic people have a crease just above the bulb of the nose from chronic rubbing or one nostril will be stretched in the direction of the rub)
- inflamed tonsils and recurrent throat infections
- skin rashes, eczema
- diarrhea, gas, constipation, nausea, bloated stomach, heartburn, stomach aches, etc.
- excessive sweating
- headaches, dizziness
- extreme salivation
- joint and muscle pain
- fatigue
- poor memory or fogginess

- bedwetting in children
- mood swings

Causes

Our immune system is causing the allergic symptoms in its bid to rid the body of what it sees as invaders. This is not a normal response and occurs only in those who have a hyperstimulated or overly sensitive immune system. In an allergy-prone person, when the immune system encounters an allergen such as pollen, the T-helper-2 cell releases an immune factor called interleukin-4 (IL-4). Interleukin-4 causes B cells to secrete IgE antibodies that then attach to mast cells. Mast cells release a cascade of chemicals, including histamine, which promote allergic symptoms. Gamma-interferon is also reduced in allergic persons and gamma-interferon is responsible for stopping IL-4. Without adequate gamma-interferon, the allergic reaction is not inhibited. Histamine is responsible for many of the symptoms experienced, such as watery eyes, itchy skin, and more. In asthmatics the situation is even worse because not only does the immune system release interleukin-4 but also an immune factor called interleukin-6 (IL-6). In asthmatics interleukin-6 causes lung tissue damage and if not controlled, can lead to reliance on steroid medications and puffers. The key to halting allergies in their tracts is stopping interleukin-4 from being released in the first place and controlling interleukin-6.

Important Research

Plant sterols and sterolins halt the release of IL-4, so histamine is not released and allergies are controlled. As well, sterols and sterolins normalize the release of interleukin-6 and protect lung tissue from further destruction. See Chapter 5 for the latest research on sterols and sterolins and allergy.

Prescription for Health

NUTRIENT	DOSAGE	ACTION
Moducare sterols and sterolins	Adults: two capsules three times daily for one week then one capsule three times daily thereafter. Children: birth to five years old, one capsule daily; five to twelve years old, two capsules daily; and 12 and older, the adult dose	Stops allergic response before it begins; decreases IL-4 and IL-6 activity; is excellent for all allergies
RespirActin	2 oz (56 g) twice daily	Works as a natural antihistamine, opens congested airways
Quercetin	500–1000 mg two to three times daily (children five and up: half the dosage)	Stops histamine release; is antiallergenic and antioxidant; especially effective for those sensitive to airborne allergens

NUTRIENT	DOSAGE	ACTION
Vitamin B_{12}	500 mcg twice daily or 1000 mcg injection with folic acid once weekly for four weeks	Reduces or stops asthmatic symptoms associated with allergies
Vitamin C	1000 mg twice daily	Reduces severity and occurrence of allergy attacks
Magnesium	500 mg three times daily	Acts as a bronchodilator and antihistamine; reduces stress
Reduced L-glutathione	45–100 mg daily	Increases intracellular glutathione; is excellent for inhalent allergies and chemical sensitivities
Evening primrose oil	500 mg twice daily	Is anti-inflammatory
Digestive enzymes	One or two capsules with each meal	Aids digestion; is important for food allergies and to repair leaky gut
Lactobacillus acidophilus	1 tsp (5 mL) daily	Improves intestinal flora; helps those with food allergies and asthma
Pantethine	300 mg twice daily	Reduces sensitivity to aldehydes
Stinging nettle (*Urtica dioica*)	300 mg twice daily	Is effective in allergic rhinitis
Omega-3 fatty acids	1–2 Tbsp (15–30 mL) of flaxseed oil daily or 3–5 g of fish oil; I like Eskimo-3 by Tyler	Reduces inflammation in the long run; deficiency upsets immune system balance
Women's Whey or Proteins+ supplement	One to two scoops daily	Contains amino acids important for repair in the body
Multimune containing A, B_6, C, E, selenium, glutathione magnesium, coenzyme Q10, lipoic acid, and zinc	Three capsules daily	Provides support for the immune system

Health Tips to Enhance Healing

- Avoid allergens whenever possible. Avoid foods that contain sulfites. Beer and wine commonly contain sulfites.
- Drink at least 8 to 10 glasses of pure, filtered water because it controls histamine production. For every juice or caffeinated beverage you drink, add another glass of water.
- See Chapter 1 for tips on how to digest foods properly to avoid leaky gut syndrome, which is associated with food allergies.
- Rotate the foods you eat. Never eat the same foods every day. Consume a diet that emphasizes natural, whole foods such as

legumes, fresh fruit and vegetables, fish, healthy fats and oils, and nuts and seeds. Avoid processed or junk foods as they are nutritionally void and contain chemicals that stress the body. Use cayenne, onions, and garlic liberally as they are high in quercetin.
- See "Allergy Detection and Elimination," page 140.
- Stress can aggravate allergies so get plenty of rest and relaxation.

Other Recommendations

- If you smoke, stop—*now*. If you don't smoke but are exposed to secondhand smoke, remove yourself from the situation or ask people to butt out. Secondhand smoke has 4000 chemicals in it, including known carcinogens. Smoke that wafts from the lit end does not go through a filter and is more poisonous than what is inhaled by the smoker. Children raised in smoking environments are more prone to allergies and asthma.
- If attacks are brought on by airborne allergens, make your living environment as allergy-proof as possible. Wash all bedding and blankets weekly; vacuum and dust with a damp cloth often; do not allow pets on the furniture. Furniture should have washable slipcovers. You may also want to have your home checked for environmental hazards such as lead and asbestos.
- Studies on the herbal mixture Saiboku-tu have shown it effective in reducing the need for steroids. While prevalent in Japan, China, and Korea, it is not available in North America, although RespirActin, a North American combination, has been shown clinically to be effective in controlling allergies and asthma. The two most active ingredients in Saiboku-tu are Baikal skullcap and magnolia, and both are found in RespirActin (see Asthma for research).
- When using herbal remedies, keep in mind that the herbs may belong to the same plant family as your allergens; for example, if you have an allergy to legumes, you may have a reaction to red clover, soybean extracts, or astragalus.
- Men with mustaches may aggravate airborne allergies because allergens build up on the surface of the mustache.
- See Asthma, Candidiasis, and Leaky Gut.

Health Fact

A report out of Long Island Hospital College, New York, stated that dark cats are four times more likely to induce severe allergy attacks than light-colored cats. The conclusion was derived from 321 questionnaires that were completed by cat owners who also suffer from allergies. The researchers believe that more dander resides on dark cat hair (*New Scientist*, November 4, 2000, Volume 168, issue 2263).

ALOPECIA (HAIR LOSS)

Alopecia simply means hair loss. Male pattern baldness is the most common form of alopecia. Inflammation, psoriasis, and fungal infections of the scalp are also associated with hair loss.

Alopecia areata is an autoimmune disorder whereby a person's immune system prevents hair follicles from producing hair fiber. Men and women are affected equally with this autoimmune disorder. According to the American Autoimmune Related Diseases Association, it is estimated that roughly 2 million people have some variation of alopecia. The condition can strike at any time, and may begin as early as childhood. This section, although focusing on autoimmune hair loss, provides treatments for all types of hair loss.

Symptoms

Alopecia areata, the mildest form of the condition, is marked by hair loss that is partial or patchy on the scalp or other parts of the body. In a more severe form called alopecia totalis, all facial and/or scalp hair may be lost. The most extreme case is called alopecia universalis and the entire body loses its hair. Sometimes hair loss is permanent; at other times, it may grow back. Those with alopecia may notice other symptoms such as brittle nails or onychogryposis, a condition where the nails have thickened with increased curvature. Often alopecia areata is seen along with other auto-immune disorders, particularly Hashimoto's thyroiditis, lupus, Addison's disease, vitiligo, and diabetes.

Causes

Organ-specific autoantibodies are increased in those persons with alope-cia areata. Although no specific autoantibody has been found specific to the hair follicles, researchers believe alopecia is an autoimmune disorder because of genetic predisposition; there is usually the presence of other autoimmune disorders and a positive response to corticosteroid therapy.

Nutritional deficiencies in biotin and zinc have been found to contribute to alopecia.

Many women experience alopecia postpartum, during menopause, and as a result of taking birth control pills, which suggests a hormone connection.

Testosterone supplements have been associated with increasing hair loss. Testosterone is converted to dihydrotestosterone (DHT). DHT is known to inhibit the growth and development of hair in the follicle. As well, high-fat diets cause an increase in free testosterone and as such are also implicated in hair loss. People with high blood levels of insulin-like growth factor-1 (IGF-1) have higher rates of baldness. There is an interplay between androgen hormones, insulin, and other hormones in the body. One factor alone does not seem to promote alopecia.

Research has shown that smoking may also increase hair loss by increasing the production of androgen hormones. It is also thought that smoking has a direct effect on hair follicles by killing the hair fiber-making cells.

Several research papers have suggested that alopecia in men may be related to heart disease. Researchers believe that increased rates of heart disease in those with alopecia may be due to elevated cholesterol. Cholesterol is converted into androgen hormones in the body.

In women hair loss has been associated with low iron levels. When iron stores returned to normal, hair regrowth occurred. Conversely, iron overload has also been shown to cause hair loss, especially in men. Hemochromatosis is a genetic disease whereby the individual's body stops breaking down and removing iron from the bloodstream, which promotes hair loss.

Tamoxifen, a drug used in treatment for breast cancer, has been demonstrated to cause alopecia. Withdrawal of the drug stops the condition; however, hair may or may not grow back. Chemotherapeutic agents may also cause hair loss.

Prescription for Health

NUTRIENT	DOSAGE	ACTION
Biotin	1–1.2 g	Has been shown to restore hair growth over six months
High-potency B-complex	Two to three capsules daily	Reduces stress; is required for healthy hair
MSM	500 mg twice daily	Supports manufacture of keratin
Zinc with copper	60 mg daily	Has been shown to restore hair growth especially in women.
Iron	15–30 mg daily	Iron should be taken only by those with marked deficiency; when iron is restored, reduce dose to 10 mg per day. Use caution as iron overload can cause hair loss as well especially in men.
Moducare sterols and sterolins	One capsule three times daily	This is the key to stopping the autoantibody production seen in autoimmune disorders and to control inflammation.
Melatonin	1–3 mg daily	Has a regulatory effect on T-helper cells important for those with autoimmune alopecia
Multimune containing vitamins A, B$_6$, C, E, selenium, coenzyme Q10, zinc, lipoic acid, magnesium, and glutathione	Three capsules daily	Improves circulation, protects against free radical damage, enhances immune function, is anti-inflammatory, switches from bad T-helper-2 to good T-helper-1

NUTRIENT	DOSAGE	ACTION
CoQ10	100 mg daily	Oxygenates the cells
Evening primrose oil	500 mg twice daily	Controls autoimmune and inflammatory processes
Protein powder, Women's Whey, or Proteins+	One to two scoops daily	Proteins improve strength and growth of hair and provide amino acids, and act as a precursor to glutathione, a powerful antioxidant.

Health Tips to Enhance Healing

- Stress reduction is the most important factor in fighting hair loss. Practice deep breathing exercises to increase oxygen intake. Get plenty of restful sleep, at least eight hours a night, and try to get up after 7:30 in the morning. Early risers have higher levels of cortisol, increasing the immune factors associated with promoting autoimmunity.
- A double-blind study showed that 44 percent of those who used the following essential oil tonic every day for seven months had new hair growth. Massage scalp every day to promote blood flow and nutrients to the scalp. Add two to three drops of each of the following to 20 mL grapeseed oil and 3 mL jojoba oil base: cedrus atlantica, lavandula augustifolia, rosemarinus officinalis, and thyme vulgaris. Do not take internally; for topical treatment only.

Other Recommendations

- Have your physician test you to rule out thyroid, estrogen, or adrenal conditions that may promote hair loss.
- Use an antifungal shampoo with tea tree oil.
- Get a hair analysis done to evaluate possibilities of heavy metal poisoning.
- When supplementing with biotin, refrain from consuming any food, drink, cough syrup, or medication that contains alcohol or caffeine. They compromise the nutrient's maximum efficacy and absorption in the body.

Health Fact

Double-blind, placebo-controlled trials in Germany using Moducare for the treatment of enlarged prostate discovered a marvellous side effect. After several months of treatment, men reported that their hair was beginning to grow back. Regular use of sterols and sterolins stops the conversion of testosterone to dihydrotestosterone (DHT). DHT promotes male-pattern baldness. Further research has shown that sterols and sterolins also control autoantibody production, thereby controlling the autoimmune process.

ANEMIA (PERNICIOUS, AUTOIMMUNE, OR IRON-DEFICIENCY)

There are several types of anemia, whereby the number of red blood cells, or the amount of hemoglobin they carry, is low. A reduction of either limits the amount of oxygen available to the lungs and other areas of the body. A simple blood test can determine anemia.

Iron deficiency anemia is the most common. When red blood cells are lost due to excessive bleeding, a deficiency of iron occurs. Normally iron is recycled to make new red blood cells but when excess bleeding has occurred there is not enough iron to rebuild red blood cells in the bone marrow. Iron supplements are used with success to correct iron deficiency anemia.

Vitamin B_{12} and folic acid are also used by the bone marrow to make red blood cells. A deficiency of one or both causes pernicious anemia. Vegetarians, and those with malabsorption syndromes caused by gut problems or autoimmune disease, such as Crohn's or autoimmune gastritis, must use vitamin B_{12} and folic acid injections to correct this anemia.

Vitamin C deficiency causes small red blood cells, which also promotes anemia.

Pernicious anemia is also associated with autoimmune disease; it develops at the last stage of autoimmune gastritis, due to the immune system destroying the gastric mucosal lining, and also develops out of autoimmune hemolytic anemia, where red blood cells are attacked and destroyed. The body is unable to use vitamin B_{12}, and as a result, digestion is compromised, as is the body's ability to produce red blood cells. Ten to 15 percent of those with autoimmune gastritis have pernicious anemia.

Two percent of the Western population over 60 years of age is deficient in vitamin B_{12} and has pernicious anemia. Pernicious anemia can easily be treated with vitamin B_{12}.

Symptoms

Signs of anemia are fatigue, shortness of breath, depression, diarrhea, paleness, rapid heartbeat, chest pains, inability to exercise even moderately, and abdominal discomfort. Stomach acid is extremely low, making digestion difficult or impossible. Iron deficiency can cause cravings for dirt and ice. Cracks at the sides of the mouth and spoonlike fingernails are also a sign of anemia. If vitamin B_{12} deficiency is left unaddressed, neurological problems can arise. Many elderly people have undiagnosed B_{12} and folic acid deficiency, leading to anemia.

Causes

The cause of pernicious anemia is still unknown, but two factors are acknowledged. First, there is a genetic inheritance leaning towards northern Europeans and those with genetic markers for fair skin, blue eyes, and blood group A. It is very rare in southern Europeans and "almost nonexistent" in Asians and Africans. Second, it coexists with other autoimmune disorders, such as Hashimoto's thyroiditis, primary Addison's disease, Type I diabetes, vitiligo, myasthenia gravis, premature graying, and primary ovarian failure. A lack of intrinsic factor needed to absorb B_{12} is often the cause of pernicious anemia. Intrinsic factor is secreted by the cells of the stomach, which are often damaged by disease; or intrinsic factor is not released due to low HCl and the pancreatic enzyme trypsin.

Vitamin B_{12} deficiency can be caused by poor nutrition, a strict vegetarian or vegan diet, and any digestive disorder, such as malabsorption syndrome, Crohn's disease, leaky gut, or by gastric surgery.

Prescription for Health

NUTRIENT	DOSAGE	ACTION
Vitamin B complex	100 mg per day	Supports B vitamin supplementation
Vitamin B_{12}	Injection 1 g weekly for six weeks or until anemia is reversed, then once monthly. Those with pernicious anemia need B_{12} for life. Oral methylcobalamin, the active form of B_{12}, in sublingual tablets, 2000 mcg per day for one month or until anemia is reversed and 1000 mcg thereafter.	Essential for blood cell formation
Folic acid	1000 mcg daily	Required for blood cell formation
Lipotropic factors Choline and inositol	250 mg Choline daily 75 mg inositol daily	Maximizes assimilation of B_{12}
Vitamin B_6	50 mg per day	Elevates hemoglobin
Vitamin C	1000 mg three times daily	Maximizes assimilation of B_{12} and eliminated iron-deficiency anemia
Floradix Iron Tonic	One to two capfuls daily	Does not constipate, enhances iron
Lactobacillus acidophilus	1 tsp (5 mL) containing 1–2 billion active organisms daily	Improves intestinal flora required to manufacture nutrients
HCl	See below	HCl deficiency common in anemia
Digestive enzymes, including pancreatic enzymes	One to two capsules with meals; pancreatic enzymes	Maximize digestion
Moducare sterols and sterolins	One capsule three times per day	Controls autoimmunity, enhances DHEA, anti-inflammatory,

Health Tips to Enhance Healing

- See also Celiac, Bowel Disease, Leaky Gut, and Malabsorption.
- If you suspect you have low stomach acid, take one capsule (600 mg) of hydrochloric acid before a large meal. If symptoms worsen, stop—you do not have low stomach acidity. If you feel the same or better, increase your dosage by one capsule at your next meal. Keep increasing dosage up to a maximum of seven capsules, or until you feel warmth in your stomach. When you feel the warmth, cut back your dosage. For some people, two capsules may be adequate; for others, it may take a maximum of seven. Use fewer capsules for smaller meals.
- Avoid alcohol, coffee, tobacco, birth control pills, and topical steroids—they inhibit vitamin B_{12} absorption.
- Take digestive enzymes before a meal, but do not drink fluids while eating, as they will dilute digestive enzymes.
- Eat calf liver.
- Eat plenty of dark green leafy vegetables.

Other Recommendations

Proper digestion is important, so do all you can to make your meals pleasant. Do not stand at the sink or eat on the run. Sit down in a relaxing atmosphere. Eat slowly, chew often, and do not drink fluids while you eat.

Health Fact

Marie Curie, the first woman to win the Nobel Prize and a recipient of two Nobel Prizes, died July 4, 1934, of pernicious anemia brought on by her lifetime exposure to radium.

ARTHRITIS
(OSTEOARTHRITIS AND RHEUMATOID ARTHRITIS)

Millions of people suffer from one form of arthritis or another and, contrary to popular belief, it is not a disease affecting only the elderly. Some forms of arthritis strike toddlers still in diapers, while thousands are stricken in the prime of their lives. Arthritis is the most prevalent chronic condition affecting women, particularly between the ages of 20 and 40. The National Institute of Arthritis and Musculoskeletal and Skin Diseases reports that one in seven have some form of arthritis.

Arthritis (*arth* meaning joint, *itis* meaning inflammation) consists of over 100 different conditions from gout to rheumatoid arthritis (see chart for a partial list). Although most of these disorders occur with joint or muscle

Types of Arthritis

Ankylosing Spondylitis
Gout
Infective arthritis
Juvenile chronic arthritis
Osteoarthritis (the most common type)
Polymyalgia rheumatica
Pseudo gout
Psoriatic arthritis
Reiter's disease
Reynaud's phenomenon
Rheumatoid arthritis
Sjogren's syndrome
Systemic lupus erythematosus

inflammation, many (like lupus) involve the skin, lungs, and kidney. Inflammation, swelling, and pain are hallmarks of arthritis.

Osteoarthritis, the most common form of arthritis, is a gradual wearing away of the cartilage that cushions the joints to prevent the bones from scraping against each other. New research is also finding that osteoarthritis results when the ability to regenerate normal cartilage is impaired. Repetitive activities and sports injuries are associated with the development of arthritis.

Rheumatoid arthritis (RA), the second most common form, is an autoimmune disease whereby the immune system produces antibodies that destroy the synovial membranes around the lubricating fluid in the joints. RA may begin in fits and starts, taking months or years to progress, but for about 25 percent of sufferers it begins abruptly and severely. In the case of RA, correcting the immune system abnormality is paramount.

Symptoms

Osteoarthritis: Usually osteoarthritis appears after the age of 40 and is characterized by joint pain and stiffness that increases in severity over a long period of time. The joints become swollen and lose their mobility. After much of the cartilage has been worn away, bone spurs develop in the joint spaces.

Rheumatoid Arthritis: The joint pain and stiffness of RA is more noticeable in the morning, and like osteoarthritis, the joints become swollen. Unlike osteoarthritis, however, RA can strike suddenly in some cases and at any time of life, even in childhood (juvenile rheumatoid arthritis). Other symptoms include fatigue, fever, depression, anemia, weight loss, and night sweats. When the joints are inflamed, they take on a purplish color and as the disease progresses the hands and feet become deformed. RA attacks symmetrically, afflicting both wrists, ankles, or both knees.

When diagnosing RA, four out of seven criteria must be met: morning stiffness that lasts more than an hour; the arthritis is symmetrical; three joint areas are simultaneously inflamed (not just bony overgrowth);

arthritis is present in any of the hand joints; nodules lie under the skin on bony prominences; serum rheumatoid factor levels are abnormal; and erosions or decalcification are detected by X ray.

Causes

Osteoarthritis: Better known as "wear and tear" arthritis, osteoarthritis can arise from repetitive use or abuse of the joints from heavy labor, sports, and injuries. Obesity aggravates arthritis because greater strain is put on the joints. Poor nutrition and dehydration, as well as food and environmental allergies, can contribute to the condition. Although aging is usually cited as a factor (70 percent of the elderly have it), there is an assumption that it is an inevitable aspect of aging. This is not true. If care is taken to address the other factors, then you may live a long life without osteoarthritis.

Rheumatoid Arthritis: Stress and its ability to disrupt hormones that promote inflammation, allergies, heredity, obesity, nutritional deficiencies, vaccines, a hyperactive immune system, and even viral or bacterial infections, are just a few of the potential causes of RA. Ten years ago rheumatologists would have disagreed that these factors play a role in promoting arthritis, but new research has shown otherwise. If you are taking immunosuppressant drugs like methotrexate or prednisone, do not stop your medications. The following recommendations are to be used in conjunction with your medication. Have your autoantibodies checked by your physician and he/she will recommend reducing your medication as your autoantibodies are reduced (for about four to six weeks).

Prescription for Health

NUTRIENT	DOSAGE	ACTION
Moducare sterols and sterolins	Two capsules three times daily for one week. One capsule three times daily thereafter.	Lowers IL-6, stops autoantibody and inflammatory processes from the immune system; naturally increases DHEA level
Glucosamine sulfate	Take 500 mg three times daily.	Promotes cartilage repair and regeneration
Chondroitin	Chondroitin 400 mg three times daily	A building block for cartilage
Green-lipped mussel (a rich source of glycosaminoglycans)	Green-lipped mussel as directed	Helps repair cartilage
Boswellia	Standardized dose of 400 mg three times daily	Anti-inflammatory as effective as NSAIDs
Multimineral supplement	Choose a multimineral supplement containing trace minerals and follow directions on bottle.	Supports muscle, cartilage, and bone development, and helps regulate some hormones

NUTRIENT	DOSAGE	ACTION
Vitamin A	5000 IU daily	Helps control IL-1
Vitamins B_3, B_5, B_6, and folic acid	Choose a high-potency B-complex and follow directions.	Reduces the effects of stress, and increases blood flow
Vitamin B_{12}	Sublingual B_{12}, 500 mcg daily	Improves digestion and supports nerves
Vitamin D	200 IU daily	Helps absorb calcium
Vitamin C	1000 mg daily	Helps synthesize collagen, the glue-like substance in cartilage; reduces pain
Vitamin E	400–800 IU daily with mixed tocopherols	Mobilizes the joints
MSM	1–2 g daily	Anti-inflammatory
Evening primrose oil	500–2000 mg	Relieves pain and inflammation
Feverfew	Standardized to 0.6 percent parthenolides	Suppresses prostaglandin production, eases pain and inflammation
Devil's claw	1–2 g of standardized devil's claw should be taken daily.	Anti-inflammatory
Turmeric	Three 400 mg doses daily	Anti-inflammatory
Willow bark	Standardized willow bark is available and dosages range from 200–1000 mg	Reduces pain and inflammation
SAM-e (S-adenosylmethionine)	200 mg twice daily	A sulfur compound that reduces pain and inflammation, and promotes proteoglycan production
DHEA	Have your doctor give you a DHEAS test to see if you are deficient. 5–10 mg of DHEA daily or (in Canada) take Moducare to naturally enhance DHEA.	Reduces IL-6, normalizes cortisol, and stops inflammatory processes
Wobenzym or Bromelaine	Wobenzym: use as directed. Bromelain: take 2000 to 6000 mcu (1200 to 4000 gdu) on an empty stomach. Do not take if you are allergic to pineapple.	Contains sulfur and proteolytic enzymes, anti-inflammatory, improves joint mobility and reduces swelling

Health Tips to Enhance Healing

- Drink eight to ten glasses of pure, clean water every day to prevent your joint cushions from becoming dehydrated. For every juice or caffeinated beverage that you consume, you must have another glass of water.
- Stress reduction is key, especially in rheumatoid arthritis (see Chapter 6 on stress and autoimmune flare-ups).
- Avoid these substances to prevent flare-ups: citrus fruit, milk, red meat, sugar products, salt, paprika and cayenne pepper, tobacco, and any member of the nightshade family (potatoes, eggplant, tomatoes, peppers, etc.).
- Focus your diet on sterol- and sterolin-rich natural, whole foods: fresh fruit, vegetables, legumes, eggs, whole grains, healthy fats

and oils, seafood, and fresh fish (see chart, page 78). They are the key to halting inflammation at the source. Eat foods with a high sulfur content, including garlic, onions, and asparagus, which will help remove metals from the body.

- Non-weight-bearing exercise like water aerobics, swimming, stationary cycling, and yoga should be performed. Be careful not to overburden joints or cause pain and inflammation.
- Lose weight—even an extra 10 lb (4.5 kg) can cause an additional 40 lb (18 kg) of pressure on arthritic knee and ankle joints.

Other Recommendations

- Use hot or cold compresses on the area to alleviate pain and inflammation. Take hot baths or saunas to keep the joints warm.
- Rule out hydrochloric acid deficiency (see page 159 for more information).
- Topical ointments may help. Look for products that contain capsaicin, dimethylsulfoxide (DMSO), or quaternary amines. Look for capsaicin creams containing 0.025–0.075 percent capsaicin (avoid contact with eyes).
- See "Allergy Detection and Elimination" in this chapter.
- Beware of taking non-steroidal anti-inflammatory drugs (NSAIDs), Celebrex, and acetaminophen (see Chapter 1, "No NSAIDs," page 13).

Health Fact

If you are taking methotrexate you must supplement with B vitamins and folic acid as the drug reduces these nutrients, promoting nausea and diarrhea. Anemia develops if this is not addressed.

ASTHMA

According to the American Lung Association, an estimated 16 million Americans are affected by asthma, a chronic lung condition characterized by inflammation of the airways. Among chronic illnesses in children, asthma is the most common, affecting twice as many boys as girls. Asthma severity may range from mild to life threatening, and over 6000 people in North America die annually from the disease.

Symptoms

Asthma is characterized by increased respiratory distress of the bronchi, which narrow and inflame the airway. Attacks begin with an excessive production of mucous, coughing, difficulty breathing, and wheezing. The narrowed airway makes it extremely difficult for air to move in and out of the lungs. Recurring asthma attacks promote an abnormal thickening and hardening of air passages. Our immune system also responds by secreting dangerous immune factors, namely interleukin-6, which eventually destroy delicate tissues lining our airways. Between asthma attacks, an asthmatic will generally seem healthy.

Causes

Allergic reactions to foods or environmental triggers are present in over 50 percent of asthmatics. Heredity, allergens, nutritional deficiencies, and an increase in the use of antibiotics in infants all contribute to the development of asthma. Car exhaust, petrochemicals, cigarette smoke, animal dander, molds, dust mites, flower and tree pollens, and rising levels of air pollution are at the top of the environmental list of asthma triggers. The most common food allergies for asthmatics are wheat, milk, eggs, tomatoes, and the sulfites found in beer and wine.

Antibiotic/Asthma Connection: Three or more courses of antibiotics in the first year of life are associated with a fourfold increase in the risk of asthma. Researchers at the University of Antwerp, Belgium, have found a link between the use of antibiotics in the first year of life and an increased risk of later developing asthma and allergic disorders in children who have a family history of allergy. Immunologists think that the proper development of our immune system and protection from allergies may be related to early exposure to certain natural infections, like colds and flu (see Health Facts on page 167 for further information).

What Triggers Asthma? Most asthmatics have an allergy to some offending agent. This allergy then acts as the trigger that starts the inflammatory, lung-damaging asthma process to begin. It is easy to diagnose an allergy that presents itself quickly and clearly in the form of a runny nose and itchy eyes as a result of exposure to a particular agent such as cats or peanuts. It is much more difficult to discover the trigger for an allergy that has vague symptoms or takes hours to display its effects (called delayed-onset allergy). (See Allergies for more information.)

Several studies have looked at airborne allergen exposure during infancy in relation to asthma. It is very interesting that children raised in areas of low altitude have significantly higher rates of asthma. Moreover, children born during the high-pollen months have a higher incidence of asthma and allergic rhinitis compared to those born during non-pollen-production months. If you have a strong history of allergy or asthma, choosing low-pollen months for the birth of your baby may be an important factor in protecting your child from future allergies.

Dairy allergy in children can cause ear infections that are unsuccessfully treated with repeated antibiotic therapy. Antibiotics create gut problems that eventually lead to leaky gut syndrome, whereby undigested food particles enter the bloodstream through damaged areas of the gut, causing allergic reactions. Antibiotics are also associated with causing *Candida albicans*, yeast overgrowth that further exacerbates allergic symptoms. It becomes a vicious cycle of allergy, leaky gut problems, ear infections, antibiotics, and candida overgrowth with the cycle repeating over and over again.

Babies born to parents with food allergies should be breast-fed for as long as possible. If there is a family history of dairy or wheat allergy, a breast-feeding mom should avoid eating the allergy-causing foods to ensure that the baby does not react to the antigens in breast milk. Chronic ear infections in young children are a good indicator of dairy allergy. Eliminate all dairy products and test for other allergies and see if ear infection rates decline.

Exercise-Induced Asthma: Some asthma attacks are triggered by exercise. Excessive coughing during exercise is an early warning sign that you may have asthma. Exercise should not be eliminated entirely, but milder forms of exercise should be adopted, such as walking during pollen-reduced days. Breathe through the nose instead of the mouth, and take extra vitamin C before physical activity.

Prescription for Health

Note: If you are currently taking medication (including inhalers), do not stop treatment. Once you start taking the nutrients below and adopting the protective measures, your symptoms will appear less often and with less intensity, requiring less medication.

NUTRIENT	DOSAGE	ACTION
Moducare sterols and sterolins	Two capsules three times daily for one week; one capsule three times daily thereafter. Children: Birth to five years, one capsule per day; five to 12 years, two capsules per day; 12 and over, the adult dose.	Decreases inflammation, controls secretion of IL-4 and IL-6 both associated with the onset and severity of asthma. Regulates cortisol.
RespirActin	56 g (2 oz) twice daily	Works as a natural antihistamine
Vitamin B$_6$ (taken in the form of P-5-P with a B-complex)	50 mg daily	Repairs mucous membranes damaged by allergy, reduces allergic reactions

NUTRIENT	DOSAGE	ACTION
Vitamin B_{12}	500 mcg orally twice daily or 1000 mcg injection with folic acid, one weekly for four weeks	Reduces or stops wheezing
Vitamin C	1000 mg twice daily	Reduces severity and occurrence of allergy attacks, protects against exercise-induced asthma
Lycopene	30 mg daily	Protects against exercise-induced asthma, is an antioxidant
Quercetin	500–1000 mg two to three times daily (children five and up: half the dosage)	Works as an antihistamine, antiallergenic, and antioxidant; is especially effective for those sensitive to airborne allergens
Magnesium	500 mg three times daily Children five and up: 100 mg twice daily	Stops attacks, acts as a bronchodilator and antihistamine; also required to replace magnesium, which is depleted during an attack
Omega-3 fatty acids	1–2 Tbsp (15–30 mL) of flaxseed oil or fish oil (Eskimo-3)	Reduces inflammation, protects mucous membranes
Lactobacillus acidophilus	1 tsp (5 mL) daily	Improves intestinal flora; reduces allergic reactions
Ginkgo biloba	120–140 mg standardized extract daily (children five and up: 30–60 mg)	Reduces wheezing, coughing, shortness of breath, and frequency of attacks
Multimune containing vitamins A, B_6, C, E, selenium, zinc, magnesium, reduced L-glutathione, lipoic acid, and coenzyme Q10	Three capsules daily	Supports immune function, is an antihistamine, prevents free radical damage, eliminates toxins, and reduces chemical sensitivities
Ma huang	Follow directions carefully (unless standardized for 10 percent alkaloids, then 125–250 mg three times daily is sufficient). *Caution:* Not safe for children.	Opens the air passages; use for emergencies only and do not take more than the recommended dose

Health Tips to Enhance Healing

- See "Allergy Detection and Elimination" in this chapter.
- Drink eight to ten glasses of pure, clean, filtered water every day because it controls histamine production (see Chapter 4).
- Stop smoking. See Allergies for more information on secondhand smoke and asthma in children.

Other Recommendations

- Stay fit and lose those extra pounds. Carrying extra weight, especially on the upper torso, can decrease lung capacity and make it more difficult to breathe.
- Ninety percent of asthmatics breathe through the mouth (versus breathing from the nose, which is the normal breathing pattern), making it easier for pollution, organisms, and cold air to get into the lungs. Those with asthma are often poor at exhaling the air from their lungs completely. Practice taking deep breaths in through your nose and then slowly expel all the air out through your mouth. Do this exercise five times and repeat several times throughout the day.
- In North America, double-glazed windows, central heating, and energy-efficient homes result in an overabundance of dust mites and molds, which exacerbate allergic asthma. Fresh air is essential and an attempt to have an allergen-free home can help reduce asthma attacks. See Allergies for additional tips.
- When using herbal remedies, keep in mind that the herbs may belong to the same plant family as your allergens.
- Inhalers are intended for emergency use only and do not prevent asthma. If an asthmatic is using two inhalers per month, they are at a higher risk for a lethal asthma attack. Misuse of inhalers is a serious concern. As inhaler use increases so must the dosage as the body becomes tolerant over time. Excessive reliance on inhalers increases the risk for heart problems, including high blood pressure and stroke.

Health Facts

Research Confirms RespirActin's Action: Leigh Broadhurst, Ph.D., has used a traditional liquid herbal blend called RespirActin to successfully treat allergies and asthma. It contains rosemary, honey, witch hazel, fenugreek seed, black seed, king solomon seed, ginseng powder, damiana leaves, marshmallow, sage, juniper berries, chamomile flowers, cloves, cinnamon, spearmint, and thyme. These herbs have antioxidant, expectorant, anti-asthmatic, antiallergenic, antihistamine, and bronchial-dilating effects.

The *Medical Chronicle* (October 2000) reported that Canadian researcher George Luciuk, MD, a certified allergist and clinical immunologist, completed a double-blind, crossover clinical trial of RespirActin in 11 adult asthma patients, confirming Dr. Broadhurst's reports. The study showed that patients with more symptomatic asthma had significant improvement within a few days to two weeks in lung-function markers and quality of life assessments. Some patients had a significant beneficial bronchodilating effect with their first dose. The benefits appear to be beneficial over time. Most importantly,

RespirActin has the ability to reverse small airway obstruction, which until now was deemed almost irreversible, especially with standard metered-dose, inhaler-delivered medication. Researchers believe that the oral administration of RespirActin allows better perfusion and delivery to small airways in the lung that have been hard, if not impossible, to reach adequately. Reversing this area of obstruction can make a big difference to how asthmatic patients feel. Many asthmatics have become so used to having reduced lung capacity that when it is restored they are shocked at how much better they feel. With this research in mind, it is also thought that RespirActin may enhance lung function in athletes and racehorses to achieve a competitive edge. It definitely benefits those suffering from exercise-induced asthma.

Researchers in this study believe that RespirActin works by reducing the production of potent chemical mediators called arachidonic acid (AA). Arachidonic acid is released from cell membranes and converted to either prostaglandins or thromboxane by the enzyme cyclooxygenase or into the leukotrienes by 5-lipoxygenase. RespirActin's active botanicals block the components of both of these pathways and as a result:

- control mucous gland hypersecretion in the airways, reducing bronchial tube plugging and nasal congestion
- reduce bronchial smooth muscle contraction, opening narrow airways and improving breathing
- halt inflammation; researchers stated that "RespirActin has 5-lipoxygenase activity preventing the inflammatory cascade thereby reducing destruction of airways."
- reduce asthma-induced coughing by 34 percent

RespirActin combined with Moducare should be the basis for your asthma treatment program (2 oz/60 g twice per day for four to six days, then reduce to 1 oz/30 g twice per day). RespirActin is safe for children as young as six months. Infants six months to two years should take 1½ tsp (7 mL) morning and evening. Children aged two to ten should take 1 Tbsp (15 mL) morning and evening.

Stomach Flu May Stop Asthma

Paolo Matricardi stated in *The British Medical Journal* that stomach infections early in childhood may help people avoid respiratory allergies and asthma later in life. Researchers believe that food-borne bacterial infections in childhood may help the immune system build up a resistance to allergies.

Many scientists believe that environmental poisons and pollution are only partly responsible for the increase in asthma. Matricardi and his research team showed that 1659 air force cadets who had stomach flu early in life and exposure to food-borne bacteria and the common stomach bacteria *Helicobacter pylori* were less likely to suffer asthma and upper respiratory infections.

Our fear of bacteria and obsession with cleanliness has gone overboard. Matricardi stated that "we must improve hygiene to reduce the impact of infectious diseases but at the same time, we must learn how to safely train our immune system, especially during infancy, in order to prevent allergy." We must realize that childhood illnesses are the training ground for our immune systems. In order for the immune system to develop properly, a few illnesses in early childhood may be a good thing.

BOWEL DISEASE

The American College of Gastroenterology says that over 50 million Americans are suffering with irritable bowel syndrome (IBS). The International Foundation for Bowel Dysfunction says that IBS is second only to the common cold as a cause of absenteeism from work. Over 1.1 million North Americans suffer from inflammatory bowel disease (IBD), and it is thought that Canada has one of the highest rates of IBD in the world.

Irritable Bowel Syndrome (IBS)

Irritable bowel syndrome, also called spastic colon, is when the large intestine spasms and prevents the passage of waste (constipation) or moves it along too quickly (diarrhea). Women are twice as likely as men to have IBS. IBS is often confused with colitis or Crohn's disease, which are inflammatory bowel diseases (IBD), but IBS does not have the inflammation associated with IBD, nor is it as serious. IBS is an annoying disorder, but it is not a disease requiring surgery or strong medication.

Inflammatory Bowel Disease (IBD)

Symptoms of IBD include inflammation of the bowel, which causes anemia, fever, and weight loss. It occurs in men and women equally, and tends to strike between the ages of 16 and 40. Three thousand cases of Crohn's disease are diagnosed every year in North America. In people with IBD, the immune system is unable to down-regulate the inflammation and the Th-1 response is allowed to carry on. The inflammation injures the epithelium, resulting in gastric distress (among other symptoms) and damage to the tissues.

Colitis, also called ulcerative colitis, is an inflammation of the colon, causing a continuous need to eliminate (diarrhea), which can be mild to severe.

Symptoms

Although each bowel disease is different, the symptoms are so similar that a proper diagnosis can be difficult, especially as the symptoms are not unusual and we have all experienced them at some time. However, if you

Sterols, Sterolins, and Gut Health

By Patrick J.D. Bouic, Ph.D.

Many inflammatory diseases of the gastrointestinal (GI) tract involve the cells of the immune system and an immunological response to an offending agent. The diseases may be grouped as follows:

- *"Allergic" in nature:* such as celiac disease or gluten allergy (also called gluten-induced enteropathy)
- *"Inflammatory" in nature:* such as inflammatory bowel disease (IBD) which includes ulcerative colitis or Crohn's disease
- *"Autoimmune" in nature:* such as pernicious anemia (where vitamin B_{12} uptake is inhibited due to the presence of an antibody)

Irrespective of whether the disease is purely inflammatory in nature or has an underlying autoimmune component, the end result is damage to the mucosal lining of the GI tract, and a state of chronic inflammation. Certain bacteria or viruses may cause the initial onslaught but once the immune response has been set in motion, it becomes a self-perpetuating cycle of inflammation, tissue damage, more inflammation and so on. It is therefore imperative to break the cycle by avoiding certain foods and by using supplements that stop the inflammation.

Research using sterols and sterolins has shown that these important molecules have potent immune-modulating properties. This means that they can intervene at the level of the immune cells, getting these cells under control, either by switching off the secretion of factors which promote inflammation, or by switching on other factors which control the release of "bad" factors. It has been shown that sterols and sterolins are able to stop the release of inflammatory factors such as Interleukin-6 and TNF-alpha, both of which are involved in the tissue damage to the mucosal membrane of the gut. Also, sterols and sterolins are able to enhance the activity of the Th-1, T-helper cells, cells that control autoimmune processes. These same cells are also underactive in cases of allergies (including gut allergies): due to this underactivity, the cells, which release allergic factors, go uncontrolled.

Although clinical studies have not been conducted using sterols and sterolins, based on the above science it is foreseeable that taking sterols and sterolins in cases of IBD or celiac disease, or even pernicious anemia, will result in controlling the immune onslaught taking place on the mucosal surface. Sterols and sterolins will decrease the release of the inflammatory factors, get the good T-cells to secrete the good factors, and induce a state of balance in the immune response. By so doing, it will allow repair mechanisms to kick in and recovery from such chronic conditions to take place.

have a regular history of heartburn, nausea, diarrhea, gas, bloating, belching, abdominal cramps, constipation, or bowel movements that are in ribbons or small balls, these problems should be addressed to prevent more serious damage. Consult your physician immediately if you have rectal bleeding, fever, sharp abdominal pain, or intestinal obstruction.

Causes

The exacerbation of bowel diseases and disorders is inextricably linked to fried, greasy foods, a low-fiber diet, a diet too high in processed foods, and overeating. When we treat our stomach like a garburator by eating junk foods and not chewing our food properly, the small and large intestines suffer the consequences. Stress aggravates the situation. In IBS, the cause is unknown, but depression, stress, and food allergies are the main triggers. See Chapter 1 to learn more about ways to heal gut problems.

Irritable bowel disease is promoted by our immune system. New evidence has found that the inflammatory factors secreted by the immune system (IL-1, IL-6, and IL-8) are associated with damage to the intestinal wall and increased inflammation in bowel disease. At this time it appears that increased IL-6 is associated with Crohn's disease, while higher levels of IL-8 is more characteristic of colitis. In the case of Crohn's disease, a researcher at St. George's Medical School near London declared that it is caused by a mycobacterium infection from drinking contaminated milk (see Chapter 1, page 7, for more information).

Prescription for Health

NUTRIENT	DOSAGE	ACTION
Moducare sterols and sterolins	Two capsules three times daily for one week, one capsule three times daily thereafter	See research on page 170; also supports immune function and controls inflammation in the gut
Vitamin B-complex	Use as directed	Supports digestion, and neuronal activity as well as being important for repair mechanisms.
Folic acid	1–5 mg per day until diarrhea subsides	Stops chronic diarrhea. Not to be taken in doses higher than 400 mcg by those with epilepsy
Vitamin D$_3$	400 IU per day	Restores deficiencies that could lead to bone disease
Vitamin C with quercetin	1000 mg vitamin C and 500 mg quercitin	Prevents inflammation and boosts immunity
Omega's Hi-Lignan Nutri-Flax	1–3 tsp (5–15 mL) daily with plenty of water	Increased fiber controls diarrhea, corrects constipation, and soothes intestinal lining.
Calcium and magnesium	1000 mg calcium, 500 mg magnesium	Restores possible deficiencies and helps to prevent colon cancer
Plant digestive enzymes with food	Two capsules with meals	Aids proper digestion
Iron	10 mg daily	Use only if diagnosed with anemia

NUTRIENT	DOSAGE	ACTION
Lactobacillus and *Bifidus acidophilus*	1 tsp (5 mL) daily	Improves intestinal flora, reduces diarrhea, irritable bowel, diverticulosis, and constipation
Multimune containing vitamins A, B_6, C, E, selenium, zinc, magnesium, lipoic acid, coenzyme Q10, reduced L-glutathione	Three capsules daily	Supports immune function, controls allergic reactions, is an anti-inflammatory
L-glutamine	1000 mg daily	Supports health of villi, the surfaces that facilitate absorption in the intestine
Omega-3 fatty acid	1–3 Tbsp of flax oil daily	Reduces inflammation; EPA is thought to suppress the leukotriene responsible for signaling inflammation in the mucosal membrane
Evening primrose oil	500 mg twice daily	Reduces inflammation by inhibiting inflammatory mediators; prevents zinc deficiency
Colostrum	1 tsp (5 mL) daily	Contains lactoferrin and enhances immunoglobulins in the gut
Peppermint oil enteric-coated capsules	Three to six capsules daily	Reduces cramps, relieves gas, and increases bile; used mostly in IBS

Health Tips to Enhance Healing

- Eliminate allergens.
- See Chapter 1 tips for heartburn.
- Eliminate refined carbohydrates, as they promote diarrhea.
- Aid digestion by taking digestive plant enzymes with every meal. If gas, bloating, and bowel movements don't improve, you may not be producing enough stomach acid to break down your food properly. Hydrochloric acid supplements with meals may alleviate this condition.
- Don't dilute your stomach acid or enzymes by drinking during your meal.
- Eat seven to ten half-cup servings of organic fruits and vegetables every day. If you don't eat raw vegetables regularly, start by steaming your vegetables and don't forget the digestive enzymes. Cut out the white pasta, white rice, and white flour and opt for natural whole grains instead.
- Eat one half cup of plain yogurt with active cultures every day unless you are lactose intolerant. Lactose intolerance is a common cause of bowel problems. Stop all dairy products for six weeks and see if your gut distress is relieved. Soy and rice milk make great alternatives and they come in many flavors.

- Drink eight to ten glasses of pure filtered water a day, but do not drink during meals or else you will dilute your digestive enzymes. For every cup of a caffeinated beverage that you drink, add another cup of water.
- To spark your digestive juices, add fresh-squeezed lemon juice to a cup of herbal tea 15 minutes before your meal. Coffee aggravates the gut, so switch to herbal tea, or try green tea, which has a third of coffee's caffeine and is rich with antioxidants. Effective herbs to soothe your tummy include ginger, peppermint, and fennel. Take them alone or in combination. If bile production is underactive, try the bitter herbs such as dandelion, plantain, yarrow, wormwood, or gentian.
- Big meals are hard to digest, so try eating small meals throughout the day. Not only will it help heal stomach problems, it will keep your blood sugar in a healthy range. Sit, relax, and enjoy your food—remember, digestion begins in your mouth.

Other Recommendations

- See Constipation and Leaky Gut.
- Do whatever it takes to reduce your stress levels. Meditation, yoga, breathing exercises, and/or a walk in the park can help reduce the intestinal effects of stress.
- Using non-steroidal anti-inflammatory drugs (NSAIDs) increases your risk of upper gastrointestinal ulcer, bleeding, and digestive difficulties. There are many safe alternatives to NSAIDs. *Nature's Pain Killers* by William Cabot, MD, and Carl Germano, RD, recommends willow bark, boswellia, turmeric, and Pycnogenol®.
- Avoid diet drinks because they usually contain aspartame, a substance containing known toxins. Sorbitol, sucralose, and other artificial sweeteners can create gas, bloating, and increased diarrhea. White sugar depresses immunity. Try using the herbal sweetener stevia instead. It comes in liquid drops and tablet and powder form.
- Exercise regularly. Yoga or tai chi are great for improving circulation, reducing tension, and promoting healthy digestion and elimination. Stretching exercises in which you must touch your toes or draw your knees up to your chest are also good to get the bowels moving.
- A chiropractor may be able to provide some relief if there is a misalignment in your spine.
- An acupuncturist may be able to provide relief to reduce need for surgery.

Health Fact

Sherry Rogers, MD, in her book *No More Heartburn*, says that 90 percent of gut problems can be alleviated with simple dietary changes, the elimination of allergy-causing foods and *Candida albicans*, stress reduction, and immune enhancement.

BRONCHITIS

Bronchitis occurs when the main air passages of the lungs, the bronchi, become inflamed.

Acute bronchitis is most often a result of viral infection and occasionally bacterial chlamydia infection in the lower respiratory tract. If the condition is not addressed, the inflamed bronchi provide a cozy habitat for secondary bacterial infections such as pneumonia. Chronic bronchitis is largely a result of smoking or other airborne agents, such as chemicals or fumes. Smokers are especially prone to chronic obstructive pulmonary disease and emphysema.

Symptoms

A bout of acute bronchitis begins with a runny nose, sore throat, an irritating cough, and eventually produces green or yellow mucous. Fever and chills follow, then a shortness of breath and fatigue. The chest feels heavy or is in pain. The coughing is the most noticeable factor of bronchitis at its peak; the coughs produce mucous and are deep, painful, and hoarse sounding and can come in such quick succession that a bout of coughing can go uninterrupted for a few minutes, making it very difficult to breathe. There is also wheezing and shortness of breath, especially after coughing. Even after the worst of the illness is over, coughing may continue for many weeks.

Causes

Acute bronchitis occurs when respiratory viral infections such as the rhinovirus (common cold) flourish in the respiratory tract and attack the bronchi. Less commonly, bacteria *Chlamydia pneumoniae* and *Mycoplasma pneumoniae* are responsible for bronchitis. Chemicals, fumes, or asthma can injure and inflame the bronchial wall causing bronchitis.

Smoking brings on 80–90 percent of all chronic bronchitis cases. Other airborne irritants, such as pollution and allergies, can also trigger chronic bronchitis. A previous infection of acute bronchitis sensitizes the bronchi to any airborne irritant and if caution is not taken to reduce this type of exposure, repeat infections can occur, leading to chronic bronchitis.

Prescription for Health

NUTRIENT	DOSAGE	ACTION
Vitamin A (Micel A)	100,000 IU or one full dropper daily until symptoms abate. Then take 5,000 IU daily for maintenance	Fights infection and heals mucous membranes
Vitamin C with bioflavonoids	1000 mg vitamin C with 500 mg bioflavonoids three times daily	Fights infection and strengthens collagen along the bronchi; reduces histamine
Vitamin E	400 IU daily	Heals tissues and acts as an antioxidant
Women's Whey or proteins+ protein powder	One or two scoops daily	Provides amino acids for repair mechanisms in the body
Reduced L-glutathione	45 mg daily	Is lung tissue specific and repairs airway damage; improves immune function
N-acetylcysteine (NAC)	250 mg three to four times daily	Thins out the mucous, making it easier for expulsion
Echinacea and goldenseal tincture	20 drops in a glass of water taken three times daily	At the first sign of a cold, it may stop the cold from developing into bronchitis. Goldenseal soothes mucous membranes and acts as an antibiotic against chlamydia.
Reishi, shiitake or maitake, cordyceps mushroom extract	600 mg twice daily	Strengthens immunity and acts as an antiviral
Cherry bark	Use as directed	Eases cough
Astragalus	200 mg three times daily	Enhances immune function, source of selenium
Moducare sterols and sterolins	Two capsules three times daily until symptoms abate, then one capsule three times daily for maintenance	Increases T-cell activity to fight infection and reduces inflammation in the bronchial tubes
Pycnogenol or grape seed extract	500 mg three times daily	Is a powerful antioxidant and removes toxins
Multimune containing vitamins A, B$_6$, C, E, selenium, zinc, magnesium, reduced L-glutathione, coenzyme Q10, lipoic acid	Three capsules daily	Supports immune function

Health Tips to Enhance Healing

- Stop smoking—*now*. If you don't smoke but are exposed to secondhand smoke, remove yourself from the situation or ask people to butt out. Secondhand smoke has 4000 chemicals in it, including known carcinogens. Smoke that wafts from the lit end does not go through a filter and is more poisonous than what is inhaled by the smoker. Children raised in smoking environments are more prone to lung disorders such as bronchitis.

- Avoid sugar and dairy products—even fruit—as their natural sugar content is high. Sugar depresses the immune system and dairy products promote the formation of mucous.
- The important thing to remember about bronchitis is that you want to expel the mucous that is sitting in the bronchial tree. Do not take commercial decongestants or antihistamines because they dry up the mucous lining, making it more difficult and painful to expel. To facilitate the drainage process, Michael Murray, MD, suggests applying a hot water bottle, heating pad, or mustard poultice to the chest for twenty minutes. Remove the hot pack and lean over the bed so that the forearms support the whole torso. Stay in this position for five to 10 minutes, coughing up phlegm into a wastebasket or onto a newspaper on the floor.
- Use Weleda Husten Elixier as an effective expectorant cough syrup.
- Get outside and enjoy the fresh air. Too much time is spent at the office indoors, inside the car, and in the home. Trapped air is stale and loaded with airborne germs.
- Practice deep-breathing exercises to improve oxygen intake.
- Maintaining a regular exercise program when you are not suffering from bronchitis will encourage deep breathing and circulate oxygen.
- Get plenty of rest. Too much stress and not enough sleep or relaxation takes its toll on the immune system, making it easier for infections to occur.
- Drink 8 to 10 glasses of pure, filtered water every day. For every juice or beverage with caffeine you consume, have another glass of water.

    Caution: Do not take antibiotics if you have a virally induced bronchitis. Antibiotics only work on bacterial infections (such as pneumonia) and will destroy the good infection-fighting bacteria in your intestinal tract.

Other Recommendations

- See Allergies. If you have recurring bronchitis it may be due to allergies.

CANCER

Within the scope of this book I can provide you with only a fraction of what is possible in the prevention and treatment of cancer. It is heartening to note that unlike decades past, there are more natural options available to replace or complement the methods of chemotherapy, radiation, and surgery. I highly recommend one of my favorite reference books, *Definitive Guide to Cancer*, published by Burton Goldberg.

Cancer is the second leading cause of death in the United States, exceeded only by heart disease. The five states with the highest rates of cancer are (in descending order) District of Columbia, Rhode Island, Florida, Pennsylvania, and Massachusetts. In Canada, the five provinces with the highest rates are Ontario, Quebec, British Columbia, Alberta, and Manitoba. It is expected that over 550,000 Americans and 65,000 Canadians will die of cancer this year.

Normal, healthy cells go through a series of steps to ensure life. They grow, divide, and create new cells in a carefully performed, predetermined symphony. During this highly complex reproductive process, the cell's genetic code or DNA is duplicated and transferred to new cells. Normally this process takes place without error but every once in a while, approximately one in 1000 divisions, a mistake may occur. Most mistakes are quickly repaired but on occasion a mistake may miss detection and cells will be allowed to perform differently than they were intended.

Normal cell conduct organizes cells into their correct location, turns growth off and on as required, and ensures that cells do not crowd each other. Due to this set of rules, normal cells do not travel to incorrect areas of the body and they do not form abnormal structures such as tumors. Cancerous cells, on the other hand, do not follow any hard and fast rules. They mutate as often as possible to avoid detection and survive at all cost even if they kill their host.

Cancer begins from normal cells that become renegade. These abnormal cells turn the immune system against itself, multiply unchecked, steal nutrients, and reroute blood supplies away from normal body functions. Because these turncoat cells are similar to other healthy cells, often the immune system fails to detect and kill them. Or if the body's defense system is not functioning optimally it can also miss these marauding cells.

The assumption that governs conventional approach to cancer is to cut, burn, or poison the tumor. This has been the basis of cancer treatment for 60 years, and yet in less than 100 years the death rate has increased by 800 percent. Stephen Langer, MD, wrote in his book *Pocket Guide to Natural Health* that the incidence rate for cancer was one in five when he began to practice medicine. Today it is one in three. The alternative approach to cancer treatment is to look at the patient as a whole and view the illness as systemic.

There are five classes of cancer: carcinoma, sarcoma, leukemia, lymphoma, and myeloma. Carcinomas are the solid tumors that are found on organs, mucous membranes, glands, and skin. Sarcomas are solid tumors, but they form in the bone, connective tissue, and muscles. Leukemias are cancers in the blood. Lymphomas are found in the lymphatic system. Myelomas affect the plasma cells in tissues and bone where antibodies are produced.

People can have two types of tumors, benign and malignant. Benign tumors are generally harmless and they are surrounded by fiber protecting other body structures from invasion. Malignant tumors are cancerous and are often not encapsulated, so they are free to spread. Localized cancers are cancers that remain in the area from where they evolved. If the cancer cells move to other areas of the body, the cancer is described as metastasized.

Over the last decade much discussion has focused on antioxidants and whether they are appropriate for supplementation during chemotherapy. Conventional medicine feels that antioxidants would interfere with types of chemotherapy that are believed to utilize oxidative damage as part of their anticancer action. There are many studies that attest to the contrary. Varying trials with rats and humans as subjects suggest that antioxidants do not compromise the efficacy of chemotherapy, but either enhance its action, reduce the toxic side effects, or have no noticeable effect at all.

Symptoms

Cancer-related symptoms vary depending on where the cancer is in the body. The signs that you should look for are changes in moles or warts (especially if they bleed or grow), a lump or dense feeling in the breast or testicles (or any noticeable change such as swelling, soreness, itchiness), unusual bleeding or discharge, and chronic fatigue. Other signs are sores that won't heal, a persistent sore throat or cough (or coughing up blood), changes in urination and bowel habits (pain, bleeding, color, other difficulties), weight loss and changes in appetite and digestion (or difficulty swallowing).

Causes

Poor diet, environmental toxins, lack of antioxidants, viruses, chronic stress, and feelings of hopelessness are some of the possible reasons why the body allows cancers to grow.

Viruses are known factors in your risk of certain cancers. *Helicobacter pylori* is now thought to be a causative agent for stomach cancer; human T-cell lymphoma virus is responsible for T-cell lymphoma; human papilloma viruses are involved in cervical cancer and the hepatitis virus is linked to liver cancer. A healthy immune system will deal with viruses in a vicious way. Yet the viruses mentioned above are able to circumvent the body's defenses and cause serious cancers to develop.

Although genetics or a family history is a predisposition to acquiring cancer, it can be factored out if super nutrition is adopted. Regardless of your genetic makeup, if you keep your toxic load under control and boost your immunity, cancer can be avoided.

It is also believed that due to environmental and nutritional factors, natural killer cell function is depressed, resulting in an inability of the immune system to recognize cancerous cells. Without a method of recognizing cancer cells as foreign, the immune system cannot deal with them.

Cancer can develop in any tissue of the body and it is thought that a cell's

DNA may become damaged by any one of the following: radiation exposure, ultraviolet damage from the sun, free radicals, chemical toxins, viruses, hormones, tobacco, and alcohol. Each one of these potential DNA-damaging substances can be neutralized with specific nutritional treatments.

Cancer is a complicated disease. Each type of cancer has different traits. Some are slow growing and easy to treat, while others are aggressive and require a much more diverse treatment approach. Treatments that work for one cancer may not have any effect on another. Similarly, each person has unique biochemistry and this must be factored in when treating a patient. Several different treatments combined with a wide range of immune nutrients should be adopted.

The *Definitive Guide to Cancer* lists 33 factors that can trigger cancer or promote cancer once it has begun to replicate. An abbreviated version of that list includes environmental pollution, radiation, toxic metals, chemicals in products, tobacco and smoking, immunosuppressive drugs and hormonal therapies, nutritional deficiencies/poor diet, pathogens, viruses, emotions, weakened immune system (poor nutrient absorption, detoxification, and infection-fighting abilities), and heredity.

Blood Test for Breast Cancer

According to the American Cancer Society's 1999 Surveillance Research, breast cancer is the second most common cancer among women (after skin cancers) and accounts for nearly one of every three cancers diagnosed in American women. In 1999, it was estimated that approximately 175,000 new cases of invasive breast cancer were diagnosed in the United States, along with an estimated 40,000 additional cases of *in situ* breast cancer. More than 91 percent of these cancers were diagnosed in women over 40 years of age. The American Cancer Society reported over 183,000 new cases of invasive breast cancer and over 40,000 deaths from the disease in 2000. Only lung cancer accounts for more cancer deaths in women.

One in eight women will be diagnosed with breast cancer in their lifetime. Currently mammography and breast self-examination are the only tools used to detect a breast mass or lump. When one is detected, a biopsy is done to rule out or confirm a diagnosis of breast cancer. Mammography has its limitations. It does not determine the risk of developing breast cancer, but detects lumps and masses that have already developed. In women under the age of 40, mammograms are difficult to interpret because of dense breast tissue, fibrocystic, or benign breast disease. According to the National Cancer Institute's web site (www.nci.nih.gov), a mammogram has a 15 percent rate of false negatives and even higher rate of false positives. When undergoing the procedure, women are exposed to radiation and each successive mammogram increases breast cancer risk. It is uncomfortable at best and many woman find it very painful.

Breast Cancer Surgery—Timing Is Everything

If you must have a lumpectomy, biopsy, or mastectomy, the timing of your operation may be a matter of life or death. A research study performed at the clinical oncology unit at Guy's Hospital in the U.K. found that the timing of operation and the menstrual cycle played a role in the recurrence and survival of premenopausal women with breast cancer. The records of 249 women treated between 1975 and 1985 were broken down into two groups. Group one had their surgery between three to twelve days after their last menstrual period. Group two had surgery between zero to two days or 13 to 32 days after the last menstrual period. At the 10-year mark, those women in the second group had a recurrence-free survival rate of 84 percent, whereas those in the first group had a 54 percent survival. The effect was independent of other factors, including node status and both estrogen receptor positive and negative tumors. Researchers determined that the phase in the menstrual cycle at the time of the operation is very important for the long-term survival of women with breast cancer.

To address the need for an accurate method to identify those women at risk of developing breast cancer, a simple blood test called the Mammastatin Serum Assay™ (MSA) is now available. Mammastatin is a protein produced by normal healthy breast cells and has been shown to inhibit breast cancer cell growth. The test measures the amount of mammastatin present. Mammastatin levels are higher in healthy women as compared to breast cancer patients, and levels are low in many women considered to be at high risk or who have breast cancer according to established criteria.

The Mammastatin Serum Assay™ not only identifies woman with breast cancer but also identifies those at risk of developing breast cancer before it is detected by traditional means. This test will help reduce the emotional trauma associated with false positive mammograms and the resultant unnecessary biopsies.

Early detection is the key to survival. The percentage of patients who are alive five years after diagnosis is called the five years relative survival rate. Determining the "stage at diagnosis" is the process of finding how far the cancer has spread. This is very important because the treatment and the outlook for recovery clearly depend on the stage of the cancer. In general, the lower the number, the less the cancer has metastasized or spread. A higher number, such as Stage IV, means a very serious cancer. Women diagnosed at Stage I have a 98 percent chance of survival five years after diagnosis; an 88 percent chance at Stage IIA; a 76 percent chance at Stage IIB; a 56 percent chance at Stage IIIA; a 49 percent chance at Stage IIIB; and a 16 percent chance of survival at Stage IV. The blood test is able to detect breast cancer long before it is visible on a mammogram and it can also tell whether you are at low, moderate or high risk.

The Mammastatin Serum Assay™ has a 98 percent accuracy in determining that a woman does not have breast cancer and an 84 percent overall accuracy in determining that a woman has or is at high risk of breast cancer. Every woman should have the test annually from the age of 25 onwards. Young women are developing breast cancer at an alarming rate, but mammograms are normally not performed on women under the age of 40 and few young women are performing breast self-examinations. This type of diagnostic test can help women prevent cancer by understanding their true risk.

Ask your doctor about the Mammastatin Serum Assay™. For more information, contact Genesis Bioventures at 1-877-BIOLABS (246-5227) or go to the web site (www.breastbio.com).

Prescription for Health

When choosing your alternative or complementary cancer therapies, choose what you can afford, what you can do every day, and do not switch treatments every month. Stick to your protocol and do it until your cancer is in remission. Many people make the mistake of changing their supplement routine every month. Work with your alternative medical doctor. Contact the American College for Advancement in Medicine ACAM at 1-800-532-3688 or email at acam@acam.org for an alternative medical doctor near you or go to www.findahealthdoctor.com.

NUTRIENT	DOSAGE	ACTION
Vitamin A	10,000 IU daily	Boosts immunity and acts as an antioxidant
Vitamin B_6 (in the form of P-5-P with a B-complex)	50 mg daily	Protects against mutagenesis, carcinogens, and tumor initiation
Folic acid	1–10 mg daily; doses of 10 mg per day should only be taken upon recommendation by your physician. 1 mg per day for maintenance	Deficiency can promote cervical dysplasia and increase risk of cervical cancer.
Beta glucans (any one of), reishi, maitaki, cordyceps, shiitaki	600 mg twice daily	Enhances immune function, NK cells, gamma-interferon, and macrophage function
Vitamin C	1000 mg or to bowel tolerance daily	An anticancer nutrient, reduces pain associated with cancer, and inhibits free radicals
Vitamin E	400–800 IU daily	Acts as an antioxidant and protects against cancer
Zinc	30 mg daily	Supports cancer-killing T-cells
CoQ10	300–400 mg daily	Increases IgG antibody production and natural killer cell activity, and inhibits metastasis of tumors
Magnesium	500 mg daily	Supports overall immune function

NUTRIENT	DOSAGE	ACTION
Selenium	100 mcg daily	Prevents cancer and restores deficiencies
Lycopene	100 mg daily	Protects against cancer
Multimineral with trace minerals	Use as directed	Supports all body systems
Lactobacillus acidophilus	1 tsp (5 mL) daily or 1 cup (250 mL) of acidophilus-rich yogurt daily	An antibacterial, improves intestinal flora, and aids digestion
Omega-3 fatty acids	1–2 Tbsp (15–30 mL) of flaxseed oil daily	May delay onset of malignancy
Moducare sterols and sterolins	Two capsules three times daily until cancer abates	Increases NK cell activity, gamma-interferon, T-helper cells, cytotoxic T-cells, IL-2. Most importantly, it stops hair loss, nausea, and mouth sores from chemotherapy.
Carnivora (pressed juice of the venus fly trap plant)	Use as directed	Has antitumor activity, improves well-being
Pau d'Arco, tahebo	250 mg with meals	Shrinks tumors, reduces nausea and vomiting
Mistletoe (*Viscum album*) by Weleda	Iscador injections administered by physician	Increases NK cell activity, cytotoxicity, macrophage function, T-cells and the cytokines they secrete
PSP or PSK from *Coriolus versicolor*	1–2 g three times daily	Inhibits or reverses tumor growth, extends survival rates
Curcumin	750 mg daily	Reduces the lesions and pain of skin cancer, protects against the carcinogenic affects of cigarette smoke
Ginger	One capsule for nausea as needed	Controls nausea during chemotherapy
Panax ginseng	200 mg twice daily	Inhibits cell cancer growth
Milk thistle	175 mg three times daily (at least 80 percent standardized extract of silymarin)	Promotes healthy liver function
Green tea	Drink throughout the day	Acts as an antioxidant and anticarcinogen
Isoflavones	25–50 mg daily	Reduces excess estrogens
Astragulus	1–4 g daily	Reduces side effects of chemotherapy and radiation and enhances their effectiveness
Women's Whey or proteins+	One to two scoops daily	Ensures adequate protein for cell repair
Garlic	Two capsules of Kyolic daily and plenty of fresh garlic in foods	Boosts immunity, protects against carcinogens, blocks the formation of nitrosamines, reduces the risk of stomach and esophageal cancers.
Wobenzym	Three to five tablets daily	Is powerful enzyme to disable cancer cells

Health Tips to Enhance Healing

- Quit smoking. If you haven't started, don't. Every puff of smoke contains 4000 toxins and 43 known carcinogens. The contents in tobacco damage cells and increase mutation. In some cases, damaging effects may be reversible if smoking is stopped at an early enough stage.
- If you have *H. pylori*-induced stomach ulcer, have it treated aggressively as this bacteria is associated with a greater risk of gastric cancers.
- Drink eight to ten glasses of pure, filtered water daily—not from the tap. For every cup of liquid with caffeine that you drink, add another cup of water. In 1999 the *New England Journal of Medicine* published a 10-year study that found men who drank more water had less likelihood of developing bladder cancer.
- Enjoy sunshine regularly, but in small doses; remember that the sun burns hottest between 10 a.m. and 2 p.m. Wear a hat. Protect your children from excessive exposure; one serious sunburn involving blistering of the skin dramatically increases the risk of melanoma, a virulent form of skin cancer.
- Fighting cancer means paying special attention to plant-based diets. Eat at least seven to ten servings of fruits, vegetables, seeds, and nuts daily. Drink fresh-squeezed vegetable and fruit juices. Avoid the bad fats (see Chapter 4) and red meat, which are associated with colorectal, breast, and prostate cancer. Investigating plant-based diets that are rich in sterols and s terolins has led researchers to believe they reduce hormone-related cancers and reduce the mortality rate of these cancers. Studies of cell cultures that were supplemented with beta-sitosterol showed 66 percent fewer breast cancer cells.
- Choose organic fruits and vegetables to avoid a toxic load of herbicides and pesticides as well as heavy metals. Buy free-range poultry raised without antibiotics and hormone therapy.
- Avoid caffeine and alcohol. Consume herbal teas regularly: red clover, Jason Winters tea, dandelion, pau d'arco, black radish, and echinacea.

Other Recommendations

- Do *not* take iron supplements unless you have been diagnosed with anemia. People with excess iron in their body have higher incidences of cancer. The body prevents cancer cells from getting iron and it was reported in the *New England Journal of Medicine* that excess iron inhibits macrophage activity and meddles in the function of the T-cells and B-cells.

- Avoiding constipation should be a priority. Do not eat processed, refined, or fried foods. Avoid products based on white flour, sugar, salt, and bad fats. Do not eat luncheon meat, hot dogs, smoked or cured meat at all. Restrict, but do not eliminate, intake of dairy and soy. Occasional consumption of yogurt, kefir, and soy products is fine.
- Avoid eggs, especially fried eggs. (See "The Dangers of Dairy and Eggs" in Chapter 4, page 68.)
- Avoid exposure to chemicals, paints, fumes, pesticides, aerosols, and so on, to protect the immune system from further contamination.
- Get plenty of fresh air and inhale deeply to get oxygen into your system.
- Exercise is very important. (See Chapter 6 for more information.)
- Do not wear constrictive clothing. For men this may mean tight underwear or pants; for women this means any type of binding, especially bras. Bras worn too tightly and for too many hours of the day prevent the flow of lymph that is so important to clearing out the toxins. It is theorized that one of the reasons why women are so susceptible to breast cancer is that many lymph nodes are situated along the top of the shoulder and under the arm—exactly where the bra constricts. *Dressed to Kill*, written by Sydney Ross Singer and Soma Grismaijer, describes an original experiment that was spurred on by Soma's discovery of a lump in her breast.
- Reduce stress and practice relaxation techniques such as biofeedback, yoga, qigong, and deep breathing. Maintaining a positive attitude while fighting cancer is paramount. Participating in a support group may give you the freedom to express emotions that you may not otherwise feel you can share with friends and family (see Chapter 6).

Health Fact

An observation of cancer patients was made by W.B. Coley, MD, of Sloan Kettering Hospital, that the patients who developed postoperative infection fever were more likely to go into remission than those who did not. It appeared as if the fever "turbo-charged" the immune system.

Since 1972, incidences of brain cancer in children has increased 26 percent. Incidences of testicular cancer in males aged 15 to 30 years has almost doubled.

CANDIDIASIS

Candida albicans is one of many candida fungi, or yeast, that exist in our intestinal tract; in women it is also found in the vagina. It resides quite peaceably in the intestines and the genital area unless there is a disturbance in their environment that allows candida to grow out of control. When candida does proliferate, yeast infections occur and manifest in many areas of the body (see Fungal Infections). It can affect men as well as women, but women are four times more likely to suffer candida overgrowth.

Candida organisms can produce hormone-like substances that mimic human hormones. Also, some types of candida have receptors for hormones on their surface. Most people with candida overgrowth have some serious nutritional deficiencies, most likely because the gut is damaged, promoting malabsorption of our nutrients. The immune system may also be producing antibodies against the candida, promoting an allergy response to this organism that is inherent to the body and normally not harmful.

Conventional medicine acknowledges that there is a harmless, irritating level of yeast problems such as thrush or vaginal yeast infection, as well as life-threatening *Candida septicemia* in people with compromised immune systems, but conventional practitioners are reluctant to view allergies, chronic fatigue syndrome, bowel problems, and other conditions as related to candida yeast.

Symptoms

Over 50 symptoms have been identified as indicators of candida in the body, including chemical sensitivities, allergy, asthma, mood swings, fatigue, headaches and migraines, muscle pain, rectal itching, irritability, dizziness, depression, insomnia, and lack of concentration. Candida has been associated with low stomach acid, so intestinal disorders including diarrhea, constipation, cramps, and foul-smelling stools, breath, and urine are very common. The symptoms are so similar to other illnesses that diagnosis can be missed. Chronic candida can also be a symptom of other illnesses such as chronic fatigue syndrome and HIV. Vaginal yeast infections are apparent by the presence of a white cheesy discharge with a distinct odor, itching, and irritation, and it can be painful to urinate. Men may also experience genital candida as a urinary tract infection (UTI) or an itching or burning sensation at the head of the penis. Dark circles under the eyes, a thick white coating on the tongue, and fungal infections around the nails are also signs of candida overgrowth.

Causes

Yeast becomes invasive in the body when there is not enough "good" intestinal flora to keep it in balance. Antibiotics are the most well-known culprits for killing the "good guys" in the gut and allowing a hospitable environment for candida. Birth control pills, steroids, and chemotherapy can also contribute to candida overgrowth. Food allergies, alcohol, dairy products, or diets low in fiber and high in sugar and refined carbohydrates that are a smorgasbord for yeast can also be responsible for creating the perfect environment for candida. Other triggers can be smoking, stress, multiple pregnancies, and a weakened immune system. Serious illness, such as HIV, increases vulnerability to systemic candidiasis, where candida can proliferate anywhere in the body. If it reaches the bloodstream, it can act as poison, resulting in *Candida septicemia*.

Prescription for Health

NUTRIENT	DOSAGE	ACTION
Vitamin C with quercetin	1000 mg vitamin C with 500 mg quercetin three times daily	Vitamin C is anti-inflammatory, antibacterial, and controls allergic reactions
High-potency B-complex	Two to three capsules daily	Protects against deficiency and improves digestion, reduces stress
Magnesium	500 mg twice daily	Deficiency is common; required for over 300 reactions in the body and promotes detoxification
Multimune containing vitamins A, C, E, P-5-P, zinc, selenium, magnesium, reduced L-glutathione, coenzyme Q10, and lipoic acid	Three capsules daily	Gives immune support, is antihistamine, promotes detoxification, is antiallergy
Vitamin K	60–80 mcg daily	Restores imbalance caused by antibiotics
Essential fatty acids (Udo's Choice or Omega Essential Balance)	2 Tbsp (30 mL) daily	Protects the integrity of cells, is anti-inflammatory
Caprylic acid (enteric-coated)	1–2 g daily with meals	Acts as an antifungal
Oil of oregano	Two drops three times daily in juice or water	Is a powerful antifungal
Tea tree oil (must be diluted before application)	Local application of 40 percent solution for a maximum of five days	Is effective for candida vaginitis. Do not apply to broken skin. If irritation occurs, discontinue.
Omega's Hi-Lignan Nutri-Flax fiber supplement	1–2 tsp (5–10 mL) daily, drink two glasses of water for every teaspoon of flax fiber	Prevents constipation
Goldenseal	400 mg three times daily. Ensure it has an 8 to 10 percent berberine content.	Acts as an antifungal
Lactobacillus acidophilus	1 tsp (5 mL) providing 1–2 billion live organisms	Replenishes and boosts intestinal flora

NUTRIENT	DOSAGE	ACTION
Garlic	1000 mg daily of Kyolic	Garlic is a natural antifungal
Echinacea	Forty drops daily for two weeks	Research shows a 40 percent drop in the recurrence of candida vaginal infections
Moducare sterols and sterolins	Two capsules three times daily for one week; one capsule three times daily thereafter	Enhances immune function to fight excess candida; your immune system should keep candida in balance.

* Pregnant women should consult their naturopathic doctor for treatment of candida overgrowth.

Health Tips to Enhance Healing

- The best prevention and offense against candida is to boost the immune system. Eat plenty of fruits and vegetables, 7 to 10 half-cup servings daily. Legumes, fish, whole grains, nuts, seeds, and their oils will provide your body with balanced nutrition. Avoid eating simple carbohydrates such as white bread, cake, cookies, and chips, and too many citrus fruits, which allow candida to flourish.
- If candida is a recurring problem, switch to a diet that excludes all yeast and sugar (that means fruit too). Any food that has been aged or fermented should also be eliminated, so no cheese, soy sauce, pickles, raw mushrooms, vinegar, or alcohol, to name a few. Avoid gluten and eat millet, quinoa, and brown rice instead.
- If you are not lactose intolerant, eat plenty of plain organic yogurt to increase the good bacteria population in your intestines. Half a cup to one cup every day will ward off yeast infections and restore balance to the body. If you are taking antibiotics, it is especially important, but if you do not like the taste of yogurt, you can always supplement with probiotics.
- Do not eat animal or dairy products that have been injected with antibiotics. Dairy also has a high level of milk sugar.
- Drink at least eight to ten glasses of pure, filtered water daily. For every juice, caffeinated, or alcoholic beverage you consume, have another glass of water.
- Do not overeat; it suppresses the immune system.
- Stop smoking.
- Take one or two digestive enzymes before every meal. Do not drink while eating or else you will dilute your enzymes.
- If you suspect you have low stomach acid, see the introduction to this chapter.
- See "Allergy Detection and Elimination" in the introduction to this chapter.

Other Recommendations

- Wear loose white cotton underwear instead of synthetic and leave the pantyhose in the drawer. Change undergarments daily, and wash them at high temperatures.
- After going to the toilet, wipe front to back to avoid spreading the fungus back to the vagina.
- Take baths instead of showers to ensure that the genital area is washed thoroughly. Make sure that you dry off very well.
- Avoid taking oral contraceptives or steroid medications; they can alter your body's environment to encourage yeast growth.
- Although there is still the need for more research in this area, sexual transmission is being investigated for its role in yeast infections. To be safe, use a condom during sex so you don't infect your partner, who may then infect you again.
- Reduce your exposure to chemicals, perfumes, dyes, fragrances, and scents. When fighting an infection, don't use bubble bath, douches, perfumed toilet paper, deodorized tampons, etc. Soap should be natural as well.
- Mercury toxicity can make the body vulnerable to yeast overgrowth. Have a hair, urine, and blood analysis done to determine if that is a factor. If so, avoid exposure to mercury and have dental amalgams removed. (See Toxic Metal Poisoning for more information.)
- If you are having four or more vaginal yeast infections in a year, consult your health-care practitioner.
- Not all infections in the vagina are yeast problems, so have sexually transmitted diseases ruled out.
- See also Fungal Infections.

Health Fact

Some forms of candida, such as *Candida krusei* and *Candida parapsilosis*, produce an enzyme called thiaminase that destroys thiamine (vitamin B_1) before you have a chance to absorb it so ensure your B-complex contains thiamine.

CARPAL TUNNEL SYNDROME

Carpal tunnel syndrome is a painful disorder of the wrist where the median nerve is pressed alongside ligaments and the eight little bones they pass through. While this condition may seem fairly minor, the U.S. Bureau of Labor Statistics estimates that there are 400,000 to 500,000 cases per year, costing $2 billion annually.

The average cost per worker is $12,700 to $12,900. Less than half that cost is attributed to medical expenses, while the rest is in terms of lost productivity. Surgery is often performed to relieve the pressure on the nerve when symptoms persist for up to six months, but often it does not cure the problem and there is a risk of nerve damage and a reduction in grip strength. Recurrence is common.

Symptoms

When the nerve is compressed, the hand feels weak and it is difficult to grasp things. While not performing the repetitive task, the forearm, wrist, and fingers may burn, tingle, or ache as the nerve relaxes and swells. Over time it becomes far more painful, and the nerve becomes so irritated that it will be impossible to make any movement at all.

Causes

It is most common in people whose work entails repetitive, strenuous motions with their hands such as typists, grocery clerks, carpenters, machinists, and athletes engaged in racket sports. Carpal tunnel syndrome can be brought on by arthritis, nerve disorders, bad posture (the median nerve goes all the way up to the neck) and a deficiency in vitamin B_6 (the nervous system vitamin).

Prescription for Health

NUTRIENT	DOSAGE	ACTION
Vitamin B_6 in the form of P-5-P with a B-complex	50 mg three times daily P-5-P with a B-complex containing 50 mg B_2	Studies have shown B_6 to be an effective treatment for carpal tunnel. Allow three months for results.
Multimune containing vitamins A, B_6, C, E, zinc, magnesium, selenium, coenzyme Q10, lipoic acid, reduced L-glutathione	Three capsules daily	Reduces inflammation, is an antioxidant and detoxifier, enhances immune system
Wobenzym	Two capsules daily on an empty stomach	Reduces inflammation and eases pain
Omega-3 fatty acid, flaxseed oil	1–2 Tbsp flaxseed oil	Reduces inflammation, lubricates joints, repairs cell membranes
Moducare sterols and sterolins	Two capsules three times daily for one week, then one capsule three times daily thereafter	Decreases inflammation of the nerve

Health Tips to Enhance Healing

- Stop repetitive activity. If you use a computer, ensure that the keyboard and mouse are at the correct height so as not to overextend muscles and ligaments.
- Avoid salty foods to reduce water retention.
- Drink eight to ten glasses of pure, filtered water daily. For every juice, alcoholic, or caffeinated beverage you drink, add another glass of water.
- Take up yoga. It has been shown to be effective in reducing the pain and inflammation of carpal tunnel syndrome.

Other Recommendations

- Try taking breaks as often as you can when you are performing the repetitive tasks. Shake out the hand and fingers, and move them in an opposite way from what the work requires.
- If possible, learn to use the opposite hand for some tasks so that you can rest the overused one. I'm right-handed, but I use the mouse with my left. Initially it took me a little longer to do things, but within a week I was comfortable with it and up to speed.
- The best way to combat carpal tunnel syndrome is to prevent it from happening in the first place. Learn ergonomic safety for your occupation and apply those measures on a daily basis.

Health Fact

The *Journal of the American Medical Association* reported that 22 people who experienced carpal tunnel syndrome and took eight weeks of yoga classes felt significant relief of symptoms compared to a similar group using wrist splints. Iyengar yoga was practiced in two-hour classes. Compared to the control group, the group practicing yoga felt less than half the pain and increased their grip strength by almost fourfold. Improving grip strength was observed to be integral to relieving symptoms.

Researchers did not have conclusions about why yoga has this effect on carpal tunnel syndrome, but initial observations suspect that it helps by increasing awareness of posture and improving upper body alignment.

CELIAC DISEASE

Celiac sprue, also referred to as celiac disease, is one in a group of disorders that falls under the umbrella of gluten-sensitive enteropathy. It is an auto-immune disease that causes damage to the small bowel because of a reaction to protein fractions in barley, oats, wheat, and rye. Other gluten-sensitive disorders are transient gluten intolerance, IgA nephropathy (kidneys), and dermatitis herpetiformis (skin).

People who are susceptible to celiac disease cannot digest the protein fraction in certain grains. The undigested proteins promote allergic and inflammatory reactions, causing damage to the lining of the small bowel. In severe cases, absorption of essential nutrients is inhibited, causing malabsorption and wasting syndromes (see Chapter 1). More women are affected by celiac disease than men, and it can strike at any age, although it occurs more frequently in adulthood. Transient gluten intolerance resembles celiac disease and appears in children under the age of two.

Celiac disease was first described in 1888, but the role of protein fractions in certain grains was not discovered until 1953 by a Dutch pediatrician, William Dicke. Until proper diagnosis and management of the disease was developed, celiac disease was often fatal.

Symptoms

Because so many of the symptoms are similar to irritable bowel syndrome, celiac disease is often misdiagnosed. The extent of the symptoms can depend on the severity of the damage to the small bowel and include anemia, bloating, chronic fatigue, constipation or diarrhea (or alternating between the two), weight loss, intolerance to dairy products, weakness, muscle cramps, and pain in the bones. The skin, kidneys, and other organs are often involved in celiac disease.

Those with celiac disease may show signs of osteoporosis, milk intolerance, chronic fatigue, osteomalacia, infertility, dementia, neuropathy, short stature, and defects in dental enamel. Children may have projectile vomiting, diarrhea, and a bloated abdomen. They may also fail to grow. Recent studies conducted on children with Down's syndrome found that 10 percent of them had celiac disease. Celiac disease can be the underlying condition responsible for severe migraines that do not seem to respond to standard treatment. When anemia is being investigated, celiac disease serology should be used as gluten sensitivity can go undetected with current testing methods.

Causes

Celiac disease has a genetic predisposition and it is crucial that the disease be detected early before gut damage is too advanced. When gluten is ingested, an allergic response from lymphocytes inflames the membranes of the intestine and causes the villi (minute, hair-like structures that absorb nutrients) to atrophy (shrink). Villi cannot regenerate after they have been destroyed. Losing the villi makes the stomach and intestinal lining more fragile and easily damaged, causing leaky gut syndrome.

Antibodies are produced by the immune system against gluten peptides or connective tissue. These antibodies can be detected in the saliva and serum of most celiac sufferers, although they do not have to be present to diagnose the disease. Once the intestinal lining is damaged, it becomes difficult to absorb nutrients, in particular fats and fat-soluble vitamins. The inability to absorb nutrients results in nutritional deficiencies, malabsorption syndrome, and other disorders.

Prescription for Health

Successful treatment requires lifelong avoidance of wheat, oats, barley, and rye. Make sure that all the supplements you purchase are gluten and allergy free. Copper levels should be checked by a physician and if deficient, a copper supplement should be added.

NUTRIENT	DOSAGE	ACTION
Vitamin B₁₂	1000 mcg injection per week as absorption is impaired in those with bowel problems	Offsets deficiency caused by damage to the walls of the intestinal tract
Vitamin B-complex	Two to three capsules daily	Supports all B vitamin supplementation
Folic acid	1-5 mg daily, dosages of 10 mg have been used to treat chronic diarrhea under a doctor's guidance. Once diarrhea is gone take 400 mcg daily	Stops chronic diarrhea
Moducare sterols and sterolins	Two capsules three times daily for one week, then one capsule three times daily thereafter	See article on page 170, written by Prof. Bouic; also supports immune function and controls inflammation in the gut
Vitamin D₃	400 IU daily	Restores deficiencies that could lead to bone disease
Vitamin C with quercetin	1000 mg vitamin C and 500 mg quercitin	Prevents inflammation and boosts immunity
Omega's Hi-Lignan Flax	1–3 tsp (5–15 mL) daily with plenty of water	Controls diarrhea, corrects constipation, and soothes intestinal lining
Calcium and magnesium	1000 mg calcium, 500 mg magnesium	Restores possible deficiencies and helps to prevent colon cancer
Plant digestive enzymes	Two capsules with meals	Aids proper digestion
Iron	10 mg daily	Use if diagnosed with anemia
Multivitamin with minerals	Use as directed	Restores possible deficiencies
Lactobacillus and *Bifidus acidophilus*	1 tsp (5 mL) daily	Improves intestinal flora, reduces diarrhea, irritable bowel, diverticulosis, and constipation

NUTRIENT	DOSAGE	ACTION
Multimune containing vitamins A, B_6, C, E, selenium, zinc, magnesium, lipoic acid, coenzyme Q10, reduced L-glutathione	Three capsules daily	Supports immune function, controls allergic reactions, is anti-inflammatory
L-glutamine	1000 mg daily	Supports health of villi, the surfaces that facilitate absorption in the intestine
Omega-3 fatty acid	1–3 Tbsp (15–45 mL) of flaxseed oil daily or 500 mg twice daily of fish oil (Eskimo-3)	Reduces inflammation; EPA is thought to suppress the leukotriene responsible for signaling inflammation in the mucosal membrane
Evening primrose oil	500 mg twice daily	Reduces inflammation by inhibiting inflammatory mediators; prevents zinc deficiency
Colostrum	1 tsp (5 mL) daily	Contains lactoferrin and enhances immunoglobulins in the gut
Peppermint oil enteric-coated capsules	Three to six capsules daily	Reduces cramps, relieves gas, and increases bile, with its most prevalent use in IBS

Health Tips to Enhance Healing

- Eliminate all gluten from the diet starting with wheat, oats, rye, and barley. Read labels carefully—be wary of packaged foods because they usually contain gluten. Some examples include: condiments (ketchup, soy sauce, mustard, etc.), hot dogs, luncheon meat, sausages, white vinegar, baked beans, soups, and nutritional supplements. Gluten is also known by the names malt, modified starch, hydrolyzed vegetable protein, hydrolyzed plant protein, texturized vegetable protein, and natural flavorings.
- Drink eight to ten glasses of pure, filtered water every day. For every juice or beverage with caffeine you consume, have another glass of water.
- Rule out lactose intolerance. Many celiacs are intolerant to dairy products because they lack the enzyme to break down lactose.
- Avoid any foods or drinks that will aggravate the small intestine, such as dairy products, alcohol, caffeine, sugar, and other refined carbohydrates or processed foods.
- Follow a diet that is rich in natural, whole foods to ensure that fiber requirements are met. Eat plenty of fresh fruits and vegetables, legumes, nuts, and seeds. Also include fresh fish, lean meat and poultry, healthy fats and oils, and soy products. Choose organic produce, wild fish, and free-range meat

whenever possible. The fewer toxins you introduce to an ailing intestine the better.

Other Recommendations

- Aid digestion by taking digestive plant enzymes with every meal.
- Big meals are hard to digest, so try eating small meals throughout the day. Sit, relax, and enjoy your food—
remember, digestion begins in your mouth.
- Children as young as six months have been known to get celiac disease, so if you notice sores or blisters on the body, consult a professional. Eliminate all gluten and milk products to see if symptoms disappear.
- Reduce stress and improve immune function.

CHOLESTEROL (HIGH)

Despite the resources that have been spent educating the North American public about the dangers of total fat and high cholesterol foods in their diet, heart disease is still the number one cause of death. What is shocking is that the majority of fatalities could be prevented with simple modifications to diet and lifestyle.

According to both the American Heart Association and the Canadian Heart and Lung Association, 40 percent of the adult population have high cholesterol levels, the leading risk factor for heart disease. However, more attention is beginning to focus on the role of high triglyceride levels as a better predictor of heart attack risk.

Cholesterol has been given a bad reputation. The fact is that cholesterol is essential to our health. It allows our body to make repairs, insulate our nerves, form cell membranes, and produce certain sex hormones. Cholesterol is found not only in many of the foods we eat, but it is also produced in the liver. Most people have a feedback mechanism that moderates their cholesterol levels. If we eat too much cholesterol, the liver makes less and if we eat too little, the liver makes more. For some, however, their cholesterol levels must be maintained by making simple changes in the diet and taking nutritional supplements. Although we hear plenty about high cholesterol, many are not aware that very low levels of cholesterol can be an indicator of other health concerns. Cholesterol levels below the normal range are often associated with cancer. Low cholesterol is also common in those who are very thin and rarely exercise.

There are two types of cholesterol: low-density lipoprotein (LDL) cholesterol and high-density lipoprotein (HDL) cholesterol. LDL carries cholesterol and triglycerides from the liver to the cells. When there is too much LDL, known as the "bad" cholesterol, plaque slowly accumulates on the blood vessel walls. The arteries become narrower and the heart must work harder to pump blood to the body. If there is too much plaque, the blood and oxygen cannot reach the heart and there is a pain in the chest (angina). With narrower arteries, a small piece of debris, such as a blood clot, can completely obstruct the artery and cause a heart attack.

HDL cholesterol is the "good" cholesterol because it transports LDL cholesterol away from the cells and back to the liver, thus preventing the arteries from hardening. HDL is also responsible for breaking down cholesterol into fatty acids, which are essential for strong cell membranes.

Triglyceride levels also play a part in heart disease and may be a better predictor of heart disease than high cholesterol. Triglycerides are the most prevalent type of fat existing in the body and, when present in excess, can damage the arteries by encouraging arteriosclerosis. The perfect level for triglycerides would be 140 mg/dL (milligrams per deciliter), but 140–160 mg/dL is considered normal.

Increasing HDL blood cholesterol while reducing LDL and triglycerides can have a profound effect on your risk of heart disease and stroke. The Heart and Stroke Foundation states that "for every 1 percent drop in LDL cholesterol a 2 percent reduction in risk of heart attack occurs and for every 1 percent increase in HDL levels, the risk of heart attack drops 3 to 4 percent." By following a healthy diet, taking supplements, and making a few modifications to your lifestyle, you can prevent or delay the need for cholesterol-lowering medication.

Symptoms

Symptoms may include angina or chest pain. A fatty tissue buildup under the skin, especially on the eyelids, indicates poor cholesterol metabolism. In severe cases pain in the legs may occur when walking. The following are the accepted guidelines for determining your level of risk.

Total Cholesterol:
Desirable: less than 200 mg/dL
Borderline to high: 200–239 mg/dL
High: 240 mg/dL or higher

LDL:
Desirable: less than 130 mg/dL
Borderline to high: 130–159 mg/dL
High: 160 mg/dL or higher

HDL: Higher than 35 mg/dL

Triglycerides: Less than 150 mg/dL

Causes

As mentioned earlier, high cholesterol is largely a product of poor habits. Following a diet that is high in bad fats and refined carbohydrates, low in fiber, and devoid of fresh fruits and vegetables is the main problem. Excessive stress, a sedentary lifestyle, smoking, and genetic predisposition compound the problem. Hypothyroidism has also been linked to high cholesterol and if (subclinical) hypothyroidism (see page 22 in Chapter 2 for more information) is the instigator, low-cholesterol diets and supplements to lower cholesterol will have no effect on your cholesterol levels.

Prescription for Health

If you are on Coumadin or Statin cholesterol-lowering medication, talk to your naturopathic physician before embarking on this protocol. The following will lower cholesterol in less than 90 days in most cases, so your medications will need to be adjusted accordingly.

NUTRIENT	DOSAGE	ACTION
Inositol hexanicotinate (nonflushing niacin)	500–1000 mg three times daily with meals. If using just niacin, increase dosage slowly over three weeks until using 3000 mg daily to avoid the harmless flushing of the skin.	Lowers LDL cholesterol and triglycerides while raising HDL cholesterol. Have liver enzymes and cholesterol checked every three months if using plain niacin.
High-potency B-complex	Two capsules daily	Normalizes homocysteine levels, aids digestion, and protects nerves
Vitamin B_5, pantethine	300 mg three times daily	Lowers LDL and triglycerides and raises HDL
Vitamin C with bioflavonoids	1000 mg twice daily	Reduces LDL and increases antioxidant activity
L-carnitine	500 mg three times daily	Stimulates the breakdown of fats, improves cardiac function
Garlic, standardized Kyolic	4000–5000 mcg allicin content daily	Lowers cholesterol and blood pressure
Gugulipid (standardized extract of mukul myrrh tree)	500 mg three times daily (standardized for 25 mg guggulsterone)	Increases the liver's metabolism of LDL cholesterol, lowers LDL cholesterol and triglyceride levels, and raises HDL cholesterol levels; also shown to prevent atherosclerosis and reverse pre-existing plaque
Essential fatty acids, from flaxseed, Omega Essential Balance, or Udo's Choice oil	1-3 Tbsp (15–45 mL) daily	Decreases triglyceride level, raises HDL level and improves transportation of cholesterol to liver for metabolism
Phytosterols	1–2 g of plant sterol daily	Plant sterols fill the receptor sites in the small intestine and reduce the absorption of cholesterol. Do not eat sterol-enriched margarines.

Health Tips to Enhance Healing

- See Cardiovascular Corruption, page 17.
- See High Blood Pressure and Low Thyroid, page 21.

- Simple diet changes alone can reduce cholesterol by 20 percent. Eat plenty of fresh fruits and vegetables. Enjoy the whole rainbow of colors, not just the pale green ones. Include carrots, yams, broccoli, squash, tomatoes, eggplant, dark green leafy vegetables, berries, cantaloupe, and citrus fruits.
- Increase your intake of dietary fiber, including plenty of soluble fiber (oats, legumes, beans, and apples), and watch cholesterol levels decrease. Oat bran and oatmeal were responsible for some of the greatest drops in total serum cholesterol.
- Eat fish often because they are rich in good fats that are good for the heart. Broil, sauté, or steam them.
- Avoid animal fats and hydrogenated oils and margarines, and decrease your egg consumption to one a day (each egg contains approximately 200 mg of cholesterol). As well, eliminate the following foods because they contain oxidized cholesterol and trans fatty acids, which also increase triglycerides and cholesterol: store-bought baked goods, coffee whiteners, crackers, cookies, powdered milk and eggs, bread machine and cake mixes.
- According to Dr. Julian Whitaker, eating two medium-sized carrots every day can drop your cholesterol by 50 points in as little as 21 days.
- Plant sterols are a must in cholesterol-lowering diets. Found in fruits, vegetables, nuts, seeds, and soy products, about 0.25 g of plant sterols and 0.3 g of cholesterol occur naturally in the daily diet. A vegetarian diet gives you twice the amount of plant sterols consumed daily. Plant sterols reduce the absorption of cholesterol from foods by about half to one-quarter.
- Stop eating margarine and use the "better" butter mentioned in Chapter 8 (see page 107). Margarine and hydrogenated vegetable oils raise LDL cholesterol and lower the protective HDL cholesterol. Or, better yet, skip the butter and consume only the essential fatty acid-rich nut and seed oils that are cold-pressed and unrefined.

Other Recommendations

- Get your body moving, your blood flowing, and your heart pumping. Start an exercise program even if it means walking to the corner of your street and back, or parking your car a block or two away from your destination. Studies show that low-intensity exercises such as walking, hiking, or slow jogging use up triglycerides. The enzyme activity used to break down the triglycerides is stimulated by regular exercise.
- Stop smoking.
- Reduce your consumption of alcohol and caffeine. Alcohol raises triglyceride levels.

- Don't skip breakfast. A national survey evaluated the nutritional practices of Americans and discovered that those who ate whole-grain cereal for breakfast had the lowest serum cholesterol levels, but the people who ate breakfast foods that were high in cholesterol still had lower total cholesterol than those who skipped breakfast altogether.
- Although the "niacin flush" is completely harmless, it makes some people slightly uncomfortable or nauseous. Try increasing dosages gradually. For those who really have a low tolerance for it, you can take inositol hexanicotinate, usually sold as nonflushing niacin. If you have liver disease or diabetes, have your physician monitor your liver enzymes and cholesterol levels every three or six months while on niacin. When your cholesterol and triglycerides get in the healthy range, reduce intake to a maintenance dosage.
- Subclinical hypothyroidism should be ruled out before treating cholesterol levels. It is more difficult to detect than hyperthyroidism and often goes undiagnosed.
- If you are taking medication for your cholesterol, talk to your pharmacist because statins to lower cholesterol reduce your coenzyme Q10 to dangerously low levels.

Health Fact

In September 2000 the U.S. Food and Drug Administration gave phytosterols a recognized health claim for reducing the risk of coronary heart disease. See the chart on page 78 and add many of the sterol-rich foods to your diet.

CHRONIC FATIGUE SYNDROME

Chronic fatigue syndrome (CFS) is an immune system disease that affects millions of North Americans. After contracting CFS, many cannot continue to work, some are bedridden, and others can work only part time. Chronic fatigue syndrome produces a profound fatigue state including weakness, swollen glands, fever, problems with balance, brain lesions, flu-like symptoms, depression, and a severe lack of energy lasting up to several years in serious cases. Women account for the majority of those affected. It is also called myalgic encephalomyelitis.

A new study from DePaul University estimates 800,000 Americans suffer from chronic fatigue syndrome, and about 75 percent are young, white, professional women.

Symptoms

So diverse and transient are the symptoms of chronic fatigue that it has been maligned and misdiagnosed as depression and other mental illness. Some sufferers have been labeled as hypochondriacs for their many visits to endless numbers of physicians and specialists. To put an end to the difficulty in diagnosing CFS, the Center for Disease Control created criteria to be used in evaluating this unusual syndrome. It states that "onset of debilitating fatigue must persist in a steady or recurring state for at least six months and halt normal daily activities over fifty percent of the time. Low grade fever, sore throat, chills, muscle and joint aches and weakness, sleep problems, mental confusion and emotional imbalance are also included in the criteria."

Other symptoms noted with CFS are depression, fevers, chills, brain lesions, allergies, and emotional imbalance. Antibody levels are down-regulated in people with CFS, and they have few natural killer cells. Those with CFS also secrete less gamma-interferon, IL-2, and tumor necrosis factor. As well, elevated T-cell to suppressor T-cell ratios, interleukin-4, and elevated B-cells and autoantibodies are seen. Over 65 percent of CFS people have allergies and high histamine.

Causes

Some researchers believe that viruses may be at the root of these disease states and many feel that chronic fatigue may also be sourced from viral infections as well. It is thought that Epstein Barr virus (EBV), cytomegalovirus, herpes simplex virus (both oral and genital), and herpes Type 6 virus may be the cause of CFS and the subsequent dysfunction of the immune system. We know that viruses have the ability to alter normal immune function in order to maintain their survival and even subvert normal attack mechanisms so they can lie dormant for years, even decades. It is thought that these dormant viruses replicate when the immune system stops functioning properly, encouraging the syndrome of chronic fatigue.

A suppressed or dysfunctional immune system is at the root of CFS. Over time the body's immune system is gradually weakened due to lack of sleep, too much work, poor nutrition, chronic stress, lack of exercise, pollutants, and food contaminants. Then along comes a significant stress event, such as the death of a loved one, and the immune system is at an all-time low. A viral infection takes hold and flourishes. The immune system is too weak to destroy the virus, so it then lies within our cells undetected until the next flare-up, creating a cycle of disease and a vast array of symptoms. Improving immune function, controlling overactive antibodies and histamine, while increasing gamma interferon and IL-2 is the basis for the following recommendations.

Plant Sterols and Sterolins for CFS

Sterols and sterolins have been shown in research to enhance gamma-interferon and interleukin-2 while decreasing the inflammation and allergy-promoting cytokine IL-4. It also enhances NK cell and cytotoxic T-cell activity. Both these cells are important for destroying virus-infected cells. Sterols and sterolins also increase DHEA naturally and regulate cortisol.

Prescription for Health

NUTRIENT	DOSAGE	ACTION
Vitamin A	25,000 IU daily for 6 weeks, then reduce to 5000 IU for maintenance	Helps regulate the immune system
High-potency B-complex	Two capsules daily	Supports adrenal function, metabolism, and energy production
Vitamin C	To bowel tolerance (see Chapter 5, "Nutritional Supplements," page 86)	Stimulates T-cells and increases the release of interferon
Multimune containing vitamins A, B_6, C, E, selenium, zinc, magnesium, lipoic acid, reduced L-glutathione, and coenzyme Q10	Three capsules per day	Supports immune function, controls histamine, is a potent antioxidant, increases energy production
CoQ10	100 mg twice daily	Increases natural killer cell and antioxidant activity
Astragulus	One capsule (500 mg) twice daily	Improves stamina and stimulates antibody production and white blood cell activity
Licorice DGL	1 g daily	Increases blood pressure in those with low blood pressure (commonly seen in CFS)
Acetyl-L-carnitine	1 g three times daily	Improves energy production
Moducare sterols and sterolins	Two capsules three times daily for six weeks, then one capsule three times daily for maintenance	Increases gamma-interferon and IL-2, stops autoantibody production, decreases inflammation and IL-4 implicated in allergies
Women's Whey or proteins + protein powder	One to two scoops daily	Provides adequate protein for repair
Lactobacillus acidophilus	Dosage containing 1–2 billion active organisms	Improves intestinal flora; is especially good if candida is present

Health Tips to Enhance Healing

- Follow the diet recommendations in Chapter 4 and avoid all sugar. As little as 1 tsp (5 mL) of sugar causes our virus-fighting cells to be inactive for hours.

- Drink eight to ten glasses of pure, filtered water daily. For every other beverage (with the exception of herbal tea) that you consume, drink another glass of water.
- Eliminate alcohol, cigarettes, and caffeine. Alcohol suppresses your nervous system, smoking makes your body work harder to eliminate toxins, and caffeine may give you a short-term boost, but the subsequent crash is much harder for those with CFS than in healthy individuals.
- Get regular exercise, but don't overexert yourself. This may seem like an impossible feat, but gentle moderate exercise improves your circulation and overall well-being. Be sure to rest. Work up to 20 to 30 minutes of walking, at least five times a week.

Other Recommendations

- Keep a positive frame of mind. It would be very easy to let this disease bring you down, but don't let it take control of your life. Adopt the strategies mentioned in Chapter 6.
- If you are supplementing with iron, monitor your intake carefully. Iron deficiencies can cause fatigue and impair the immune system, but excess iron will feed the bacteria and yeast that require it for their replication, thus also hindering the immune system.
- Identify and eliminate food allergies. Have your physician give you the ELISA test.
- Have dental amalgams removed (see Toxic Metal Poisoning).
- See Candidiasis.

Health Fact

In 1995 the U.S. Department of Veterans Affairs supported precursory research into the relationship between Gulf War veterans and incidences of CFS. In a self-administered postal survey, none of the 1611 respondents indicated signs of CFS prior to going to the Gulf War. After returning from the Gulf, 16 percent of the respondents met enough of the markers to qualify as having CFS. As the study was conducted via post and did not include a diagnostic exam, further research was recommended for validation; however, the incidences were high enough to cause concern.

CONSTIPATION

Most alternative doctors have stopped asking their patients if they are regular because they always say yes, regardless if they have a bowel movement once a day or once a week. North Americans spend almost $1 billion per year on laxatives. Each of us has been constipated at one time or another, but 20 percent of us are chronically constipated. Few discuss the problem and what little knowledge that is gained usually comes from advertisements and laxative packaging.

Constipation occurs when waste is not eliminated from the body in an appropriate amount of time and it becomes necessary to strain in order to remove hard feces. You should have at least one large bowel movement a day, or two to three smaller ones (about 12 in/30 cm of waste should be excreted in total). The feces should be soft, bulky, and easy to pass.

Symptoms

Infrequent, small, hard, and dry bowel movements that are difficult to pass is the main symptom. Constipation often results in hemorrhoids, skin problems, headaches, body odor, and fatigue, as well as irritability, depression, obesity, insomnia, and diverticulitis. Waste that is left in the colon too long causes toxin buildup and can lead to more serious bowel disease and cancer.

Causes

When disease is not present, constipation usually arises when we don't drink enough water or eat enough fiber, eat too much protein and highly processed food, or when we don't make enough time to have a bowel movement. A change in routine, business travel, and restaurant eating can all lead to constipation. The typical Western diet does not encompass enough whole natural food and relies far too much on what is convenient, either fast foods or store-bought packaged foods that are devoid of fiber and processed to ensure a long shelf life. Packaged foods are also high in sugar, sodium, artificial flavors, and chemical colorants that lead to constipation.

Other factors that can contribute to constipation are a lack of exercise, prolonged use of laxatives or antacids, nutritional deficiency, pregnancy, parasitic infection, and yeast overgrowth. Constipation is also seen in people with low thyroid function and food allergies, and in those who take prescription medications or iron supplements.

Prescription for Health

NUTRIENT	DOSAGE	ACTION
Vitamin C	Determine amount just under bowel tolerance; as a preventative, 500 mg twice daily. See Chapter 5 to learn how to take vitamin C to bowel tolerance.	Softens stools, promotes elimination and strengthens intestinal capillaries
Vitamin B-complex	Two or three capsules daily	Aids metabolism, improves digestion

NUTRIENT	DOSAGE	ACTION
Calcium with magnesium	1000 mg calcium and 1000 mg magnesium daily. Increase magnesium if constipation persists.	Always supplement magnesium with calcium to aid elimination.
Flaxseed oil and Omega Hi-Lignan Flax Seed	1–2 Tbsp (15–30 mL) of the oil and powder daily. Make sure to drink two glasses of water for each Tbsp of ground flaxseed	Soothes intestinal lining and promotes elimination
Moducare sterols and sterolins	Two capsules three times daily for one week, then one capsule three times daily thereafter	Reduces inflammation of the intestinal tract and venous system
Lactobacillus acidophilus	1 tsp (5 mL) twice daily containing at least 1–2 billion live bacteria	Improves intestinal flora and reduces harmful bacteria
Artichoke	160–320 mg three times daily with meals, assuming standardized to contain 13–18 percent caffeolquinic acids calculated as chlorogenic acid	Increases bile formation and flow to digest and absorb fats
Cascara sagrada	Tea or capsules containing 250 mg for several days. Do not use continually.	Improves peristaltic action of the colon
Pantothenic acid	250 mg daily	Improves peristaltic action of the colon

Health Tips to Enhance Healing

- Take time each day to have a bowel movement, preferably the same time every day. Do not be rushed; eventually the body will respond at the same time each day.
- Drink eight to ten glasses of pure, filtered water daily, but do not drink during meals or else you will dilute your digestive enzymes. For every juice, alcoholic, or caffeinated beverage that you drink, add another glass of water. A study in Italy found that drinking eight glasses of water daily and eating a high-fiber diet was more beneficial than eating a high-fiber diet alone.
- Do not use commercial laxatives because they promote dependence and chronic constipation. High-fiber foods such as prunes or other dried fruit, whole grains, or seeds (especially ground flaxseed or psyllium seed), and sauerkraut (or sauerkraut juice) are far more effective in alleviating constipation and support the body's functions naturally.
- Eat vegetables or fruits at every meal—seven to ten half-cup servings per day. If you haven't been eating raw veggies regularly, start with steamed as it is easier on the digestive system. And remember—if your food comes from a box, it's bad for your bowels.
- Get plenty of exercise. Yoga or tai chi are great for improving circulation, reducing tension, and promoting healthy digestion and elimination. Stretching exercises in which you must touch your toes or draw your knees up to your chest are also good to get the bowels moving.

- Avoid deep-fried foods, food that is high in sugar, and other refined carbohydrates (like white bread), caffeine, alcohol, and dairy (except yogurt).
- If you suspect you have low stomach acid, see the introduction to this chapter.

Other Recommendations

- Get tested for food allergies or low thyroid function.
- When eating, ensure that the atmosphere is relaxed and pleasant. Don't work through lunch or dinners, or eat hunched over the coffee table or while standing over the sink. The benefits of spending 15 to 20 minutes of sitting and enjoying your meal far outweigh the time saved eating on the run.
- For quick relief, magnesium oxide taken before bedtime will flush out your system the next morning. It turns stools to liquid and cleans trapped waste out of the small pockets in the intestines.
- If you need to take additional iron, try a liquid iron supplement like Floradix. It is non-constipating.
- See Chapter 1 on digestive problems.

Health Fact

Before you say "It's just easier to use a laxative," consider this: not only do over-the-counter laxatives not address the problem of why you are constipated, they actually make the problem worse. Regular use of laxatives disturbs the body's natural rhythm. In essence, the body forgets how it is supposed to eliminate waste. Also, laxatives are drugs that can cause nutritional deficiencies. The unnatural increase in gut motility can prevent calcium and vitamin D absorption. Some products can prevent the absorption of fat-soluble vitamins and folic acid.

DEPRESSION

More than 17 million North Americans are afflicted with some form of depression, and it occurs twice as often in women than in men. The intensity of the depression may vary from mild to severe, and it may happen once or recur throughout one's lifetime. While everyone feels down at some time or another, depression is a deep unhappiness that imposes itself on a person's state of mind and affects his or her habits and normal conduct for at least two consecutive weeks. In some cases depression can last months or even years before a diagnosis is made or treatment is sought.

Symptoms

Symptoms vary, but it is generally agreed that the appearance of at least four or five of the following symptoms indicate depression: emotions that are out of place (crying, nervousness, or anger with little or no reason, inappropriate feelings of guilt), lethargy, apathy, a change in sleeping patterns (too much or too little), difficulties with concentration, low self-esteem, lack of interest in usual pursuits, diminished sex drive, recurring thoughts about death or suicide, poor or excessive appetite, physical hyperactivity (or lack of activity), and digestive upsets. In severe cases, the sense of hopelessness, helplessness, and exhaustion are overwhelming.

Causes

A sudden trauma, such as the loss of a loved one or serious physical injury to oneself, was once thought to be trigger depression. Today we would diagnose this type of depression simply as a grieving period. Clinical depression often starts without a clear reason, is more intense, and can last for a longer period. We face sad or negative situations throughout our lives. Depression is not sadness (nor a neurosis), it is a biochemical change in the brain. People who are depressed have low levels of the neurotransmitter serotonin.

There are psychological causes for depression such as physical or sexual abuse, alcoholism or drug addiction, or an inherited biochemical imbalance. Food allergies and nutritional deficiencies can have a profound effect on the biochemical activities in the brain. The foods we eat are responsible for triggering the transmission of neurotransmitters and problems arise when we do not get enough of the nutrients we need for those signals to happen.

Thyroid disease can cause depression. Seasonal affective disorder or SAD, a condition caused by a lack of sunlight in the winter, is also thought to contribute to depression.

Prescription for Health

NUTRIENT	DOSAGE	ACTION
High-potency B-complex	Look for a supplement containing 500–1000 mcg of B_{12}, 800 mcg folic acid, 100 mcg biotin and 50–100 mg of each of the other B vitamins or take individually to obtain optimal dosage	Required for brain and nerve function
Inositol hexanicotinate (nonflushing niacin)	1000 mg twice daily	Inositol improves mood and niacin has been used to treat depression.

NUTRIENT	DOSAGE	ACTION
Multimune containing Vitamins A, B_6, C, E, selenium, zinc, lipoic acid, reduced L-glutathione, Q10 and magnesium	Three capsules daily with food	Provides immune support and protects against free radicals
5-HTP precusor to tryptophan, which helps make serotonin	100 mg three times daily	Increases serotonin; as effective as prescription SSRIs (selective serotonin reuptake inhibitors)
St. John's wort	300 mg three times daily (standardized to 0.3 percent hypericin); allow six weeks for improvement	Relieves depression and anxiety. Do not combine with prescription antidepressants or lithium without a physician's advice.
Ginkgo biloba	80 mg three times daily. I like Nature's Way ginkgo.	Is effective in treating depression in the elderly
SAM-e	400 mg three times daily on an empty stomach	Acts as an antidepressant, enhances dopamine and serotonin
Moducare sterols and sterolins	Two capsules three times daily for one week, then one capsule three times daily thereafter	Modulates cortisol, enhances DHEA
Udo's Choice oil or Omega Essential Balance	1–3 Tbsp (15–45 mL) daily	Supports proper neuron transmission

Health Tips to Enhance Healing

- Exercise regularly, even if it is just a walk around the block, and inhale deeply through the nose. Studies have proven that low-to-moderate physical activity can put you into a good mood and offset feelings of anxiety or depression.
- Laugh—it has been clinically proven that laughter and humor can keep illness at bay, and is especially important in cases of depression when negative thoughts have got you in a downward spiral. Rent videos, read books, or go out to movies or comedy clubs regularly.
- Eat a well-balanced diet that focuses on natural, whole foods: legumes, fresh fruits and vegetables, fresh fish, nuts, and seeds. Ensure that you get enough fresh fish and healthy fats and oils to keep up your levels of omega-3. Sixty percent of the brain is composed of fat; DHA is one-fourth of that.
- Avoid processed and junk foods, caffeine, and alcohol. Not only are these foods nutritionally void, they contain unwanted chemicals and bad fats that can aggravate depression. Caffeine and alcohol provide false stimulation, and leave you feeling worse afterwards.
- Spend as much time outside on sunny days as you can, or if you live in a wet climate, replace all the bulbs in your home with full-spectrum lightbulbs.

- Develop a positive attitude. It may sound easier said than done, but in fact the majority of the things that we tend to worry about are not life-threatening, and worry inspires negativity. Try to see the good side of bad situations. A mistake is only a mistake if we don't learn from it. Encourage a positive attitude by setting moderate goals, reciting positive affirmations, or seeking help from a professional. And don't reproach yourself about needing help, we all need it at some time in our lives—even Superman has friends.

Other Recommendations

- Reduce stress by spending time with friends and family.
- If your work environment makes you unhappy, consider a career change. It may seem drastic, particularly if you've spent several years training for your job, but remember that at least one-third of your life is spent working, and that is a lot of time to be miserable. Make a plan that makes you feel confident about your choice. Seek alternative training, scale back spending habits, and talk to your loved ones about how you feel.

Health Fact

"Runner's high" occurs when the production of endorphins and other neurotransmitters is increased because of an increase in activity, but you don't need to train for a marathon to benefit. A study conducted with seniors who had major depression revealed that 15 minutes of exercise three times per week worked as effectively as the antidepressant Zoloft. After six months, those who took Zoloft were more likely to have a relapse than those who only exercised.

DIABETES

Diabetes is a serious condition whereby the body does not convert sugars and too much sugar builds up in the blood. Diabetics can either secrete little or no insulin, and/or their body does not respond appropriately to insulin, meaning it cannot transfer glucose from the bloodstream into cells and maintain blood glucose balance. It affects 10 million Americans and is the seventh leading cause of death. There are two major types of diabetes.

Type I, insulin-dependent diabetes mellitus (IDDM), or juvenile diabetes, accounts for 10 percent of all diabetics and affects men and women equally. In Type I diabetes the pancreas is unable to produce the hormone insulin, and in over 85 percent of those cases, it is an autoimmune process whereby the immune system destroys the pancreatic insulin-secreting beta cells. The inability of the pancreas to produce insulin causes glucose to build up in the bloodstream and be excreted. Because glucose is not transferred to our cells, the body "starves" to death.

Type II diabetes, or adult-onset diabetes, also called non-insulin-dependent diabetes mellitus (NIDDM), accounts for 90 percent of diagnosed diabetics. Type II diabetics tend to be over 40 and overweight, although there have also been cases of it diagnosed in young children who are overweight. In Type II diabetes, although the pancreas may produce low or normal amounts of insulin, the peripheral organs and tissues have become resistant to insulin's effects.

Complications that arise for both types of diabetes are a result of long-term elevations of either glucose or insulin. If blood glucose levels and blood insulin levels are allowed to vary outside of normal levels for extended periods of time, inflammation results and complications including nerve damage (neuropathies), blindness (retinopathies), kidney disease, and heart and circulatory problems occur.

Gestational diabetes occurs only during pregnancy. Those who developed gestational diabetes are at risk for diabetes later in life.

Symptoms

The tell-tale signs of diabetes are a constant, excessive hunger and thirst, a frequent need to urinate, and weight loss. There can be feelings of deep fatigue, lightheadedness, depression, irritability, numbness or tingling in the toes, and recurring vaginal yeast infections. The skin may itch excessively and vision may be blurred. Type I diabetics can develop a serious side effect of the disease called ketoacidosis, which makes them thin, whereas Type II diabetics rarely develop this disorder and are often overweight. Symptoms of Type II diabetes appear gradually over years. So insidious are these symptoms that most people do not notice them creeping up. Type II diabetics can experience bladder or vaginal infections as well.

Because insulin is required for the transportation of vitamin C into the cell, diabetics are frequently deficient in vitamin C even if their diet is high in this important vitamin. High cortisol and low DHEA (immune and antiaging hormone) accompany many cases of elevated insulin in Type I and Type II diabetes, and signals the liver to produce inflammatory proteins. Arteriosclerosis and poor wound healing are also common in both types of diabetics.

Causes

Researchers believe that cow's milk allergy to albumin triggers an autoimmune reaction against the pancreas, promoting the destruction of beta cells. Clinical research has shown that breast-fed infants appear not to develop Type I diabetes as severely as those who are fed cow's milk formula. Viruses may also play a causative role in developing Type I diabetes. Whooping cough virus, hepatitis, rubella, coxsackie, Epstein Barr, cytomegalovirus, and herpes virus are thought to induce autoimmune reactions. Observations have also been made correlating a rise in diabetes after major flu epidemics. Low thyroid function is also linked to the onset of diabetes.

Type II diabetes is a result of diets that are too high in fat and sugar and too low in fiber and complex carbohydrates. This type of diet usually indicates other compounding problems such as nutritional deficiencies (especially chromium and phytonutrients), being overweight, a lack of exercise, and too much stress. A cause for concern is that the number of children who are overweight increases every year, leaving them at risk for Type II diabetes.

Prescription for Health

NUTRIENT	DOSAGE	ACTION
Vitamin B-complex	Two or three capsules daily	Required for digestion and metabolism, supports adrenals and nerve function
Multimune containing Vitamins A, B$_6$, C, E, zinc, selenium, magnesium, Q10, lipoic acid and reduced L-glutathione	Three capsules daily with food	Supports immune function, contains vitamins A, B$_6$, C, E, selenium, zinc, lipoic acid, reduced L-glutathione, coenzyme Q10, magnesium; protects against neuropathies and retinopathies
Vitamin C (buffered with mineral ascorbates, i.e., calcium ascorbate)	2000–3000 mg daily in divided doses	Prevents vitamin C deficiency and reduces sorbitol and aldose reductase, an enzyme that causes many diabetic complications. High levels of sorbitol can damage sensitive tissues in the eyes, causing retinopathies. Vitamin C protects against retinopathy.
Chromium picolinate	200 mcg twice daily	Improves blood sugar levels
Multimineral without iron	One or two capsules daily	Supports nutrient absorption and repairs deficiency
Reduced L-glutathione	500 mg twice daily	Increases insulin sensitivity and prevents depletion of intracellular glutathione stores, allowing the cells to continue normal functions even in the presence of stressors. For the diabetic, this means that in spite of imbalanced insulin levels, glucose levels, and hormonal levels (DHEA, cortisol, adrenaline, etc.), cells making up delicate tissues such as the eyes, nerves, pancreas, liver, and circulatory system can function well and begin to repair themselves.
Alpha lipoic acid	300 mg twice daily	Converts glucose to energy, protects against free radical damage, improves insulin sensitivity, recycles vitamin C and stops neuropathies
Moducare sterols and sterolins	One capsule three times daily	Increases DHEA, inhibits inflammation by IL-6 and decreases the B-cell antibody production against pancreatic tissues; in the remaining cases of Type I and Type II diabetes, works to control inflammation reducing nerve damage, kidney failure, and infections.

NUTRIENT	DOSAGE	ACTION
Omega-3 fatty acid	One capsule of fish oil (EPA/DHA) three times daily	Lowers blood pressure, increases levels of good cholesterol, reduces the level of bad cholesterol and lowers the levels of fibrinogen, a protein that makes blood thicker and stickier; is also necessary for the formation of prostaglandins
Evening primrose oil	1000 mg capsule three times daily with meals	Improves diabetes-related peripheral nerve dysfunction and increases the enzyme activity on omega-6 that is inhibited by abnormal blood glucose and insulin levels
Gymnema sylvestre (studies used GS4, a water-soluble extract of the leaves)	400 mg daily GS4 or 75–150 mg of standardized Gymnema extract daily	Research studies in humans showed that blood glucose was lowered; insulin increased, a reduction in medication was required, and there were no side effects. A rat study found an increase in the number of islet and beta cells of the pancreas, and the pancreas increased in weight by 30 percent.
Bitter melon	Either fresh, unripe bitter melon or in capsules as recommended	Normalizes blood glucose
Women's Whey or proteins+ protein powder	1 scoop daily	Ensures adequate amino acid consumption and helps to maintain sugar levels.
Milk thistle Nature's Way Thisilyn	Two capsules daily	Protects the liver

Health Tips to Enhance Healing

- I recommend you read *Syndrome X* by Jack Challem, Burton Berson, MD, and Melissa Smith. Their book is full of information on preventing and reversing insulin resistance.
- Eat small, frequent meals high in protein. Dietary changes are an absolute priority for diabetics. Adopt the simple rule of not eating any white foods, white sugar, white flour, white pasta, white rice, white potatoes, etc. Eat brightly colored fruits and vegetables because they are high in vitamins and minerals. A 1999 study in the U.K. found that regular consumption of fruits and vegetables reduced the risk of diabetes.
- Consume less milk since it is high in milk sugar.
- In addition to avoiding white foods, pay attention to the level of dietary fiber in the diet. No more than 40 g of fiber should be eaten daily by diabetics.
- To beef up your intake of EPA and DHA, add regular servings of fish such as salmon, herring, or mackerel to your diet.
- Eliminate white sugar and artificial sweeteners (aspartame) and use stevia.
- Avoid alcohol.

Other Recommendations

- Regular exercise, along with an excellent nutritional program and the addition of diabetic-specific nutrients, will help control insulin levels and promote healing (see Chapter 6). Studies have demonstrated that doing yoga every day for 40 days could normalize blood glucose levels and reduce medication.
- Have your physician check you for hypothyroidism. Supplementation with dessicated thyroid in those with hypothyroid can prevent, delay, or even reverse the complications associated with diabetes.
- A 1992 study conducted at the University of Wisconsin used biofeedback therapy and demonstrated success in improving blood flow to areas endangered by neuropathy (which could lead to amputation). It was also shown to control blood sugar.

DIARRHEA

Diarrhea is classified as frequent, loose, and watery stools accompanied by an extreme sense of urgency to get to the bathroom. It predominantly affects babies and young children, but we have all been affected at one time or another. Diarrhea is the leading cause of death in infants worldwide. In severe, prolonged diarrhea, body chemistry is disrupted.

Symptoms

Symptoms of diarrhea include frequent (more than three a day) bowel movements of watery stools and can be accompanied by cramps or abdominal pain. There may or may not be control of the bowel movements. Due to the amount of water passed, there is an increase in thirst. Sometimes a fever may be associated with it and in extreme cases there may be vomiting.

Causes

There are an abundance of causal factors that can contribute to diarrhea because it is not just an illness itself, but also a symptom of other illnesses such as cancer, diseased pancreas, irritable bowel syndrome, food allergies, grief, stress, Crohn's disease, colitis, or any other intestinal disorder. Food poisoning due to ingestion of uncooked meat, unripened fruit, or mishandling of food during preparation is quite common. When the body fights an infection of viruses, bacteria (E. coli, salmonella), or parasites, it may try expelling them as forcefully as it can.

Stress can cause waste to move through the intestines more rapidly than normal. Partially undigested food can also promote intestinal irritation promoting diarrhea. Foods or chemicals that the body is allergic to or cannot tolerate may be treated in the same manner. Another common instigator of diarrhea is a sudden change in the water we drink or food we eat because we are in a different country. This does not only occur when traveling through developing countries where sanitation may be an issue, but includes industrialized countries as well. Your body may be sensitive to differences in water purification methods.

Prescription for Health

NUTRIENT	DOSAGE	ACTION
Lactobacillus acidophilus	1 tsp (5 mL) twice daily containing 1–2 billion active organisms. Yogurt should be eaten every day unless there is an allergy to dairy products or lactose intolerance.	Increases friendly bacteria and reduces harmful bacteria
Teas containing tannin (green or organic black tea or red raspberry)	Drink strong clear tea throughout the day. Green tea contains theophylline, a muscle relaxant, reducing intestinal motility.	Slows and/or halts diarrhea
Bilberry	Standardized extract to 25 percent proanthocyanidins, 400 mg daily	High in tannins and anthocyanidins to restore bowel motility
Citrus seed extract	Two drops in ½ cup (125 mL) of water twice daily	Effective against parasite- or bacterial-induced diarrhea
Oil of oregano	Two drops in ½ cup (125 mL) water twice daily. My family uses oil of oregano when we travel to Mexico and no one gets Montezuma's revenge.	Effective against parasite- or bacterial-induced diarrhea

Health Tips to Enhance Healing

- The greatest danger with diarrhea is dehydration. Be sure that you drink plenty of water.
- To ease cramps and abdominal discomfort, drink herbal teas containing blackberry bark or root, fennel, chamomile, ginger, or raspberry leaf.
- Take digestive enzymes to ease the digestive process.
- Eat soluble fiber daily such as fresh apples, ground flaxseeds (2 Tbsp/30 mL), or cooked cereal to add bulk to the stools so they will travel more slowly through the intestines and minimize dehydration.

Other Recommendations

- A hot water bottle applied to the abdominal area can ease pain and cramping.

- Avoid dairy products—the enzyme to digest lactose is temporarily inhibited during diarrhea.
- Avoid eating foods that are difficult to digest such as fats. Bananas, rice, cooked potatoes, and applesauce are easy on the stomach. Do not drink apple juice as this can exacerbate the situation.
- Homeopathic remedies can be beneficial. *Sulfur* is for sudden diarrhea. *Podophyllum* is for watery stools. For diarrhea that is burning and aggravated at night, try *Arsenicum album*.
- If any of these symptoms are present, consult your physician: diarrhea is still present after two days, there is a fever over 101°F (38°C), stools are bloody or look like tar, there is severe rectal or abdominal pain, dehydration is visibly noticeable or urination has stopped.
- See Chapter 1 (carbohydrates and diarrhea) and related conditions, Candidiasis, Celiac Disease, Crohn's Disease, Diverticulitis, and Irritable Bowel Syndrome.

Health Fact

Anti-diarrhea medications are designed to plug you up by slowing the muscles of your intestines or by absorbing extra water. The toxins that your body is trying to eliminate will get absorbed along with the water; with regular use, these remedies will also change your body's natural rhythm of waste elimination by slowing things down and increasing the time food is left putrefying in the intestines.

DIVERTICULITIS

Diverticulitis is an inflammatory condition of the colon or large intestine whereby small pouch-like areas called diverticula are formed. These pouches become impacted with fecal matter and become inflamed and infected, causing pain and fever. Years of constipation weaken the mucous membranes of the colon and straining to pass hard stools produces the pouches. The pouches are not a problem until they become impacted and fecal matter putrefies, causing infection and inflammation. It is a common condition in those over 50. In severe cases, pouches can rupture, promoting infection in the abdominal cavity, which requires emergency treatment.

Symptoms

Typical symptoms of diverticulitis include cramps, nausea, constipation or diarrhea, and abdominal tenderness. You may feel tender on the left side of the abdomen, but are relieved from it by passing gas or having a bowel movement. If you have blood in the stool, advise your doctor immediately.

Causes

Constipation, stress, a poor diet high in fatty food and sugars while low in fiber, and obesity have the greatest influence on developing diverticulitis. Other conditions that can aggravate diverticulitis are allergies, gallbladder disease, and coronary artery disease.

Prescription for Health

The basis for treatment is fiber and dietary changes. There is an African expression: "Where the people have large stools, they have small hospitals."

NUTRIENT	DOSAGE	ACTION
Omega's Hi-Lignan Nutri-Flax	1–2 tsps (5–10 mL) daily with a high-fiber cereal	Soothes gut lining and promotes good elimination
Omega-3 fatty acid	1–2 Tbsp (15–30 mL) of flaxseed oil or 500 mg three times per day of fish oil (Eskimo-3)	Reduces inflammation of the intestinal lining and promotes elimination
Lactobacillus acidophilus	1 tsp (5 mL) twice daily containing 1–2 billion active organisms	Improves intestinal flora and reduces harmful bacteria
Moducare sterols and sterolins	One capsule three times daily	Reduces inflammation of the intestinal tract, improves walls of the venous system, increases T-cell activity to fight infection
Peppermint oil	One or two enteric-coated capsules three times daily between meals (0.2 mL active agent per capsule)	Reduces cramps, relaxes esophageal sphincter (reducing pressure from stomach), increases bile flow
Vitamin C	1–3 g daily	Stops inflammation, promotes healing of diverticula, strengthens colon wall

Health Tips to Enhance Healing

- If you suspect you have low stomach acid, see the introduction to this chapter.
- Take digestive enzymes before every meal. Do not drink while eating as it dilutes the enzymes.
- Follow a diet that is high in fiber and be sure to drink eight to ten glasses of pure, filtered water to prevent constipation (see Constipation). For every juice, alcoholic, or caffeinated beverage that you drink, add another glass of water.
- Do not eat foods that contain seeds until your digestive system is working well again. Eat all vegetables steamed until soft.
- For quick relief of constipation, magnesium oxide taken before bedtime will flush out your system the next morning. It turns stools to liquid and cleans trapped waste out of the small pockets in the intestines. Or take vitamin C to bowel tolerance (see page 94).

- Herbal teas can be soothing to an overactive stomach and an overactive mind. Taken alone or in combination, effective herbs include ginger, peppermint, fennel, valerian, and lemon balm.
- If symptoms are aggravated after a fatty meal, your bile production could be underactive; stimulate gastric juices with bitter herb teas such as dandelion, plantain, yarrow, wormwood, or gentian.

Other Recommendations

- Get tested for allergies (see Allergies).
- Get regular exercise to improve the flow of oxygen and blood, as well as to reduce weight.
- If you know that gallbladder or heart disease may be contributing to diverticulitis, see Gallstones and Gallbladder Disease or Heart Disease.

ECZEMA (ATOPIC DERMATITIS)

Eczema is predominantly an allergic condition whereby abnormalities in the immune system promote an overproduction of inflammatory and allergic reactions in the skin, and there is poor resistance to skin bacteria and viruses. It is estimated that 10 percent of North Americans suffer from eczema. It is common in infants and toddlers and often appears when children are teething or after they have been immunized. There are five types of eczema: atopic (allergic), infantile seborrheic, adult seborrheic, occupational irritant contact dermatitis, and allergic contact dermatitis.

Symptoms

Eczema is intensely itchy and the skin may be flaky, thick, or scaly; there may also be weeping, crusting, or a change in color. The skin inflammation commonly appears on the wrists, ankles, face, and the creases of the knees, ears, between the fingers, and elbows. Skin thickening often occurs due to scratching and rubbing the skin; bacterial or viral infections are also common.

Causes

Children are more likely to develop eczema if there is a history of asthma, eczema, or hay fever in the family. Triggers include stress, infections, and climate changes. Stress is a major factor in adult eczema flare-ups. Those with eczema often have allergies that have been confirmed by allergy tests and elevated IgE levels, as well as a family history of these conditions. Common allergens are food additives and preservatives, milk, eggs, wheat, soy, tomatoes, oranges, and peanuts. Eczema can be the result of other conditions such as candidiasis, leaky gut syndrome, and a lack of stomach acid. Severe essential fatty acid deficiency is also associated with the development of eczema, which inhibits the skin's ability to hold moisture properly.

In occupational irritant contact and allergic contact dermatitis, exposure to environmental allergens such metal alloys in zippers and jewelry, cosmetics, perfumes, rubber, latex, and poison ivy are the source of the problem. Infantile seborrhea is more commonly known as cradle cap and adult seborrhea is red, dry, flaky skin that may also appear as mild dandruff.

Prescription for Health

NUTRIENT	DOSAGE	ACTION
Moducare sterols and sterolins	One capsule three times daily. Birth to five years of age should take one capsule daily; five to twelve years of age should take two capsules daily; twelve years and older should take the adult dose.	Normalizes IgE, controls histamine release, regulates immune function, enhances the immune system's ability to fight bacteria and viruses, and regulates cortisol
Essential fatty acids, Eskimo-3, Udo's Choice Oil, Omega Essential Balance, or flaxseed oil, or evening primrose oil	Eskimo-3, 500 mg three times daily or 1–3 Tbsp (15–45 mL) daily of Udo's Choice, or Omega Essential Balance, or flaxseed oil, or lastly try evening primrose oil, 1,000 mg three times daily.	Controls inflammatory prostaglandins, ensures adequate EFA levels, maintains skin integrity
Multimune containing vitamins A, B_6, C, E, selenium, zinc, magnesium, lipoic acid, coenzyme Q10, reduced L-glutathione	Three capsules daily with food	Is anti-inflammatory, antiallergy, helps maintain skin integrity, has potent antioxidants, contains zinc needed to convert essential fatty acids
Kindervital by Flora Distributors (multivitamin for children)	Dosage as recommended	A liquid multivitamin with minerals for children to ensure adequate levels
Quercetin or grape seed extract	500 mg three times daily	Is anti-inflammatory, antiallergy, halts histamine release
Plant digestive enzyme	Two capsules with every meal	Aids digestion; those with eczema often have poor digestion, which increases allergic reactions

Health Tips to Enhance Healing

- See Allergies, Candidiasis, Thyroid, Leaky Gut Syndrome (and Malabsorption Syndrome).
- See "Allergy Detection and Elimination" in the introduction to this chapter.
- Have your thyroid checked. Low thyroid function impairs the immune system.

- Do not take immune boosters like echinacea that enhance macrophage function as they will increase inflammatory immune cells in the skin.
- Eat seven to ten half-cup servings of fruits and vegetables every day. If you haven't been eating raw veggies regularly, start with steamed; it is easier on the digestive system. Eat plenty of cold-water fish, dandelion greens (available at health food stores or pick in areas that are not sprayed by pesticides), and essential fatty acid-rich seed and nut oils. These foods help heal eczema.
- Avoid deep-fried foods, meat, food that is high in sugar and other refined carbohydrates (like white bread), caffeine, alcohol, and dairy products.
- If you suspect you have low stomach acid, see the introduction to this chapter.

Other Recommendations

- Use topical ointments that contain licorice (Simicort from Enzymatic Therapy), or Herbacort (a combination of cortisone-like herbs), and chamomile ointments (Camocare).
- Use hypoallergenic laundry detergents and rinse your bedding, towels, and clothing twice to eliminate detergent residue. Do not use fabric softeners or dryer sheets as these are often a source of skin irritation and allergy.
- Reduce stress. (See "The Immune System and Stress" in Chapter 3.)
- Drink eight to ten glasses of pure, filtered water a day.

Health Fact

Topical licorice (glycyrrhetinic acid) was better able to relieve symptoms of eczema when compared to cortisone ointments. Long-term use of cortisone ointments can cause serious side effects and skin thinning and they should not be used continuously. Avoid using them for small children and determine underlying allergies quickly before chronic skin inflammation occurs.

ENDOMETRIOSIS

The Endometriosis Association states that it is extremely rare that a woman in this day and age should ever need a hysterectomy for endometriosis, no matter how severe, yet three out of four gynecologists I visited said they would recommend a hysterectomy if they find extensive endometriosis during laparoscopy. I discovered this response when searching for a diagnosis for severe pelvic pain. The thought of a hysterectomy sent me searching for the cause of the intense pain I was experiencing. All my symptoms seemed to point to endometriosis. Finally, the fourth doctor I visited discussed diagnosis and treatment options with me without mentioning hysterectomy as a "cure." That was years ago and today I am still free of endometriosis.

Symptoms

Endometriosis is one of the most common yet misunderstood female diseases. Approximately 15 percent of women between the ages of 20 and 45 are affected with this painful and debilitating disorder. Symptoms can begin with the onset of menstruation and progressively increase with pending menopause. Dysmenorrhea (pain with menses), dyspareunia (pain with intercourse), and infertility may also be present. The pain some women experience can be devastating. Pain worse than childbirth was my only symptom, and strangely the pain radiated from my left hip into my back. Many women also experience pain when they have a full bladder or bowel. Some women experience no pain, but may have fertility, ovarian, or menstrual problems. The symptoms are many and vary from woman to woman.

Careful Diagnosis: Pelvic examinations by a highly skilled gynecologist may disclose nodules or lesions on the ovaries. Ultrasound tests will only show endometriosis if the ovaries are involved. Laparoscopy is the only diagnostic technique that can clearly determine if endometriosis is present. It is used not only to diagnose endometriosis but also if abnormal tissue is found, it will be removed to avoid having more than one surgery. This surgery, performed under general anesthetic, involves inserting a light-containing telescope through a small incision in your navel and another one or two small incisions along the bikini line for the instruments.

A laparoscopy is only as good as the surgeon who performs the exam. Removing all the endometriosis tissue requires a physician who is committed to biopsy and getting rid of all suspicious abnormalities. My surgeon was extremely meticulous and I was rid of endometriosis in one surgery.

Endometrial tissue can look like tiny blueberries or black spots, white, yellow, or reddish cysts, which can vary from blisters to large chocolate cysts up to 8 in (20 cm) in diameter. Only biopsy can confirm which tissue is truly endometriosis.

It is not uncommon for endometrial cells to grow on the ovaries, the fallopian tubes, the pelvic ligaments, the outer surface of the uterus, bladder, the large intestine, and the covering of the abdominal cavity. Women are often misdiagnosed with irritable bowel syndrome, bladder infections, appendix attack, "just" PMS, or painful cramps.

Cause

Until recently, the most predominant theory to explain the cause of endometriosis was that of retrograde menstrual flow. It was believed that blood flowing backward pushed tiny fragments of normal endometrial tissue (from the lining of the uterus) up the fallopian tubes where it took residence in the abdominal or pelvic cavity. Here this tissue acted as it would in the uterus in accordance with the monthly menstrual cycle. The blood often could not escape, however, and caused the formation of deposits and severe pain.

Our Immune System Is the Key: Other researchers believe that retrograde menstruation occurs, but only in women with altered immune function that allows the endometrial tissue to implant on other body areas. In other words, your immune system should not allow the endometrial tissue to survive where it does not belong. Once this abnormal tissue is present, the immune system may mount an antibody response and create inflammation and pain in the region involved.

New research points to a glitch in the immune system. Dr. David Redwine, world-renowned expert and director of the Endometriosis Program at St. Charles Medical Center in Bend, Oregon, believes that some women are born with abnormally located endometrial cells and that something goes astray with the immune system, causing the cells to become active. This theory has gained acceptance because endometrial implants have been found in the nose, lungs, and organs far from the uterus. Dr. Redwine has a web site where further information on his technique can be found (www.empnet.com/scmc/redwine.html) or phone 1-541-383-6904.

Environmental Pollutants Linked to Endometriosis: Convincing evidence has linked organochlorine exposure to the development of endometriosis. Organochlorines are highly persistent in our environment and do not break down, and toxic substances like DDT, PCP, and dioxins are estrogen mimickers, causing an increase in estrogens in the body. Endometriosis is thought to be higher in women who have higher than normal circulating estrogens. Carolyn De Marco, in her book *Take Charge of Your Body*, states that dioxins are a group of 75 chemicals used to make PVC plastics (our drinking water runs through pipes made from PVC in our homes), solvents, pesticides, refrigerants, and dioxins used in the pulp and paper industry. These same chemicals also persist in the fats of meat and dairy products. The EPA estimates that 90 percent of human dioxin exposure is through food, primarily meat and dairy products (see "Environmental Estrogens Linked to Increased Risk of Cancer," page 70).

Endometriosis is an insidious disorder, but it can be cured forever if you examine and reduce your stress levels, reduce the environmental toxins you are exposed to, and improve your nutrition. I stopped my endometriosis from recurring and you can too.

Seven Early Warning Symptoms of Endometriosis:

1. Menstrual cramps that increase in severity.
2. Intermenstrual pain, usually at mid-month.
3. Painful intercourse or dyspareunia.
4. Infertility of unknown origin.
5. You think you have bladder infection, but the test results are negative.
6. Pelvic pain that is all-encompassing.
7. History of ovarian cysts.

Prescription for Health

NUTRIENT	DOSAGE	ACTION
Natural progesterone cream	40–60 mg daily for day five to 28 (or whenever your normal cycle ends). I use ProgestaCare by Life Flo, which delivers 20 mg in a premeasured pump dose.	Limits the endometrial tissue buildup caused by estrogen.
Multimune containing vitamins A, B₆, C, E, selenium, magnesium, zinc, coenzyme Q10, lipoic acid, and reduced L-glutathione	Three capsules daily with food	Supports immune function, anti-inflammatory, reduces excess estrogens, controls cortisol, and regulates hormones
High-potency B-complex	Three capsules daily	Reduces the effects of stress, eases PMS symptoms, balances hormonal state, elevates mood, and controls fluid retention
Multimineral	One or two capsules daily or as directed	Required for enzymatic reactions in the body and to prevent deficiency.
Vitex (chaste tree berry)	40 drops of tincture twice daily	Relaxes the uterus and reduces cramps
Cramp bark tincture	½ tsp (2 mL) every two to four hours for acute pain	Relaxes the uterus and reduces cramps
Moducare sterols and sterolins	One capsule three times daily	Reduces inflammation, modulates cortisol

Health Tips to Enhance Healing

Find a skilled gynecologist willing to remove all of your endometriosis during laproscopy and then adopt all of the recommendations to ensure it does not return.

- Follow a vegetarian diet with no more than 20–25 g of fat each day from the good fats profiled in Chapter 4.

- The key to eliminating endometriosis is no dairy products. Dairy products promote the prostaglandins and leukotrienes, which cause inflammation and abdominal muscle cramps and pain. Dairy also contains circulating estrogens.
- Excess estrogens must be eliminated. Reduce your consumption of estrogens from pesticide-laden foods—buy organic foods whenever possible.
- Reduce stress in your life. Working women with Type A personalities are the most prone to endometriosis. Women who are constantly under stress from their job, family pressures, and personal expectations are at higher risk for developing endometriosis. In Tori Hudson's book *The Women's Encyclopedia of Natural Medicine*, she states that "Baboons who developed endometriosis in captivity were found to have higher stress levels and a decreased ability to react to stress compared to those in the wild, suggesting a stress factor."
- Get regular exercise to ensure that circulation in the pelvic area is restored. If you sit all day, your lower abdomen becomes congested.
- A special endometriosis tea formula was developed by herbalist Rosemary Slick. A healthy liver is essential for hormonal regulation because it converts active ovarian estrogen (estradiol) into the safer form (estriol). She recommends that women with endometriosis drink three to four cups of this tea per day for four to six months.

ENDO-TEA

3 parts dandelion root
3 parts wild yam root
2 parts burdock root
2 parts pau d'arco bark
1 part vitex berries
1 part Oregon grape root
½ part dong quai root
Sassafras, cinnamon, orange peel, and ginger to taste

Combine herbs. Fill a large pot with 4 cups (1 L) of cold water. Add 4–6 Tbsp (60–90 mL) of the herb mixture. Simmer over low heat for 20 minutes. Strain. You can find these ingredients at your local health food store.

Other Recommendations

- See "Environmental Estrogens Linked to Increased Risk of Cancer," page 70.

- Do not use bleached paper products containing dioxins (estrogen mimickers). This includes toilet paper, sanitary napkins, and especially tampons.
- Do not use plastic containers to store food or water. They contain estrogen mimickers. Do not microwave in plastic as the estrogens leach into the food.
- Castor oil packs are excellent at controlling pain. Take six pieces of flannel soaked in castor oil (damp but not dripping) about the size of the area you want to treat and place over the lower abdomen. Put a hot water bottle wrapped in a towel on top for 30 to 45 minutes several times a day. This will not only relieve pain but also improve circulation in the pelvic area. Castor oil packs work well for many types of pain and congestion; place the pack over any painful area.

Drug Side Effects

Because of the hormone connection, medical therapy for endometriosis has concentrated on altering a woman's hormonal chemistry with drugs. These drugs include Danazol, gonadotropin-releasing hormones (GnRH) such as Nafarelin, and birth control pills.

Drugs can be successful in alleviating endometrial symptoms (although they won't eliminate the condition), but not without side effects. They include acne, breast reduction, depression, oily skin, appearance of facial hair, and weight gain. Some may induce menopausal symptoms such as lowered libido, vaginal dryness, hot flashes, and a loss in bone density. No drug can cure the disease. Upon withdrawal, the endometriosis symptoms return. Holistic treatment that allows the body to heal itself is more effective and much safer.

FIBROCYSTIC BREAST SYNDROME

With the fear of breast cancer so prevalent today, breast lumps are a concern for many women. Fibrocystic breast syndrome (FBS), also called cystic mastitis, is a common non-cancerous condition. It can be mildly uncomfortable to severely painful, especially when breasts become swollen. Fluid that has not been drained via the lymphatic system fills in small spaces within the breast. The fluid is then encapsulated by fibrous tissue and thickens like scar tissue. The cysts may swell before and during menstruation. Although it does not increase your risk of cancer, it may make detecting cancerous tumors difficult through breast self-exams.

Twenty to 40 percent of women who are premenopausal (between the ages of 30 and 50) experience FBS with the symptoms generally disappearing after menopause. It is affected by the rise and fall of monthly female hormones.

Symptoms

Breasts are a mixture of fat, glands, and connective tissue, so their texture will always be irregular. Breast tissues are affected by a woman's monthly hormonal cycle. During the cycle milk-secreting glands enlarge with fluid and their cells multiply. Most of the excess fluid is reabsorbed or drained by the lymphatic system. This occurs month after month and year after year. In some women this process causes fibrous tissue to develop into lumps. Symptoms include breast tenderness and swelling and a lumpy feeling to the breast.

It can be very distressing to feel these lumps. The Mammastatin Serum Assay to detect breast cancer (see page 181), infrared breast scans, and/or ultrasound can help allay your fears of breast cancer to rest. If a breast lump is discovered, have your physician assess it and don't worry—most lumps are benign. Report the following to your physician immediately: lumps that suddenly grow larger and don't change with your menstrual cycle, discharge from your nipple, severe unrelenting pain, or puckered or dimpled skin.

Causes

FBS occurs when there is excess estrogen or an imbalance in estrogen to progesterone in the body due to stress, estrogen-replacement therapy, and xenoestrogens. It is also seen in young women with irregular periods. Lumps may come and go with symptoms often disappearing after menstruation has passed and hormone levels return to normal. Because of its timing, it is considered a symptom of PMS. It is not considered a major risk factor for or precursor to breast cancer.

Heavy coffee consumption has been linked to FBS along with a diet high in "bad" fats. As well, being overweight is a risk factor for FBS.

Prescription for Health

NUTRIENT	DOSAGE	ACTION
Multivitamin with minerals	Three capsules daily	Ensure adequate nutrient status
Vitamin E	200 IU twice daily	Alleviates breast tenderness
Multimune containing Vitamins A, B_6, C, E, selenium, zinc, magnesium, lipoic acid, Q10, reduced L-gluthatione	Three capsules daily	Protects against environmental toxins, is anti-inflammatory, and supports immune function
High-potency B-complex	Two capsules daily	Regulates estrogens, is a natural diuretic, reduces PMS symptoms
Iodine or kelp	Shake kelp on food; use iodine as directed	Important for thyroid activity. Deficiency of iodine promotes FBS symptoms.
Vitex (chaste tree berry)	40 drops of tincture twice daily	Balances estrogen to progesterone hormones

NUTRIENT	DOSAGE	ACTION
Evening primrose oil	Six 500 mg capsules daily	Is anti-inflammatory, controls negative prostaglandins involved in pain and inflammation
Natural progesterone cream	20 mg from day five to 28 days or until period begins	Restores progesterone level and alleviates estrogen dominant symptoms
Women's Whey protein powder	One scoop per day	Ensures adequate amino acids and protein for cell repair
Moducare sterols and sterolins	One capsule three times daily	Decreases inflammation, promotes proper immune function, reduces cortisol

Health Tips to Enhance Healing

- To reduce estrogen levels, follow a vegetarian diet and increase your soy intake. Fiber carries estrogen out of the body.
- Increase intake of seaweed and seafood as a natural source of iodine.
- Detoxification and elimination of waste is very important. Eat liver-friendly foods such as lemons, onions, garlic, leeks, kale, carrots, beets, artichokes, and members of the cabbage family (broccoli, Brussels sprouts, cauliflower).
- Avoid caffeine, chocolate, black tea, and cola drinks as they contain methylxanthines that cause FBS.
- Treat constipation to ensure elimination of toxins (see Constipation).

Other Recommendations

Have the Mammastatin Serum Assay blood test to rule out breast cancer. See page 181 for more information.
- Exercise regularly to improve circulation, help the detoxify your body, and manage weight.
- Rule out low thyroid (see page 22 for a home thyroid test).
- Do self-exams monthly to familiarize yourself with your breasts so that you are able to detect subtle changes such as thickening, lumps, etc., and when they occur or disappear.
- Avoid antiperspirants as they clog up drainage from the sweat glands and the toxins have to drain back into the breast.
- Massaging your breasts in a circular motion will improve lymph flow and circulation, while at the same time familiarizing you with their architecture. Make it a daily ritual, either during your morning shower or before you go to bed.
- To control pain use castor oil packs (see Endometriosis for how-to information).

Health Fact

Dr. John Lee stated in his book *What Your Doctor May Not Tell You About Menopause* that in every case where he prescribed natural progesterone, there was a positive outcome.

FIBROIDS (UTERINE)

Uterine fibroids (or myomas) are round, firm, benign growths on either the interior or exterior wall of the uterus. These growths are comprised of connective tissue and smooth muscle bundles and can be small (like a pea) or large (like a grapefruit), but the average size is like an egg. They usually appear in groups, not singularly, and sometimes they affect the cervix as well. Most fibroids grow slowly; if they grow quickly, they could be malignant. Roughly 20 to 30 percent of women will have fibroids at some time. They have a tendency to form eight to ten years prior to menopause.

When women go to see their doctor about fibroids, the approach conventional medicine takes is to suggest a hysterectomy. However, removing the entire uterus because of fibroids is an extreme measure. Skilled surgeons can remove the fibroids without damaging the uterus (called a myomectomy). In many cases, surgically removed tumors will return if lifestyle changes are not adopted. Lupron, a drug, has been used to promote menopause, causing fibroids to shrink small enough for surgical removal.

Tori Hudson, ND, has stated that in her practice, fibroids are the most difficult cases to treat with naturopathy, although there are notable isolated success stories. Her aim is to treat the symptoms, attempt to control the condition until menopause, and identify if the situation has progressed to where conventional treatment is appropriate. In North America over 750,000 hysterectomies are performed annually, and fibroids are the main reason for this surgery.

Symptoms

Often fibroids go undetected until they are discovered during a regular pelvic exam. For those who do experience symptoms, their periods can be heavy, irregular, or painful, or there can be bleeding between periods. Anemia, fatigue, and weakness are usually present due to the blood loss. There may also be an increase in vaginal discharge, frequent urination, pain during sex, or bleeding afterwards.

Complications can occur if the location or weight of the fibroids puts pressure on the bowels, bladder, or urethra, causing obstructions. Urinary function may be compromised, pregnancy may be jeopardized, or the uterus may drop years later when the pelvic support weakens. There may also be pain in the pelvis, back, or legs. Once a woman is in menopause, fibroids tend to shrink and symptoms disappear.

Causes

Studies have shown that women who eat a diet high in red meat and ham have more uterine fibroids than those who eat a diet rich in fruits and vegetables. Uterine fibroids develop because of estrogen dominance—estrogen stimulates cells to grow, while progesterone inhibits them. Women exposed to xenoestrogens, Type-A personalities, and those under severe stress are often estrogen dominant.

Prescription for Health

NUTRIENT	DOSAGE	ACTION
Multivitamin with minerals and iron	Two or three capsules daily	Protects against nutritional deficiency; if anemic, ensure the formula contains iron
High-potency B-complex	Two or three capsules daily	Regulates hormones, treats anemia from excessive bleeding
Magnesium	400 mg daily	Regulates estrogen
Methionine and inositol	500 mg of each twice daily	Amino acid helps to break down fats, helps eliminate excess estrogens.
Evening primrose oil	500 mg twice daily	Regulates hormones, reduces bleeding
Shepherd's purse	50 drops three times daily	Works together with evening primrose oil to reduce bleeding
DIM (diindolylmethane)	100–200 mg daily	Removes excess estrogens; 300 mg daily has improved fat burning in women
Natural progesterone	20 mg per day from day five to 28	Controls excess estrogen
Vitex (chaste tree berry)	40 drops daily	Balances estrogen to progesterone, reduces circulating estrogens
Omega's Hi-Lignan Flax	1–2 tsps (5–10 mL) daily with two to four glasses of water.	Removes excess estrogens
Moducare sterols and sterolins	One capsule three times daily	Modulates cortisol, our stress hormone, decreases inflammation, and regulates immune function, protects against the effects of stress
Women's Whey Soy Formula	One scoop daily	Soy contains phytoestrogens that balance estrogen by binding to and blocking estrogen receptors if estrogen levels are too high or enhance uptake of estrogen if too low.
Multimune, containing Vitamins A, B_6, C, E, zinc, selenium, magnesium, lipoic acid, Q10, and reduced L-glutathione	Three capsules daily with food	Is antioxidant, anti-inflammatory, eliminates toxins, protects against stress, and supports immune function

Health Tips to Enhance Healing

- Detoxification and elimination of waste is very important. Eat liver-friendly foods such as kale, carrots, beets, artichokes, lemons, onions, garlic, leeks, and members of the cabbage family (broccoli, Brussels sprouts, cauliflower).
- Follow a vegetarian diet and increase your soy and fiber intake. Fiber carries estrogen out of the body. Avoid meat products (except fish). Your diet should concentrate on whole grains, fresh fruits, and vegetables. Choose organic foods whenever possible to reduce the burden of xenoestrogens from pesticides.
- Avoid alcohol, dairy products, caffeine (including medications), sugar, chocolate, coffee, black tea, and soft drinks. Alcohol interferes with liver function and caffeine exacerbates the growths.
- There are many beneficial herbs to aid in detoxification, such as milk thistle, dandelion root, Chinese skullcap, and turmeric rhizome.

Other Recommendations

- Lose extra pounds—being overweight can increase effects of estrogen on the uterus. Exercise regularly to burn calories, improve circulation, and help the detoxification and elimination process. See Chapter 6 if you haven't been active in a while.
- Reduce stress, get plenty of sleep, and practice relaxation techniques such as visualization, biofeedback, qigong, yoga, and deep breathing exercises.
- Castor oil packs are excellent at controlling pain. Take six pieces of flannel soaked in castor oil (damp but not dripping) about the size of the area you want to treat. Place them over the area and put a towel-wrapped hot water bottle on top. Use the pack two to four times per week.
- Do not take estrogen medications, including the birth control pill.
- Avoid constipation (see Constipation).

FIBROMYALGIA

Almost 16 million North Americans suffer from fibromyalgia (FM), a multi-system disorder and common rheumatic syndrome that has also been referred to as the "invisible illness" because of its difficulty in being diagnosed. The name fibromyalgia is rooted in Latin: *fibro* meaning supportive tissue; *myo* for muscle; and *algia* for pain. The hallmark of fibromyalgia is the widespread pain throughout the muscles, stiffness, and chronic aching.

It affects women more than men and usually strikes between the ages of 30 to 60 years. It accounts for 15 to 30 percent of all visits to rheumatologists.

The pain of FM is thought to be caused by a tightening and thickening of the thin film of tissue that holds muscles together. A diagnosis of FM will be confirmed if your doctor finds pain or tenderness in 11 out of 18 trigger points located in the knees, hips, rib cage, shoulder, and neck.

Many of the symptoms of FM overlap with those of chronic fatigue syndrome (CFS). The main symptom difference between the two is profound fatigue in CFS and muscle pain in FM. Treatments for chronic fatigue syndrome focus on eliminating viruses that may be causing the fatigue, whereas FM treatments look at reducing the inflammatory factors that cause the pain and swelling of joints and muscles. Due to the many symptoms of FM and chronic fatigue, a combination of therapies may be required to get the conditions under control. (See treatments for Chronic Fatigue Syndrome as well.)

Symptoms

The symptoms of FM are varied and highly individualistic. They can include allergies, anxiety, mental confusion, fatigue, dysmenorrhea, ridged fingernails, stiffness, inability to exercise, gastrointestinal problems, depression, mood swings, headaches, irritation caused by light, sound, or odors, dizziness, anxiety, mental confusion, heart palpitations, sleep disturbances, carpal tunnel syndrome, excessively sensitive skin, swollen joints, total body aches, and pain. Non-restorative sleep is a major symptom where those affected sleep but never feel rested.

When people describe their muscle fatigue, they liken it to shoveling snow or gardening for days without a break, or as if the muscles are being stretched and torn. The unique nature of each person's symptoms makes FM difficult to diagnose. Many tests—including urine, blood, CAT scan, magnetic resonance imaging, X ray, and others—may still not indicate what is wrong with the person and often sufferers are referred to psychiatrists. Life becomes unbearable for those living with FM. It can also be difficult for family and friends to understand this disease.

Causes

No single cause can be pinpointed, but it is believed that multiple stressors, a traumatic emotional or physical event, and depressive episodes that upset the functioning of the immune system contribute to the disorder. It is suspected that there is a connection between FM and chronic fatigue syndrome as those with FM usually have a history of extreme, relentless fatigue. Viruses such as Epstein Barr or a fungus like *Candida albicans* may be factors. Heavy metal and chemical toxicity, as well as nutritional deficiencies, are also major players in the progression of FM. Allergies are also thought to be contributing factors in FM as well, and they must be diagnosed and eliminated to allow healing. Low serotonin levels and low DHEA are also seen in those with FM. Physicians must treat each symptom individually in order to eliminate this disorder.

Sterols, Sterolins, and Fibromyalgia

Sterols and sterolins should be the basis for your FM recovery program because they regulate the immune factor. Many FM sufferers have found that none of the supplements they try work. There is a good reason for this. FM is made worse by the release of interleukin-6, which causes pain and inflammation, and unless we turn off this powerful inflammatory immune factor, we are not getting to the root of the problem. Once we turn off IL-6 with sterols and sterolins, the other nutrients can do their job. Sterols and sterolins also modulate cortisol. As mentioned earlier, high cortisol levels cause our immune systems to secrete inflammatory factors, and high cortisol also causes our DHEA to drop. Those with FM generally have very low DHEA levels. DHEA is an important anti-inflammatory hormone that reduces pain effectively. Sterols and sterolins increase DHEA as they are also precursors to pregnenolone with which the body then makes DHEA.

Prescription for Health

NUTRIENT	DOSAGE	ACTION
Moducare sterols and sterolins	Two capsules three times daily for one week, then one capsule three times daily thereafter for maintenance	Controls inflammation, regulates cortisol, enhances DHEA, is antiallergy.
Magnesium (either or a combination of citrate, fumarate, glycinate, malate, succinate, or aspartate)	200 mg three times daily	Needed for 300 enzymatic reactions, calms and supports muscle function
Multimune containing vitamins A, B₆, C, E, selenium, zinc, magnesium, coenzyme Q10, reduced L-glutathione, and lipoic acid	Three capsules daily with food	Is antiallergy, anti-inflammatory, contains potent antioxidants
5-HTP	100 mg three times daily	Increases serotonin levels, reduces anxiety, muscle pain, improves sleep and early morning stiffness, enhances mood, controls appetite
St. John's wort, standardized with 0.3 percent hypericin	100–300 mg three times daily	Effective for depression and enhances serotonin levels. Do not take with prescription antidepressants without medical supervision.

NUTRIENT	DOSAGE	ACTION
Valerian	Use as directed	Improves sleep, calms nerves
Malic acid	1200–2000 mg daily	Detoxifies the body of aluminum and reduces pain of FM, works synergistically with magnesium
Melatonin	1–3 mg per night	Improves sleep
Women's Whey protein powder	One scoop daily	Ensures adequate amino acids for cell repair
L-carnitine	500 mg daily	Improves energy production and eliminates fatigue

Health Tips to Enhance Healing

- See related conditions, including Candidiasis, Chronic Fatigue Syndrome, Depression, Leaky Gut Syndrome (and Malabsorption Syndrome), and Toxic Metal Poisoning.
- A balanced diet of fresh fruits and vegetables, healthy oils, nuts, seeds, whole grains, and fresh wild fish is essential in fighting FM. Eat smaller meals more frequently throughout the day to maintain blood sugar levels.
- Avoid processed, refined foods, which are high in sugar, salt, and hydrogenated fat.
- Drink eight to ten glasses of pure, filtered water daily. For every beverage (other than herbal tea) that you consume, drink another glass of water.
- Eliminate alcohol, cigarettes, and caffeine.
- Get regular exercise, but don't overexert yourself. Gentle moderate exercise improves your circulation and enhances your mood and overall well-being. Even walking to your mailbox or sitting in a chair and raising your arms and legs can be beneficial.
- Watch your weight. Research has shown that one-third of people who are overweight have disrupted immunity.

Other Recommendations

- Laugh! Rent videos, see a stand-up comic, and hang around funny friends. Laughter and exercise can improve mood. Keep a positive frame of mind.
- Ensure adequate rest.
- Practice deep-breathing exercises (see Chapter 7) to ensure sufficient oxygen intake.
- Detoxification is extremely important. A sauna allows toxins to excrete from the skin; dry brushing before a shower or bath will increase circulation and stimulate lymph flow; and internal herbal

cleanses, combined with fiber, will eliminate waste from the intestines and support the liver and kidneys. Have an Epsom salts and baking soda bath every night (1 cup/250 mL of each in a bath run through your shower filter to ensure you are not soaking in chlorinated water).

- See "Allergy Detection and Elimination" in the introduction of this chapter.
- Have dental amalgams removed and reduce your toxic load (see Toxic Metal Poisoning).
- Massage, acupuncture, and chiropractics treatments can help speed healing.
- When you are having a bad day, rest. On your good days, enjoy them to their fullest without overexerting yourself.

Stefan Kuprowski, ND and director of the Ecomed Wellness Clinic, treats many FM patients. He believes that FM is a curable condition. "It requires a person to take responsibility for their own healing; to seek the right professional help and therapies; transform their attitude towards the illness from curse to an incredible opportunity for growth and self-trans-formation. He says, that since there are multiple causes to this illness, there are multiple cures. What works for one person, may not work for another due to biochemical individuality. Do not give up, the most important gift is the power of faith. Faith in the healing process and faith in oneself to heal."

FUNGAL INFECTIONS

Infections from fungi are quite common and can affect any part of the skin, especially moist areas with inadequate air circulation and folds and creases.

Symptoms

Fungal infections are itchy and the infected area is raised and inflamed. The itching is persistent, leading to flaky irritations and little moist, red blisters. The skin can soften and peel away. Depending where the infection is located, it can be painful as well. Infections can be located on the scalp (tinea capitis) and calloused areas of the feet (athlete's foot), in the mouth (thrush), on the nails (paronychia), groin (jock itch), posterior (diaper rash), nipples, and in the vagina (candida; see Candidiasis).

If the infection is on the nipples or in a baby's mouth, an alternating routine of infection can transpire between mother and child. Thrush is noticeable by a white creamy coating on the tongue and in the mouth. Nail infections can be difficult to treat if there is spreading underneath the nail.

Ringworm is another fungal infection that occurs on the scalp or skin, with red spots that grow to about a quarter of an inch in diameter. The centers heal first, leaving raised borders that are like scaly, red rings.

Causes

Although fungal infections are very contagious, they develop only if there is an underlying vulnerability to them brought on by a weakened immune system. Antibiotic use kills the good bacteria that promote a healthy immune system and good infection-fighting ability. Infections are more prevalent when the pH balance of the body is upset, which is easily done by using certain cosmetics, perfumed products and creams, or removing the skin's natural protective oils by bathing too much. Poor diet, illness, oral contraceptives, obesity, and excessive sweating are also contributing factors.

Prescription for Health

See Candidiasis and Influenza for treatment recommendations to enhance immunity to fight fungal infections from within.

NUTRIENT	DOSAGE	ACTION
Oil of oregano	Three drops two to three times daily in water or juice. Apply topically to affected nails.	Acts as an antifungal
Garlic (odorless)	Three capsules daily or two cloves of fresh garlic with meals	Acts as an antifungal
Lactobacillus acidophilus	1 tsp (5 mL) daily of 1–2 billion active organisms	Restores good bacteria to the intestines
Tea tree oil	Add a few drops to shampoo or soap and wash as usual (five or six drops per ounce), or use topical oil diluted directly on infected area.	Is antifungal and heals dandruff
Moducare sterols and sterolins	One capsule three times daily	Increases T-cell activity to fight fungus, reduces inflammation, restores immune function

Health Tips to Enhance Healing

- Get plenty of sleep and rest.
- Reduce sugar intake—even natural sugars like honey, maple syrup, and fruit—because they will suppress the immune system's ability to fight fungus, bacteria, viruses, and *Candida albicans*.

Other Recommendations

- Wash thoroughly and often, and avoid touching the face, mouth, nose, and eyes. Keep affected areas dry and expose to air as much as possible.
- Wear loose cotton clothing whenever possible and do not use towels or clothing more than once without washing them between uses.
- Topical ointments that contain oil of oregano, licorice, or tea tree oil are very healing.
- For nail infections, soak hands or feet in a 50/50 solution of water and white distilled vinegar with a few drops of tea tree oil for 15 minutes every day.
- Do not lend hairbrushes or toothbrushes to others. Change them every four months to prevent contamination.
- Avoid spreading the infection by touching infected areas and then healthy areas.
- Athlete's foot is common in community showers and swimming pools, so wear waterproof sandals while walking around these areas.
- Pets can carry fungi. Wash your hands after petting or handling pets.
- If fungal infection appears to worsen in spite of treatment, or if there is fever, swelling, and redness, a bacterial infection may have developed as well. See your physician.

GALLSTONES AND GALLBLADDER DISEASE

The gallbladder plays a pivotal role in digestion. It stores the bile created by the liver and releases it to the intestines to aid in the digestion of fats and fat-soluble vitamins. Bile also carries excess cholesterol from the body. Gallstones are like little rocks composed of cholesterol that can irritate the inner lining of the gallbladder and block the passage from the liver to the intestines. Their size varies greatly, from as small as a grain of sand to as big as a golf ball.

Symptoms

Gallstones can become life threatening when they leave the gallbladder and plug up ducts to other organs. Most gallstones have no symptoms, but when symptoms begin, the upper right area of the abdomen may become tender and pain may become gradually worse over time. The gallbladder will swell and become inflamed, inducing a fever and nausea severe enough to make you vomit. Like appendicitis, this attack can be fatal if not quickly addressed. Gas, bloating, heartburn, and pain may be experienced prior to an attack.

Causes

Bile is made up of water, calcium, fatty acids, and phospholipids. If there is too much cholesterol in the bile, the cholesterol begins to crystallize and more cholesterol will adhere to it until it forms a stone. When the stone becomes large enough, it can get stuck in the bile duct and symptoms precipitate. In 25 percent of gallstone cases, the cause is too much calcium.

Diet has a major influence on gallstones and for the most part they can be easily prevented. Gallstones are caused by a diet high in fat and simple carbohydrates and low in fiber. Extra weight, lack of exercise, drinking insufficient amounts of water for digestion, high coffee consumption, and food allergies all contribute to gallstone formation. Insufficient amounts of hydrochloric acid in the stomach can prevent proper digestion, leading to gallstones. Twice as many women as men develop gallstones and we know that estrogen plays a role. As well, women who are obese have at least double the risk of developing gallstones compared to thin women.

Prescription for Health

NUTRIENT	DOSAGE	ACTION
Multimune containing vitamins A, B$_6$, C, E, magnesium, zinc, lipoic acid, coenzyme Q10, reduced L-gluthatione, and selenium	Three capsules daily with meals	Important for immune support; deficiency of vitamin C and E promotes cholesterol gallstones. Other nutrients promote proper detoxification in the liver.
Taurine	1000 mg twice daily	Necessary for bile acid formation and dissolves small cholesterol stones
Lecithin	1000 mg three times daily	Decreases bile cholesterol and stone size
Lipotropic factors, choline and inositol	Two capsules daily	Helps metabolize cholesterol and fats
Turmeric	1000 mg twice daily	Stimulates gallbladder contractions and bile flow thus preventing gallstones; is approved by the German Commission E for gallbladder disease (not for use in cases with painful gallstones)
Artichoke	1–2 Tbsp (15–30 mL) of artichoke tonic daily or eat artichokes often	Increases bile
Ginger	2 or 3 cups (500 or 750 mL) of freshly grated ginger tea in place of coffee, or ginger capsules as needed	Reduces nausea
Milk thistle	420 mg daily for 30 days. Ensure you purchase a standardized extract	Minimizes stone formation by keeping bile liquid

NUTRIENT	DOSAGE	ACTION
Peppermint oil (enteric-coated capsules)	One or two capsules with meals three times daily (0.2 mL peppermint oil per capsule)	Assists in dissolving stones
Moducare sterols and sterolins	One capsule three times daily	Decreases inflammation, controls cortisol, regulates immune function

Health Tips to Enhance Healing

- Modify diet to include plenty of fresh fruits and vegetables (seven to ten half-cup servings). Apples, beets, black radish, and green leafy vegetables are especially beneficial to the gallbladder. Plain yogurt is good for building up good bacteria in the intestines; eat fresh fish instead of fatty red meat and avoid simple carbohydrates like commercial baked goods and sugar cereals. Eliminate greasy fried and processed foods.
- If the gallbladder is inflamed, avoid solid food for a few days and drink plenty of water. You may add apple, beet, and pear juices gradually and drink for three days. Then to prepare yourself for solid foods, you may eat uncooked applesauce prepared in a blender at home and raw, shredded beets with olive oil and lemon juice.
- Rule out low stomach acid. See the introduction to this chapter.
- Take digestive enzymes before a meal to help in the digestive process.
- Drink at least eight to ten glasses of pure, filtered water daily. For every juice or beverage with caffeine that you drink, add another cup of water. Do not drink while eating. Fluids dilute the strength of the digestive enzymes.
- Reduce alcohol consumption.
- Avoid legumes. One research study showed that legumes increased bile cholesterol saturation up to 169 percent.
- Eliminate coffee as it can cause the gallbladder to spasm.

Other Recommendations

- Ask for a referral to an allergy specialist and get tested for possible triggers. (See "Allergy Detection and Elimination" in the introduction to this chapter.)
- Lose extra pounds. Carefully managed weight loss by eating smaller portions of nutritious food and moderate exercise has been shown to alleviate symptoms associated with gallstones. Regular exercise can reduce the likelihood of forming gallstones.
- Extreme restriction of calories, yo-yo dieting, or fasting can increase gallstone formation.

- If you smoke, quit. Smoking constricts the arteries and causes the gallbladder to contract.
- Acupuncture can be very beneficial to an ailing gallbladder.
- During a gallstone attack, consume a glass of pure apple juice (not from concentrate) with 1 Tbsp (15 mL) of apple cider. Symptoms should subside long enough to seek medical attention to rule out heart problems or gastroesophogeal reflux disease.
- Before agreeing to surgery, talk with your physician to find out if it is absolutely necessary. Eighty percent of cases have no symptoms and do not need treatment. In some cases, non-invasive techniques may be an option.

Health Fact

An observational study published in the *British Medical Journal* was done to see if breakfast had an effect on gallstones. Women who ate breakfast were less likely to have gallstones than women who skipped breakfast or had only coffee.

GINGIVITIS

Gingivitis is a swelling or inflammation of the gum tissue. If gingivitis is not corrected, 30 percent of all cases will become periodontitis, a condition where the bacteria has spread from the gums to the bones, possibly resulting in lost teeth, an eroded jaw bone, and the need for dental surgery.

In the past gingivitis has not caused much concern, but a study conducted in 1998 found that compared to men with healthy gums, men with gum disease were four and a half times more likely to have heart disease. The connection is thought to come from the bacteria entering the bloodstream through the gums. Another study discovered that people with gum disease had 50 percent more plaque buildup in their carotid arteries than in people with healthy gums. Plaque buildup is a major risk factor for stroke. In June 2000 it was announced that a study observing 1000 pregnant women discovered premature deliveries were eight times more likely if they had gum disease.

Symptoms

The gums become bright red, tender, swollen, and will bleed readily. Gum tissue withdraws from the teeth and leads to receding gums. Continual bad breath may be present.

Causes

Bacteria that has not been removed by brushing and flossing sits under the gum line and eventually leads to infection. Other factors that can contribute to gingivitis are smoking, brushing too hard, dental work that is too loose, nutritional deficiencies, stress, a weakened immune system, and diets that are high in refined carbohydrates and sugar. Veterans who suffer from post-traumatic stress have a higher rate of gum disease, including gingivitis.

Elevated hormones during pregnancy exaggerate the body's response to plaque in the mouth, thus increasing the likelihood of getting gingivitis. If good oral hygiene is practiced, this should not become a problem. Diabetics are known to be more prone to gingivitis than non-diabetics. However, when diabetes is well controlled, gingivitis is kept in check.

Prescription for Health

NUTRIENT	DOSAGE	ACTION
Multimune containing vitamins A, B$_6$, C, E, selenium, zinc, magnesium, coenzyme Q10, lipoic acid, reduced L-glutathione	Three capsules daily with food	Enhances immune function to fight bacteria, halts inflammation, is potent antioxidant; contains 30 mg of coenzyme Q10, which is known to support and heal gum tissue
Oil of oregano	Three drops three times daily	Antibacterial and antifungal
Tea tree oil mouthwash	Gargle and swish twice daily	Antibacterial and antifungal
Goldenseal	20 drops daily ensure an 8 to 10 percent berberine content	Acts as an antibacterial
Cranberry juice (nonsweetened)	Drink throughout the day	Prevents bacteria from sticking to the teeth and gums
Sage tea	Drink throughout the day	Soothes inflamed gums, is antioxidant and anti-inflammatory
Moducare sterols and sterolins	One capsule three times daily	Regulates immune function, enhances bacteria fighting ability, decreases inflammation and reduces the effects of stress

Health Tips to Enhance Healing

- Visit your dentist once every six months to remove hidden plaque in hard-to-reach areas.
- Chew gum containing baking soda. It helps eliminate plaque and reduce gingivitis.
- Floss at least once every two days to remove plaque buildup under the gum line.
- When you brush your teeth, don't forget about your tongue. Either brush it or use a tongue scraper to remove the bacteria that are hiding in the mucous coating.

- Drink eight to ten glasses of pure, filtered water daily. For every juice, alcoholic, or caffeinated beverage that you drink, add another glass of water.
- Eat a well-balanced diet that focuses on natural, whole foods such as whole grains, fresh fruits and vegetables, legumes, nuts and seeds, and fresh fish. Avoid processed and refined foods that are high in sugar, white flour, and bad fats.

Other Recommendations

- Stop smoking. Tobacco leaves a film of tar on the tongue, teeth, and gums that can make infections worse and delay healing. It can also lead to oral cancer.
- If flossing is impossible to incorporate into your nightly routine, there is a toothbrush called Sonicare that emits acoustic energy. It cleans in areas once only reachable by flossing.
- When you can't brush, try fizzy tablets that have sodium bicarbonate, citric acid, and silicon dioxide. They bubble up to remove leftover food particles. Or use a toothpick.
- Oral piercings increase the risk of infection, so extra attention should be paid to oral hygiene.

Health Fact

Gingivitis was a common occurrence among soldiers during World War I and so it earned the nickname "Trench Mouth." The general belief was that it was caused by poor hygiene practices. While poor hygiene is a major cause, stress should not be overlooked as an important factor. Stress depresses the immune system and prevents it from reacting to the bacteria in a quick and efficient way.

GOUT

Gout's distinguishing symptom is an excruciatingly painful big toe, but it can also affect other joints. It is a common type of arthritis that affects mostly men and arises when there is a buildup of uric acid in the body that crystallizes in the joints. Uric acid is a by-product of protein metabolism, especially from eating foods high in purines, including organ meats, beans, legumes, beer, and wine. If there is too much uric acid left in the blood, it is excreted to the joints, tissues, kidneys, and tendons where it causes inflammation. Gout comes and goes and its duration can vary from a few days to a few weeks depending on how intense the causal factors were.

Pseudo gout, officially known as calcium pyrophosphate dihydrate crystal deposition (CPPD), is similar to gout except that calcium, rather than uric acid, crystallizes in the joints. The presence of these calcium crystals weakens the cartilage, inducing it to break down more easily. The body reacts by creating inflammation to rid itself of the crystals.

Symptoms

The uric acid crystals act as an abrasive, inducing pain and swelling. The initial symptom of gout is a gnawing pain in the big toe, although it can strike the joints in the hand, wrist, and knee as well. A fever or chills may accompany it. Walking can become difficult, as can sleeping if bedcovers rest on the toe. Pseudo gout also causes redness, heat, pain, and swelling in one or more joints. Left to progress, the cartilage can become so damaged that the bones rub together.

Causes

Gout has a genetic component and often runs in families. The most likely causes of gout are insufficient uricase (a digestive enzyme), too much protein and fatty food in the diet, and excessive alcohol consumption. Stress is a trigger, as can be extra weight and a lack of exercise. Excess IL-6 is produced, causing inflammation and pain. The cause of pseudo gout is unknown, but it is suspected that there is an abnormality in the connective tissue or cartilage, possibly a genetic factor.

High blood pressure and kidney disease are often seen in those suffering with gout.

Prescription for Health

NUTRIENT	DOSAGE	ACTION
Moducare sterols and sterolins	One capsule three times daily	Reduces inflammation, controls IL-6
Vitamin C	3000–5000 mg daily in divided doses	Reduces serum uric acid
Quercetin	200–400 mg daily	Inhibits uric acid, is anti-inflammatory
Magnesium	300 mg twice daily	Is especially important for pseudo gout where calcium is up-regulated
Omega-3 fatty acid	1–2 Tbsp (15–30 mL) flaxseed oil or three 500 mg fish oil capsules (I like Eskimo-3 from Tyler) daily	Reduces inflammation, so there is less stiffness in the joints
Zinc	15–30 mg daily	Deficiency is common during gout attacks
Wobenzym or bromelain	Three tablets of Wobenzym daily 500 mg of bromelain every three hours during gout attack, or 1000 mg daily for maintenance	Improves digestion of protein, acts as an anti-inflammatory

Health Tips to Enhance Healing

- Do not take niacin as it may promote a gout attack. Vitamin A is also not indicated for those with gout as it can create toxicity due to the conversion to its more toxic retinoic acid, promoted by a dysfunction in enzymes.
- With pseudo gout it is important to have iron levels checked to make sure that they are not too high (hemochromatosis). High iron levels are associated with pseudo gout. If iron is high, give blood.
- Eating at least 1/2 lb (250 g) of dark cherries or strawberries daily can neutralize uric acid. If they are out of season, cherry extract is available at health food stores, preferably sugar-free.
- Eliminate organ and red meat, mushrooms, peanuts, meat-based gravies, shellfish, sardines, herring, and mackerel from the diet during an episode of gout. Limited consumption may resume once symptoms are gone.
- Eat plenty of fresh fruits and vegetables, raw or as juices. Berries, onions, and parsley are good sources of antioxidants.
- Drink at least eight to ten glasses of pure, filtered water per day. It will help flush out the uric acid. For every juice or caffeinated beverage you drink, add another glass of water.
- Eliminate alcohol entirely. Beer and wine is known to promote gout attacks.
- Restrict consumption of refined flour and simple sugars found in commercial bread, honey, fruit, juices, and fructose.

Other Recommendations

- Avoid NSAIDs (see "No NSAIDs," page 13, for the dangers of arthritis drugs).
- It is important for gout and pseudo gout sufferers to get regular exercise, but if you are overweight, it is even more important. Begin a moderate exercise program emphasizing the cardio component to help reduce weight, as opposed to embarking on a restrictive diet. Fasting or a sudden withdrawal of foods can increase uric acid.

Health Fact

- Ninety-five percent of all gout sufferers are male. The few women who do get gout tend to be postmenopausal.

GRAVES' DISEASE

Graves' disease, also known as toxic diffuse goiter, is an autoimmune disease whereby an antibody stimulates the thyroid to produce too much thyroid hormone. Thyroid hormone is crucial for regulating the body's ability to use fuel. Conventional treatment is to block thyroid hormone synthesis, destroy thyroid tissue with radioactive iodine, or surgically remove the thyroid.

Graves' disease afflicts both men and women, but it appears more frequently in women between the ages of 20 and 40. In Europe and the United States there are almost 3 million people with Graves' disease, and 37,000 new cases are diagnosed annually.

Symptoms

The milder symptoms of Graves' disease are nervousness, insomnia, high blood pressure, intolerance to heat, increased sweating, diarrhea, and weight loss with increased appetite. Menstrual periods may become irregular or spotty and hair may gray prematurely. In more serious cases, there may be an irregular or rapid heartbeat, tremors, swelling in the legs and eyes, extreme sensitivity to light, and clubbed fingers. The distinct symptoms of Graves' are a greatly enlarged thyroid gland causing a goiter (a big bulge at the neck), bulging eyes called thyroid-associated ophthalmopathy (TAO), and a thickening of the skin over the shins. The symptoms of bulging eyes can cause an expression of constant surprise or it may look like the person is in a fixed stare.

Causes

The immune system reacts to environmental or genetic triggers to encourage the secretion of thyroid-stimulating immunoglobulins (TSIs, antibodies against the thyroid) that adhere to the thyroid gland to provoke an increase in the production of thyroid hormone. Graves' disease is associated with a hyper-stimulation of T-helper-2 cells and the cytokines IL-1, IL-6, IL-8, and IL-10, which are involved in autoantibody production and inflammation. As well, being female increases the risk of contracting Graves' and many women develop it during the postpartum period (after having a baby). Three environmental factors have been implicated in the development of Graves': stress, iodine intake, and infection. Reports of a significantly higher number of adverse life events during the year prior to the onset of Graves' disease suggests a correlation between stress and autoimmunity (see page 47 for more information on autoimmune diseases and stress). High iodine intake increases the risk of developing an autoimmune reaction against the thyroid. Certain viruses have been associated with the onset of Graves' and the development of antibodies against the thyroid. Yersinia infections have been implicated, but scientists believe that Graves' disease is more than likely the result of many viruses causing molecular mimicry toward the thyroid.

Prescription for Health

Forty percent of Graves' patients treated with antithyroid medications achieve remission. The following recommendations are complementary, so medication should not be stopped. Moducare controls autoantibody reactions, normalizes T-helper-2 cytokines, and reduces inflammation, which is essential to the treatment and control of autoimmune disease.

NUTRIENT	DOSAGE	ACTION
Moducare sterols and sterolins	Two capsules three times daily for one week, then one capsule three times daily as a maintenance dose	Essential in the control of T-helper-2 autoantibody reactions, acts as anti-inflammatory
High-potency B-complex	Two capsules daily with meals	Required for thyroid and immune function
Multimune containing vitamins A, B_6, C, E, selenium, zinc, magnesium, coenzyme Q10, lipoic acid, reduced L-glutathione	Three capsules daily with meals	Supports the proper functioning of the immune system, is an anti-inflammatory and potent antioxidant
Vitamin C	1000 mg twice daily	Regulates immunity and combats stress
Vitamin E	400 IU daily	In several studies those with autoimmune diseases had a significant reduction in symptoms
Omega-3 fish oils	1 g three times daily	A powerful anti-inflammatory and controls T-helper-2 reactions
Evening primrose oil	1 g three times daily	Essential for recurring and relapsing autoimmune disease, ensures proper function of suppressor T-cells, is anti-inflammatory

Health Tips to Enhance Healing

- Do not take immune boosters of any type. They can enhance the cytokines responsible for antibody production, thus worsening Graves' disease. The German Commission E does not recommend that those with autoimmune disorders take echinacea.
- Avoid saturated fats from red meats, pork, and deep-fried foods and lard. Research has shown that diets high in saturated fats exacerbated autoimmune disease and increased the number of flare-ups and recurrences.

- Eat plenty of fresh fruits and vegetables, legumes, whole grains, nuts and seeds, healthy oils, fresh fish, free-range poultry, and soy products. Choose organic whenever possible to minimize toxic burden to the system.
- Detoxification and elimination of waste is very important. Eat liver-friendly foods such as kale, carrots, beets, artichokes, lemons, onions, garlic, leeks, and members of the cabbage family (broccoli, cauliflower, Brussels sprouts).
- Use Weleda eyedrops to soothe inflammation in those with thyroid-associated ophthalmopathy.

Other Recommendations

- Exercise regularly to improve circulation and to help the detoxification and elimination process.
- Reduce stress. Rest and relax when you can and practice stress reduction techniques (see "Stress-Busting Tips," page 130).
- Complications are rare (about 1 in 70 out of 0.1–0.2 percent of pregnancies), but children born to women with Graves' disease should be closely monitored for the first week postpartum, both clinically and biochemically.

GUILLAIN-BARRÉ SYNDROME

Guillain-Barré syndrome (GBS) is the most common autoimmune disorder of the nervous system that causes neuromuscular problems. Axons are long, thin protrusions of the nerve cells responsible for carrying signals. The myelin sheath surrounding the axon allows rapid transmission of nerve signals and sends them over long distances. In the course of this disorder, macrophages attack the myelin sheath and strip it. As myelin sheaths are injured, nerve signals can no longer be transmitted efficiently and muscles stop responding to the brain's commands. When the damage is severe enough, nerve conduction is blocked, resulting in paralysis. Twenty five percent of GBS cases will require breathing assistance with a ventilator and 5 percent may die from respiratory failure. Vaccinations, infections, and stress play a role in the development of GBS.

Symptoms

Symptoms for Guillain-Barré are weakness (and possibly sensory loss) that may be mild throughout the illness or develop into complete paralysis. There is also a loss of reflexes and elevated spinal fluid protein (that reflects the extent of damage to the spinal nerve roots). The disease may become increasingly worse during the first four weeks and then begin to plateau.

Recovery follows, but can take anywhere from a few weeks to a year. Usually there is a complete recovery (or almost complete). However, 15 percent of those with GBS show considerable permanent neuromuscular impairment.

Causes

It is not clear why Guillain-Barré affects some people and not others, but in about two-thirds of the Guillain-Barré cases, it usually follows an infection such as *Campylobacter jejuni*, cytomegalovirus, Epstein Barr virus, or *Mycoplasma pneumoniae*. Less often, but not to be overlooked, are infections due to herpes virus (chicken pox or zoster), surgery, or transfusions.

Guillain-Barré can complicate HIV infections and usually appears before the development of AIDS. It is not known at this time if Guillain-Barré is attached to the HIV virus itself or to a reactivated virus (such as cytomegalovirus) that is stimulated by HIV.

Vaccines have also been implicated in causing GBS. In the fall of 1976, when 45 million adults were vaccinated with influenza virus vaccine, the incidence of GBS increased by a factor of four to eight. Influenza is not the only vaccine to promote GBS, mumps, rubella, hepatitis B, diphtheria, polio virus, tetanus toxoid, and more. Researchers have recommended that patients with inflammatory demyelinating autoimmune diseases not be put at risk through immunization.

Prescription for Health

GBS is a serious disease that requires prompt medical attention before it becomes life-threatening. The following recommendations are for recovery and long-term rehabilitation.

Caution: Supplements that boost macrophage function should not be given to people with GBS as the cytokines that macrophages secrete are responsible for demyelination of the neurons.

NUTRIENT	DOSAGE	ACTION
Moducare sterols and sterolins	One capsule three times daily as a maintenance dose	Essential for regulating immune function and controlling autoantibody reactions, is anti-inflammatory
High-potency B-complex	Two capsules daily with meals	Is required for thyroid and immune function
Multimune containing vitamins A, B$_6$, C, E, selenium, zinc, magnesium, coenzyme Q10, lipoic acid, reduced L-glutathione	Three capsules daily with meals	Supports the proper functioning of the immune system, is anti-inflammatory and a potent antioxidant
Vitamin C	1000 mg twice a day	Regulates immunity and combats stress

NUTRIENT	DOSAGE	ACTION
Vitamin E	100 IU per day	In several studies those with autoimmune diseases had a significant reduction in symptoms
Omega-3 fish oils	1 g three times daily	A powerful anti-inflammatory and controls T-helper-2 reactions
Evening primrose oil	1 g three times daily	Essential for recurring and relapsing autoimmune disease, ensures proper function of suppressor T-cells, is anti-inflammatory

Health Tips to Enhance Healing

- Avoid immune boosters that enhance macrophage function.
- According to the *Merck Manual of Medical Information*, corticosteroid therapy is no longer recommended because it has no proven benefit and may actually worsen the disease.
- Eat plenty of fruits and vegetables every day. Also add yogurt (with plenty of live bacteria), legumes, fresh fish, whole grains, nuts and seeds and their oils to the diet. Fiber will assist elimination and avoid constipation.
- Reduce stress, which is a major fact in the development of autoimmunity.

Other Recommendations

- To avoid contamination from food pathogens, store meat and poultry in the refrigerator or freezer quickly. When preparing meat, avoid cross-contamination and wash hands and surfaces thoroughly. Cook thoroughly.

Health Fact

Campylobacter jejuni, a major contributor to Guillain-Barré syndrome, has grown increasingly resistant to fluoroquinolone antibiotics, a trend that has been observed since 1992. Several studies on retail poultry have found high levels of *Campylobacter jejuni*. A two-year study by the Minnesota Department of Health discovered that when they sampled poultry of the local supermarkets, 88 percent of the poultry tested positive for *Camplyobacter jejuni*. Cook chicken thoroughly.

HASHIMOTO'S THYROIDITIS

The thyroid gland regulates the rate at which the body uses oxygen and metabolizes food. It also acts as our thermostat and plays an important role in growth and development. Hashimoto's thyroiditis (autoimmune thyroiditis or chronic lymphocytic thyroiditis) is an inflammatory glandular autoimmune disease in which the immune system attacks the thyroid. It is one in a group of inflammatory thyroid disorders, but it is by far the most common within the group as well as the leading cause of hypothyroidism (low thyroid) and goiter (enlarged, protruding thyroid gland) in the United States.

Although men and women of any age can develop this disease, 85 percent of cases are women, between the ages of 30 and 50. Approximately 25 percent of people with Hashimoto's develop other autoimmune diseases such as Type I diabetes, rheumatoid arthritis, lupus, Sjogren's syndrome, and pernicious anemia. Blood tests are required to determine the presence of antithyroid antibodies. Most people with Hashimoto's require thyroid hormone replacement therapy.

Symptoms

Hashimoto's symptoms can be very subtle, and while there may be an enlarged swollen or thick feeling in the neck, there is rarely any tenderness or pain. The symptoms of Hashimoto's are opposite to those of Graves' disease, with the exception that both conditions produce fatigue. The face is puffy and the eyelids may droop, the voice may be hoarse and speech slowed, and there is depression, weight gain without increased appetite, an intolerance of cold temperatures, infertility, and constipation. The skin is dry and flaky and menstrual periods can be long and heavy. There may be loss of the hair of the eyebrows, and scalp hair may be sparse, coarse, and dry. Carpal tunnel syndrome is common.

Causes

Hashimoto's is caused by the immune system producing antibodies against several different proteins in the thyroid gland. Over the past 50 years, incidence rates of Hashimoto have risen exponentially. There can be a genetic predisposition, so a family history of thyroid disease is common.

Studies have shown that in iodine-deficient regions where iodine was added to food, an increase in thyroid autoantibodies and thyroiditis occur shortly after supplementation. There is a delicate balance of iodine needed by the body—too little or too much can cause thyroid disease. Environmental toxins are also considered a cause of thyroiditis based on animal research in which they have induced Hashimoto's by exposing animals to common chemicals.

Prescription for Health

You should not stop your thyroid medication. The recommendations below are designed to support immune function and control autoanti-body production against the thyroid (see Chapter 3).

NUTRIENT	DOSAGE	ACTION
Moducare sterols and sterolins	One capsule three times daily as a maintenance dose	Essential for regulating immune function and controlling autoantibody reactions, is anti-inflammatory
High-potency B-complex	Two capsules daily with meals	Required for thyroid, metabolism, and proper immune function
Multimune containing vitamins A, B$_6$, C, E, selenium, zinc, magnesium, coenzyme Q10, lipoic acid, reduced L-glutathione	Three capsules daily with meals	Supports the proper functioning of the immune system, is anti-inflammatory and a potent antioxidant
Vitamin C	1000 mg twice daily	Regulates immunity and combats stress
Multimineral with trace minerals	Two capsules daily	Essential precursors to thyroid hormone
Omega-3 fish oils	1 g three times daily	A powerful anti-inflammatory and controls T-helper-2 reactions
Evening primrose oil	1 g three times daily	Essential for recurring and relapsing autoimmune disease, ensures proper function of suppressor T-cells, is anti-inflammatory

Health Tips to Enhance Healing

- Do not take immune boosters. They can overstimulate the immune system and increase antibody production.
- Armour thyroid extract should be taken under the guidance of your physician. In many cases it has been used in place of prescription thyroid medication.
- Avoid fluoride toothpaste and fluoridated water as they compete with iodine for absorption.
- It is not advised to supplement the diet with iodine because there is such a delicate balance required by the thyroid to function properly that too much iodine can be damaging. If you are eating too much iodized salt, switch to sea salt that is not iodized.
- Ensure you get adequate sunshine. The thyroid gland requires vitamin D to function properly. Those living in the northern hemisphere have higher rates of low thyroid and Hashimoto's.

- Detoxification and elimination of waste is very important. Eat liver-friendly foods such as kale, carrots, beets, artichokes, lemons, onions, garlic, leeks, and members of the cabbage family (broccoli, cauliflower, Brussels sprouts).
- Stress reduction is essential. (See Chapter 3 for more on autoimmunity and stress.)

HEADACHE (AND MIGRAINE)

No other condition comes in a greater variety than the headache. In their book *Prescription for Nutritional Healing*, Phyllis Balch, CNC, and James Balch, MD, identify 21 types of headaches. They can range from mild to excruciatingly debilitating, and are often a symptom of hundreds of diseases. Tension headaches are the most frequent. Migraines, the most debilitating, constitute less than 10 percent of headaches. More women than men suffer from migraines. Cluster headaches are another type of migraine that affect mostly men 30 years and older.

Symptoms

A tension headache occurs frequently, with intermittent or constant pain that does not pulse, and can start in one place and spread over the rest of the head. Generally it is associated with a tense feeling felt on the front and back of the head.

Migraines are often accompanied by pain in and around the eye or temple and the head throbs. Often the throbbing occurs only on one side of the head. Some may experience nausea, dizziness, cold hands, vomiting, and diarrhea. Migraines can hit without warning or be preceded by "auras"—blurred vision or spots, numbness, or a disturbance in cognitive function—that are the consequence of the vessel constriction. Severe migraines can last a few days.

With cluster headaches the pain can also be on one side of the head, but they are often brief, lasting one hour or less. There are generally one to three, but may be as many as 20, headaches experienced everyday for weeks or months followed by periods with no headaches whatsoever. Swelling below the eye, runny nose, and watery eyes are symptoms often seen with cluster headaches.

Causes

Headaches can be brought on by any one or combination of triggers, including stress, anxiety, depression, eye strain, change in air pressure or weather changes, poor posture or a misalignment in the vertebrae, dental problems, overexertion, smoking, alcohol, hypertension, sinus problems, hypoglycemia, skipping meals, dehydration, constipation, magnesium deficiency, and caffeine withdrawal. Other causes are food and environmental sensitivities such as nitrites, lactose, caffeine, aspartame, copper, and vasoactive tyramines that are found in particular foods (see below). Not surprisingly, migraines tend to run in families, probably due to traditional food and lifestyle.

Prescription for Health

NUTRIENT	DOSAGE	ACTION
Feverfew	250 mcg of parthenolides taken daily equal to 125 mg of dried feverfew	Alleviates pain, nausea, and vomiting associated with migraine. Reduction in recurring headache and migraine should be noted in four weeks.
Vitamin B$_6$ with a high-potency B-complex	50 mg per day	Protects against medication-induced headaches
Magnesium	400 mg daily	Reduces muscle tension, is anti-inflammatory
5-HTP	100 mg twice daily	Inhibits substance P, a pain mediator
Capsaicin	Cream up to 0.075 percent capsaicin applied to temples	Blocks substance P, a pain mediator
Ipriflavone	Use as directed	Natural estrogen-like action may help women with hormone-dependent headaches. Controls IL-1 and IL-6 pain and inflammation mediators.
Omega 3 fish oils	Three 500 mg capsules three times daily for several weeks	Research showed a reduction in frequency and intensity of migraine headaches over a six-week period.
Ginger	500 mg every four hours	Relieves headaches and nausea associated with migraines
Kava kava	200 mg	Reduces stress, relaxes muscles

Health Tips to Enhance Healing

- Aspartame is associated with an increased risk of headache. Eliminate all aspartame-containing products, especially soda pop.
- If suffering from a migraine, eliminate noise and light. Apply cold compresses and use local pressure to reduce pain.
- Chiropractic treatments may correct misaligned bones that cause headaches. Cranial sacral therapists can also help realign bones of the skull.
- Have yourself tested for food and environmental allergies. (See "Allergy Detection and Elimination" in the introduction in this chapter.) Common food allergens are chocolate, milk, corn, cheese, yeast, coffee, wheat, shellfish, citrus fruit, wine, bananas, sausages, chicken liver, pork, and beef. (See Allergies.)

- Luncheon meats, hot dogs, bacon, and dried fruit, as well as most processed and packaged food, are full of additives, preservatives, flavoring, and coloring that high on the sensitivity list. Eat natural, whole foods, preferably organic.
- Eliminate foods containing tyramine, such as chocolate, aged cheeses, red wine, and fermented foods.
- Drink at least eight to ten glasses of pure, filtered water daily. Headaches and migraines can be brought on by dehydration.
- Reduce stress. Practice stress reduction techniques at home, in the office, or in the car on the way home. (See Chapter 6.)
- Avoid constipation (see Constipation).

Other Recommendations

- Have dental amalgams removed and replaced with non-toxic fillings, Headaches have been associated with mercury toxicity.
- Too much coffee (more than two or three cups daily) can initiate headaches. However, caffeine can also stop headaches, even migraines. Dr. Julian Whitaker, author of *Health & Healing*, recommends that if you enjoy coffee, have only a cup of coffee a day to keep headaches at bay. If you drink too much coffee, cut back, or if you are caffeine-sensitive, eliminate it altogether. Coffee is not recommended if you have osteoporosis, rheumatoid arthritis, atherosclerosis, infertility, urinary incontinence, or are pregnant.
- Ensure proper lighting to avoid eye strain.
- Eat small meals often to prevent hypoglycemia (see Hypoglycemia).
- Chiropractic, massage, reflexology and acupuncture can be very beneficial in alleviating headaches.
- Do not take pain medications regularly. They only mask the problem and can worsen the situation over time. Find out the root cause for the headaches so you know how to prevent them.
- Have your physician check you for hypothyroidism, which can be related to migraines.
- If your headaches happen consistently or worsen over a period of time, consult your physician to rule out serious problems.

HEART DISEASE

Heart disease is the category for about 30 cardiovascular conditions. The five main types are coronary artery disease (atherosclerosis or hardening of the arteries), heart muscle disease (cardiomyopathy), congestive heart failure (inability of the heart to pump enough blood), valve disorders (mitral valve prolapse), and arrhythmias (heartbeat rhythm irregularities). Heart disease is the leading cause of death in North America.

Over a century ago the medical establishment thought that heart disease was brought on by infections causing inflammation, but this theory was abandoned for what were new directions at the time. Now scientists have come full circle to focus on *Chlamydia pneumoniae*. This bacterium is found in high concentrations in the blood of people who have had heart attacks. The infection theory is significant in that it points to the immune system and its failure in defending us from simple bacteria. By enhancing immunity, we may be able to prevent heart disease. See Chapters 2 and 3 for more information on bacteria, the immune system, and heart disease.

Symptoms

It is possible to have heart disease and not know it until it is too late, which is why it is called the silent killer. Common signs include bouts of indigestion, shortness of breath, an irregular heartbeat, and chest pain during exercise that abates with rest. Symptoms that require emergency attention include chest pain that persists and does not abate with rest, profuse sweating, nausea and vomiting, dizziness, irregular pulse, anxiety, a vague tightness, and pain or discomfort in the chest that may extend to the arms, shoulders, or neck. Women often ignore the warning signs of heart disease.

Causes

Heart disease actually begins in the stomach. A poor diet of packaged and processed foods high in bad fats and void of fiber and nutrients is the leading instigator of an ailing heart. Couple a poor diet with high stress, dehydration, aging, smoking, extra weight, and lack of exercise and sleep, and the risks climb even higher. Conditions such as atherosclerosis, high blood pressure, and high cholesterol compound the problem. See those conditions for specific information.

The risk for women (especially African-American women) is significantly increased if there are diabetes or hormonal imbalances. However, men are still more likely to suffer from heart disease.

Prescription for Health

If you are currently on Coumadin, high cholesterol, or high blood pressure medication, talk to your physician or pharmacist about drug–nutrient interactions. Be aware that both high blood pressure and high cholesterol medications cause depletion of coenzyme Q10, so you must supplement to ensure adequate levels. According to the *Drug-Induced Nutrient Depletion Handbook for Pharmacists*, if you are taking Lasix (flurosemide) you should also be aware that Lasix depletes calcium, magnesium, potassium, vitamins B_1, B_6, and C, and zinc. These nutrients must be replaced to prevent deficiency. If you have high blood pressure, high cholesterol, or heart palpitations, see specific treatment recommendations for each.

NUTRIENT	DOSAGE	ACTION
High-potency multivitamin with minerals but no iron	Use as directed	Ensures adequate intake of vitamins and minerals
High-potency B-complex (ensure supplement has 400 mcg of folic acid; if not, add folic acid separately)	Two to three capsules daily	Required for supplementation of B vitamins; reduces stress
Magnesium	300 mg three times daily	Alleviates arrythmias, is essential for heart muscle
Vitamin B_1	200 mg daily	Essential to prevent depletion in those taking Lasix
Vitamin C (with bioflavonoids)	1000 mg of vitamin C twice daily 500 mg of bioflavonoids twice daily	Reduces symptoms and risk of heart disease, is antioxidant, raises HDL (the "good" cholesterol), lowers blood pressure
Vitamin E (with tocopherols)	400 IU–800 IU	Improves blood flow, reduces fatty plaques, boosts the immune system and acts as an antioxidant
Coenzyme Q10	100–300 mg per day	Improves energy production in the heart muscle, significantly improves heart function in those with congestive heart failure
Hawthorn extract (standardized 1.8 percent vitexin or 10 percent procyanidin content.)	100–200 mg three times daily	Double-blind studies show improvement in those with congestive heart failure
Pycnogenol or grape seed extract	100 mg twice daily	Reduces platelet aggregation
Essential fatty acids	1 Tbsp (15 mL) of Udo's Choice oil or Omega Essential Balance daily	Reduces risk of heart disease
Moducare sterols and sterolins	One capsule three times daily	Regulates immune function, enhances bacteria- and virus-fighting capability, controls cortisol (the stress hormone), is anti-inflammatory

Health Tips to Enhance Healing

- See Blood Pressure, Cholesterol (High), Heart Palpitations.
- See Chapter 2, "The Cardiovascular System" and Chapter 3, "The Immune System."
- Drink eight to ten glasses of pure, filtered water a day. Research on 34,000 Seventh Day Adventists compared the water drinking of habits of two groups: one group drank five glasses daily, the other two. The increased hydration reduced platelet stickiness and

improved blood flow, and the scientists found that risk of stroke or heart disease for the five-glass-a-day group was half that in those who only drank two glasses a day.

- Read dietary advice for heart disease in Chapter 2.
- Adopt an exercise program (see Chapter 6).

Other Recommendations

- Reduce your consumption of alcohol, salt, and caffeine.
- Find out what nutrients are depleted by the prescription medications you are taking. An excellent book by Ross Pelton and James LaValle, called *The Nutritional Cost of Prescription Drugs*, outlines the reactions of most major types of medications.
- Reduce stress.
- Stop smoking. Many conditions are reversible if smoking is stopped at an early enough stage in a disease's progression. Tobacco contains 4000 toxins and 43 known carcinogens that enter the lungs and travel to the bloodstream with every puff (see Health Fact).
- Get plenty of sleep and fresh air. Breathe deeply through the nose and exhale through the mouth. Women are generally shallow breathers, so be sure to take a few minutes to do five deep breaths every day.
- Seek professionals to provide other beneficial therapies such as chelation, hydrotherapy, acupuncture, massage, and traditional Chinese medicine.
- Women beware: the Heart and Stroke Foundation states that there are ways that women and men can differ in their symptoms and treatment of heart attacks. Women may have more atypical symptoms such as chest discomfort, and diagnostic tests and therapies may not be as effective in women. After a heart attack, men are more likely to be referred for bypass surgery and balloon angioplasty.
- When experiencing a heart attack, the average person waits five hours before getting medical attention. *Do not delay—get medical attention quickly.*

Health Fact

A study published in the March 2001 issue of *Psychosomatic Medicine* found that women who were angry and depressed were more likely to have hardening of the arteries. Anger and depression were associated with greater occurrences of behavioral risks such as smoking, obesity, and high cholesterol. Participants who were ranked highest for displaying outward hostility also ranked higher for bad cholesterols, lower for good cholesterol levels, and were more likely to be overweight. Those who ranked highest for depression were 2.5 times more likely to smoke.

In Milan, a study was done on the effects of the graveyard shift on heart disease and found that shift workers are at a greater risk. Even though they may feel as if they have had a good sleep, their bodies' biorhythms cannot adjust to the change quickly enough. Occurrences that the heart could normally handle during the day may be more stressful when they happen during the night.

HEART PALPITATIONS

When the heart palpitates, it beats more forcefully, faster, or with an irregular beat. This is a normal response if there is exertion such as exercise or hard labor, or if under stress, but if heart palpitations occur with little or no exertion or stressors present, then heart disease may be suspected. If the heartbeat appears to skip, it is called an arrhythmia and if it happens often, it should be monitored by a physician.

Symptoms

The heart gives the sensation of flip-flopping or fluttering. This feeling of the heart being out of control can cause fear, anxiety, or panic and exacerbate the situation. Extreme episodes of heart palpitations can provoke queasiness, shortness of breath, dizziness, or a pain in the chest. If you have been hunched over and try to straighten up, symptoms may appear. Lying down will usually make them disappear or may make them more apparent because you are lying still and can feel them.

Causes

Heart palpitations are a malfunction of the heart's electrical system cells. As much as heart palpitations can cause fear, anxiety, or panic, these feelings can also induce heart palpitations. Conditions that may provoke palpitations are heart disease (such as mitral valve prolapse), high blood pressure, pregnancy, infection, and thyroid problems. Nutritional deficiencies or allergies triggered by food or the environment can cause the heart to race. Stress, caffeine, alcohol, and nicotine also affect the heart in this manner.

Prescription for Health

NUTRIENT	DOSAGE	ACTION
High-potency multivitamin with minerals but no iron	Use as directed	Ensures adequate intake of vitamins and minerals

NUTRIENT	DOSAGE	ACTION
High-potency B-complex supplement has 400 mcg of folic acid; if not, add folic acid separately	Two to three capsules daily	Is required for supplementation of B vitamins, reduces stress
Magnesium, preferably in the glycinate form	300 mg three times daily	Alleviates heart palpitations, is essential for proper heart muscle function. If you are a heavy coffee drinker, you need more magnesium.
Vitamin B_1	200 mg per day	Essential to prevent depletion in those taking Lasix
Vitamin C (with bioflavonoids)	1000 mg of vitamin C twice daily; 500 mg of bioflavonoids twice daily	Reduces symptoms and risk of heart disease, is antioxidant, raises HDL (the "good" cholesterol), lowers blood pressure
Vitamin E (with tocopherols)	400 IU	Improves blood flow, reduces fatty plaques, boosts the immune system, acts as an antioxidant
Coenzyme Q10	100–300 mg daily	Reduces heart palpitations, improves energy production in the heart muscle, significantly improves heart function in those with congestive heart failure
Hawthorn extract (standardized 1.8 percent vitexin or 10 percent procyanidin content)	100–200 mg three times daily	Double-blind studies show improvement in those with congestive heart failure. Reduces heart palpitations.
Essential fatty acids	1 Tbsp (15 mL) of Udo's Choice oil or Omega Essential Balance daily	Reduces risk of heart disease
Moducare sterols and sterolins	One capsule three times daily	Regulates immune function, enhances bacteria and virus-fighting capability, controls cortisol (the stress hormone), is anti-inflammatory
Valerian or kava kava	Use tincture as directed	Calms and relaxes nerves

Health Tips to Enhance Healing

- See Cholesterol (High), Heart Disease, and High Blood Pressure for more information if you also have these associated conditions.
- Try a little hydrotherapy. Every night before you go to bed, wash your torso and arms with cold water, or hold your hands in cold water for 30 seconds.
- Have your physician rule out hyperthyroidism.

Health Fact

One of the largest studies done on the effects of CoQ10 on heart conditions had 2664 subjects taking 50–150 mg of coenzyme Q10 daily for three months (78 percent of subjects received a dosage of 100 mg). At the end of three months, 75.4 percent of the subjects showed a decrease in heart palpitations.

HEMORRHOIDS

Hemorrhoids are swollen tissues located inside and/or outside the rectum that can become so large they protrude around the anus. They also contain veins. Veins from the anus drain into the portal vein leading to the liver and all circulatory veins. Veins in the rectum have no valves to alleviate congestion, so the condition can be aggravated quite easily.

Symptoms

Symptoms usually begin with a swelling of tissue and itchiness around the anus. If left to continue, inflammation is exacerbated, leading to bleeding, pain, seepage, and possible tearing of tissue in the rectal area.

Causes

Hemorrhoids are brought on by a weakened venous system; however, constipation and straining during bowel movements arising from a low-fiber diet, sedentary lifestyle, and insufficient water is the main factor promoting that breakdown. When congested, the liver can also promote hemorrhoids and high blood pressure is also implicated.

People who sit or stand for many hours become susceptible because of their poor circulation and the extra pressure exerted on the venous system. Pregnant women and those who are overweight are also vulnerable because of the extra weight they carry and their increased likelihood of suffering constipation.

Another culprit is over-the-counter laxatives, although marketing campaigns would have you believe they alleviate constipation. In fact, they promote it by interfering with the body's natural rhythm, its ability to absorb nutrients (potassium, vitamin D, and calcium), and they do *not* address the underlying reason for being constipated (see Chapter 1, page 4).

Prescription for Health

NUTRIENT	DOSAGE	ACTION
Omega's Hi-Lignan Flax Seed	1–2 tsp (5–10 mL) daily, drink two glasses of water for each teaspoon of flax fiber	Eliminates constipation and soothes mucous membranes of the entire intestinal tract, softens stool
Horse chestnut seed extract or Venastat	100–150 mg daily containing escin or Venastat as directed	Increases antioxidant activity, inhibits enzymes that destroy venous walls, and improves venous tone
Flaxseed oil or Udo's Choice or Omega Essential Balance	1–2 Tbsp (15–30 mL) daily	Soothes intestinal lining and promotes elimination

NUTRIENT	DOSAGE	ACTION
Moducare sterols and sterolins	One capsule three times daily	Reduces inflammation caused by IL-6 activity, promotes proper immune function
Multivitamin with minerals	Three capsules daily or as directed	Corrects nutritional deficiency
High-potency B-complex	Two capsules daily	Improves digestion and metabolism
Reduced L-glutathioine	45–100 mg daily	Detoxifies liver
Milk thistle, Nature's Way	Two capsules daily	Detoxifies liver

Health Tips to Enhance Healing

- Coffee enemas (recommended by the Gerson Cancer clinic) help to cleanse the liver, allowing for better detoxification and circulation.
- See Constipation.
- Keep rectal area clean and use soft toilet tissue to avoid unnecessary abrasion.
- Use topical ointments containing witch hazel and vitamin E.

Health Fact

Hemorrhoids do not exist in cultures where diets are high in fiber, low in refined foods, and lifestyles are more active.

HEPATITIS

Hepatitis is an acute or chronic inflammation of the liver that is contagious in varying degrees. There are three main types of hepatitis: A, B, and C, but there are also lesser known types D, E, and G. Hepatitis A is acute and the most prevalent variation; 10 percent of hepatitis B cases and 85 percent of hepatitis C cases will develop into chronic hepatitis and more serious liver disorders. Of all chronic hepatitis cases combined, 10 to 20 percent are autoimmune in nature.

Seventy percent of autoimmune hepatitis sufferers are women between the ages of 15 and 40. (See What Is Autoimmunity? page 46 for more information on autoimmune disease in general.)

Symptoms

Hepatitis usually results from one of several viruses. In hepatitis A and the other acute variations of hepatitis, it is recognized by fatigue, flu-like symptoms, muscle and joint aches, loss of appetite and sex drive, fever, vomiting, sleep disturbances, light-colored stools, and nausea. The liver is tender and enlarged, the skin is jaundiced and itches, the urine is dark, and there is an elevation of liver enzymes in the blood. Symptoms may last several weeks to months and are rarely fatal, although the elderly and those with weakened immune systems are at greater risk. There is no long-term liver damage and once you have recovered from hepatitis A, you will be immune from further infection.

Chronic hepatitis has varying symptoms that can resemble the flu or may lie dormant but cause chronic fatigue, liver damage, and death. Hepatitis B infects 222,000 North Americans every year, but most recover without consequences. For those who develop chronic hepatitis, liver cancer or cirrhosis may develop and they can infect other people if they have intimate contact. In Canada and the United States, 6000 people die from hepatitis B every year.

Hepatitis C infection may or may not present flu-like symptoms, or appear asymptomatic but lie dormant in the body. Over 4 million North Americans are infected with hepatitis C. When hepatitis C infection develops into chronic hepatitis, it can slowly destroy the liver. Five percent of those afflicted will develop liver cancer. Those with hepatitis C show higher levels of iron in the liver, which can also contribute to liver damage.

Even though autoimmune hepatitis is chronic, the symptoms may appear similar to acute hepatitis. Occurrences of hepatitis in younger people should be checked for autoimmune hepatitis, especially if there is no history of drug or alcohol use, or risk factors for viral or metabolic causes.

Causes

Hepatitis A is brought about primarily from human fecal contamination in food and water. Families and those in close contact with someone who is infected are susceptible to infection themselves. Restaurants and day care centers are hotbeds of contamination if hygiene and sanitation standards are lax. The produce or fish we buy may be infected if they were irrigated with contaminated water due to poor sewage treatment facilities.

Hepatitis B can be transmitted through fluids such as blood and blood products, sexual secretions, saliva, and during birth. Babies born from infected mothers must be closely monitored as their risk for chronic hepatitis is high. Other sources of contamination are infected instruments that can pierce the skin such as tattoo, piercing, or electrolysis needles, dental tools, razors, and toothbrushes.

The incidence of hepatitis C has surpassed that of hepatitis B, striking over 4 million North Americans. As a result of transfusions using tainted blood prior to 1992, it is estimated that hundreds of thousands of people were affected. Ten percent of transfusions lead to hepatitis C infection. Hepatitis C is also spread through bodily fluids; however, unprotected sex is not the primary transmission. Health-care workers, emergency and ambulance workers, lab technicians, and intravenous drug users are the highest risk group.

A defective immune system allows acute viral infections to become chronic infections, but in order for autoimmune hepatitis to develop, there is also a lack of tolerance against the body's liver tissue. Another condition called toxic hepatitis is triggered by chemical and environmental toxins, or drug or alcohol use.

Prescription for Health

NUTRIENT	DOSAGE	ACTION
Multivitamin with minerals	Use as directed	Prevents deficiency of vitamins and minerals
High-potency B-complex	Two to three capsules daily	Important to support liver function and metabolism
Vitamin B$_{12}$	500 mcg twice daily	Required for liver function
Moducare sterols and sterolins	Two capsules three times daily until liver enzymes and viral load normalize	Reduces Th-2 activity and IL-6, increases Th-1 activity to protect the liver cells and fight virus, enhances gamma-interferon and DHEA naturally
Licorice (*Glycyrrhiza glabra*) standardized to 22 percent glycyrrhizin	500 mg twice daily	Is antiviral, anti-inflammatory; dosages over 1 g per month should be monitored by your practitioner
Milk thistle standardized to 70 or 80 percent silymarin	400 mg per day	Is anti-inflammatory, improves liver function, protects liver from assault
Vitamin C	Intravenous therapy by a professional only	Is antiviral and in some cases jaundice can clear in six days
Phosphatidyl choline	1000 mg three times daily with food	Reduces chronic active hepatitis, enhances action of milk thistle
Taurine	1 g daily	Beneficial in acute hepatitis
Flaxseed oil, or Udo's Choice, or Omega Essential Balance	1–3 Tbsp (15–30 mL) daily with food	Is anti-inflammatory
Padma 28, an ancient Tibetan formula	Three tablets three times daily before meals	Research shows Padma 28 halts liver inflammation and is effective treatment
Multimune containing vitamins A, B$_6$, C, E, selenium, coenzyme Q10, lipoic acid, reduced L-glutathione, magnesium, zinc	Three capsules daily with meals	A potent antioxidant, supports immune function, detoxifies liver, anti-inflammatory

Health Tips to Enhance Healing

- Emphasize nutritious food, an aggressive supplementation program, regular exercise, fresh air, positive thinking, and stress reduction. Avoid any substance, activity, or behavior that suppresses the immune system and prevents it from acting at full capacity.

- Do not consume alcohol, even so-called "alcohol-free" medications.
- Avoid all hydrogenated and partially hydrogenated margarines and oils and any product with trans fatty acids. Fat consumption should come from cold-pressed, unrefined nut and seed oils that are rich in essential fatty acids.
- Eliminate all junk foods, processed or packaged foods, or any food or drink that is filled with sugar, salt, additives, colorings, preservatives, and flavorings. A study of 21 normal subjects published in the *American Journal of Medicine* found that the typical American diet that is high in sucrose (25–30 percent sucrose of total daily intake) raised liver enzymes significantly, but once the subjects were on a low-sucrose diet (10 percent of total daily intake), the enzyme levels dropped to normal. Two subjects had to be withdrawn from the experiment because their enzyme levels were too high while on the sucrose diet.
- Eat organic cantaloupe, which is a liver-supporting food.
- Take digestive enzymes before every meal to facilitate digestion. If you suspect you have low stomach acid, see the introduction to this chapter.
- Indulge in green foods like blue-green algae, spirulina, wheatgrass, and barley grass, which contain powerful nutrients, especially sterols and sterolins, important for decreasing inflammation of the liver while attacking the virus.

Other Recommendations

- A person who is infected with hepatitis A should be quarantined.
- Ensure that all fish and shellfish that you eat have been well-cooked (to at least 140°F/60°C) or were frozen below zero prior to preparation. Eat sushi only if the fish has been previously frozen or avoid it altogether.
- Try these helpful herbs, which are all indicated for hepatitis and/or jaundice: curcumin, goldenseal, schizandra, sarsaparilla, and plantain.
- Proper hygiene and sanitation are paramount when working in the restaurant industry or in care facilities (but also in the home) where you may use the bathroom or change a diaper, and then prepare food. Clothing and bedding should be washed separately, thoroughly, and often in hot water and disinfectant. Common areas such bathrooms should be disinfected often.

Health Fact

There are vaccines for hepatitis A and B, but none for C, D, or E. The hepatitis B vaccine lasts only five years. Over the past few years the efficacy and safety of vaccines has been called into question. In 1996, the U.S. National Vaccine Information Center reported that adverse reactions and deaths in children under the age of 14 who had hepatitis B vaccines were unusually high. Another government data bank, Vaccine Adverse Event Reporting System, backed up that report by stating that 827 adverse events had occurred. In that year, only 279 cases of hepatitis B in children under 14 were documented. Hepatitis B contains thimersol, a mercury derivative associated with kidney damage, among other side effects.

Given that the virus is transmitted primarily through sexual contact and blood products, children are in a low-risk group. Children can become infected if their mothers were infected at the time of birth, yet 35 states require children to have three hepatitis B shots before they can enter public facilities such as day care and schools, while only 15 states have mandatory screening for pregnant women. This makes no sense.

HERPES VIRUS INFECTION
(SIMPLEX, GENITAL, SHINGLES/ZOSTER)

There are two main types of herpes virus that cause skin blisters—herpes simplex and zoster—but there are many types of herpes viruses, including, herpes zoster, Epstein Barr, cytomegalovirus and herpes virus 8, which is thought to cause Kaposi's sarcoma in AIDS. Herpes virus causes an inflammation of the sensory nerves that can cause a wide range of illnesses. The virus remains inactive in the body or suppressed by your immune system and when your immune system falters, the virus becomes active.

Herpes simplex I produces recurring cold sores or fever blisters on the lips and skin. While annoying or embarrassing because of its prominent placement, it is not usually harmful, unless the infection affects the eyes, where it can cause inflammation of the cornea, or if the blisters are in the nose, there is a risk (although rare) of contracting herpes encephalitis. Care must be taken not to transfer it to other members of the family by the sharing of toothbrushes, linens, kissing, etc.

Herpes simplex II, or genital herpes, is transmitted sexually and can turn into a very serious condition. Some people with the infection may never know it (although they can pass it on), while others experience regular outbreaks of the blisters in their genital area. In serious cases there is inflammation of the liver, which can lead to fever, stillbirths, or brain damage. Caesarian sections are recommended for infected mothers-to-be so as not to pass the virus to their babies as they exit the birth canal. Babies exposed to the herpes virus can suffer blindness, brain damage, and death.

Herpes zoster, or varicella-zoster, causes shingles and chickenpox. If the pain lingers following a bout of shingles for several weeks to months, it is called postherpetic neuralgia and 20 percent of herpes zoster cases will experience it. After the age of 50, chances increase 15 times.

The other herpes viruses are associated with many health conditions, some serious. Herpes viruses should always be investigated by your physician as they have been known to cause death in susceptible individuals. Cytomegalovirus can induce problems with the heart and the eyes. Epstein Barr virus is responsible for mononucleosis and chronic fatigue syndrome (see Mononucleosis). Herpes 6 and 7 are being investigated for their role in autoimmune disorders. Herpes 8 is akin to Epstein Barr and is suspected in conditions such as chronic fatigue syndrome, Kaposi's sarcoma in AIDS, and bone cancer.

Symptoms

Herpes simplex begins with a tingling or burning sensation on the lips (or genital area) before it turns into a painful swelling that develops into a cluster of multiple fluid-filled blisters. It can take anywhere from two days to a week for the sores to show up after initial contact, and the area is highly contagious until it has healed. The blisters eventually erupt and crust over, usually with no scarring.

With genital herpes, women will find blisters in the vagina, and around the clitoris, rectum, and cervix. Both men and women may have a watery discharge or find urination painful. The penis and foreskin swell, with blisters located on the scrotum, penis, and groin. An outbreak may be accompanied by a low fever, muscle aches, or swollen lymph nodes.

Chickenpox is a childhood ailment that produces an itchy rash and fever. It is not likely to cause serious harm, although some children may experience secondary infections. The virus becomes latent and remains that way until conditions are such that it erupts again in adulthood, and this is what is known as shingles. Those who are immune compromised or under constant stress are at a higher risk of developing shingles. The first symptoms are fever, body aches, and chills, followed by the appearance of red, fluid-filled blisters and extreme pain. Shingles can affect any area of skin, but is more prevalent in the area under the ribs and the nerves of the face and neck. The virus reaches the tips of the nerves and signals the brain to feel itching and burning sensations and severe pain. There may also be feelings of depression, numbness, swollen glands, and headaches. After a week or two the blisters will erupt, dry up, scab over, and drop off, without scarring in mild and moderate cases. In some people, pain can linger for months, which is called postherpetic neuralgia. If there is postherpetic neuralgia, the skin can be so sensitive that wind, clothing, and bedding can be extremely painful. When shingles involves the eyes, it is an emergency, so immediately consult your physician.

In the cases of herpes simplex I and II, the virus eventually dies out with age and outbreaks are rare after 50. Herpes zoster will happen once and then there appears to be immunity, with less than 5 percent contracting it a second time. It usually attacks after the age of 50 because that age group begins to show a decrease in T-cell immunity.

Causes

The herpes simplex virus lies dormant in the nerve cells for long periods. The frequency and intensity of eruptions can usually be linked to periods of high stress—poor nutritional habits, exposure to the sun, allergens, or toxins, or difficulty in coping. Quite often an outbreak of herpes follows a minor infection or cold. High cortisol (stress hormone) levels promote herpes outbreaks. Food allergies or consuming foods or supplements high in arginine can provoke the virus to flare up by suppressing the activity of lysine, an amino acid successful in preventing herpes. Other conditions that can bring on an attack are spinal cord injuries, drug reactions, and an immune system suppressed by illness.

The inflammation of postherpetic neuralgia may lead to scarring and shrinking of the nerve endings, promoting chronic pain. It is important to treat herpes zoster as quickly as possible to reduce the likelihood of postherpetic neuralgia.

Prescription for Health

The following protocol is to be started at the first sign of eruptions.

NUTRIENT	DOSAGE	ACTION
Vitamin C	1000 mg of vitamin C every waking hour until sores are gone, then take Multimune containing vitamin C and other antioxidants for maintenance	Enhances immune function and prevents virus from replicating
High-potency B-complex and vitamin B_{12}	100 mg of B-complex three times daily, 500 mcg of B_{12} every waking hour or 1000 mcg B_{12} injection three times per week until sores are gone. Then take 500 mcg daily for maintenance	Protects against the effects of stress. B_{12} helps with postherpetic neuralgia and shrinking of blisters. B_{12} injections have been shown to shorten the duration of shingles.
Vitamin E	400 IU of vitamin E three times daily for three days and then take Multimune containing a maintenance dose of vitamin E. Do not take vitamin E if you are on Coumadin.	Shrinks and heals blisters quickly, stops postherpetic neuralgia
Bioflavonoids	500 mg every waking hour until sores are gone, then 500 mg daily thereafter	Works with vitamin C

NUTRIENT	DOSAGE	ACTION
Lysine	2000 mg daily until sores are gone, then 500 mg thereafter for prevention	Shrinks blisters, reduces recurrence, keeps arginine in balance
Moducare sterols and sterolins	Two capsules three times daily until sores are gone, then one capsule three times daily thereafter to reduce recurrence	Regulates immune function, reduces recurrence rates, controls cortisol
Zinc citrate	30 mg daily until sores are gone, then take Multimune containing 15 mg of zinc	Prevents infection and boosts immunity
CoQ10	60 mg daily until sores are gone, then take Multimune containing 30 mg of CoQ10	Helps immune system fight viruses
Homeopathic Rhus Tox 12C	Three pellets three times daily until sores are gone	Stops virus and enhances immune function
Echinacea	40 drops daily until sores are gone, then stop	Boosts immune system to fight virus
Wobenzym	Three capsules daily	Deactivates viruses
Multimune containing vitamins A, B$_6$, C, E, selenium, zinc, magnesium, coenzyme Q10, lipoic acid, reduced L-glutathione	Three capsules daily with food	Provides immune support, reduces toxins, is potent antioxidant, controls cortisol

Health Tips to Enhance Healing

- Follow diet recommendation in Chapter 4 and avoid foods that contain high amounts of arginine, including peanuts, chocolate, raisins, carob, gelatin, cereal grains, and other arginine-rich foods or nutritional supplements. Arginine competes with lysine for absorption and when lysine is low, herpes outbreaks increase.
- At the initial signs of an outbreak, apply ice to the area every 10 minutes for up to an hour. Ice can prevent the virus from traveling from the nerve to the skin.
- Reduce your stress levels. Get plenty of sleep and rest, take more time for yourself, and practice stress-reduction techniques (see Chapter 6).
- Herbs that are particularly helpful for fighting the herpes virus are cayenne and goldenseal.

Other Recommendations

- Apply a topical tea tree oil ointment (not diluted oil), lemon balm, licorice root gel, or Quantum lysine cream to the blisters as needed.
- Avoid the sun.

- Women with genital herpes are often deficient in iron. Have your iron levels checked by your doctor.
- In severe cases of Type 1 and Type 2, injections of adenosine-5-phosphate have been successfully used to control outbreaks.
- Try not to touch the infected area, but if you do, be sure to wash your hands immediately so as not to accidentally infect your eyes or pass it on to others. If your eye does become infected, seek treatment immediately.
- In cases of genital herpes, wear cotton underwear and be sure to keep the area clean and dry.

Health Fact

- Double-blind studies conducted using proteolytic enzymes (Wobenzym) versus acyclovir found that both groups experienced the same relief of symptoms, but the proteolytic group had none of the side effects.

HIGH BLOOD PRESSURE (HYPERTENSION)

Blood pressure is the force of blood as it is pushed through the arteries and arterioles. High blood pressure, also called hypertension or the "silent killer," increases your risk of heart attack and stroke. Approximately 62 million North Americans have high blood pressure. Chronic high blood pressure damages artery walls and blood vessels, promoting plaque buildup and heart attack, blindness, kidney damage, and stroke. (See Chapter 2.)

Long-term studies are indicating that hypertension medications cause side effects that actually increase the risk of heart attack. Other studies are showing that in the borderline and mild cases, drugs have no therapeutic value and only increase risks. Although medical practitioners agree that drug intervention is unnecessary at the borderline and mild stage, medication is still prescribed. Michael Murray, ND, explains in his book, *Heart Disease and High Blood Pressure*, that yearly sales of blood pressure-lowering drugs are estimated to be greater than $10 billion. As approximately 50 percent of cases are borderline or mild, the companies would lose half of their hypertension drug revenue if people were to follow natural therapies instead.

Symptoms

Often the first symptom is a heart attack, but headaches, frequent nose-bleeds, and vision problems can be signs of hypertension. High blood pressure is measured by the amount of resistance made with every heartbeat as it pushes blood through the arteries. When blood is forced through the arteries and veins, it is called systole; when the heart relaxes between beats, the blood pressure lowers to produce diastole. A normal reading is 120/80 (systolic/diastolic). High blood pressure is broken into four groups:

Borderline: 120–160 over 90–94
Mild: 140–160 over 95–104
Moderate: 140–180 over 105–114
Severe: 160+ over 115+

More than 80 percent of cases fall into the first three groups. This is good news because in most of these cases, lifestyle and diet changes can keep blood pressure under control better than prescription medication.

Causes

There are many factors that can lead to high blood pressure, including hardening of the arteries, high cholesterol, heredity, smoking, Type A personality, poor stress coping abilities, obesity, and lack of exercise. Nutritional deficiencies or a poor diet that emphasizes salt, sugar, caffeine, and refined carbohydrates elevate blood pressure. Excessive dieting or alcohol consumption can play a part, as can some prescription drugs, including birth control pills. High levels of heavy metals such as cadmium and lead have been found in those with hypertension.

Prescription for Health

NUTRIENT	DOSAGE	ACTION
Multivitamin with minerals	Use as directed	Provides general nutritional support
Vitamin B₃ (inositol hexanicotinate, nonflushing niacin)	500 mg three times daily	Aids circulation, lowers cholesterol and blood pressure
High-potency vitamin B-complex	Two to three capsules daily	Aids circulation and lowers blood pressure
Multimune containing vitamins A, B₆, C, E, selenium, zinc, magnesium, coenzyme Q10, lipoic acid, reduced L-glutathione	Three capsules daily	Is potent antioxidant, supports immune function to fight bacteria, chelates heavy metals
Vitamin D	400 IU daily	Lowers blood pressure
Vitamin C	1000 mg three times daily	Dilates blood vessels, strengthens walls, promotes excretion of lead
Vitamin E (d-alpha tocopherol)	100–400 IU daily	Slows progression of arteriosclerosis and thins blood
Calcium and magnesium	1000–2000 mg calcium daily and 750 mg magnesium daily	It can take six weeks for these nutrients to lower blood pressure
Potassium	500 mg daily, plus plenty of potassium-rich foods (see page 267)	Maintains blood pressure and reduces calcium loss
CoQ10	30–100 mg twice daily	Helps lower high blood pressure and improves cardiac function

NUTRIENT	DOSAGE	ACTION
Flaxseed oil	1–2 Tbsp (15–30 mL) daily	Improves blood circulation, prevents platelets from sticking
Garlic	2000–4000 mg of Kyolic garlic daily	Improves circulation, reduces blood pressure
Hawthorn	120–240 mg daily of standardized extract containing 1.8 percent vitexin or 10 percent procyanidins, or 240–480 mg daily of those standardized to 18 percent procyanidolic oligomers	Dilates arteries, lowers blood pressure
Moducare sterols and sterolins	Two capsules three times daily for one week, then one capsule three times daily thereafter	Decreases inflammation, enhances immune system to fight bacteria helpful in preventing infections in arteries
Coleus forskohlii	5–10 mg forskohlin	Relaxes arteries, reduces blood pressure
Taurine	500 mg twice daily between meals	Eliminates extra body fluid

Health Tips to Enhance Healing

Have your kidney function tested. Often high blood pressure is a symptom of kidney insufficiency.

- To lower blood pressure, include more fresh fruits and vegetables (7 to 10 servings daily) such as celery, onions, green leafy vegetables, and citrus fruits. Vegetarians have fewer problems with blood pressure than meat-eaters, so when choosing protein, try opting for more fiber, nuts and seeds, legumes, cold-water fish, or protein powders. Use garlic liberally with meals.
- Avoid sugar and aspartame. Use stevia, which is available from health food stores.
- A common imbalance found in people with high blood pressure is the wrong ratio of potassium to salt. Reduce sodium intake by avoiding table salt and processed foods. Increase your intake of potassium-rich foods such as bananas, apricots, tomatoes, avocados, potatoes, lean chicken meat, and fresh fish.
- Avoid eating animal fats and substitute plant fats instead. (See the recipes in Chapter 8 for lots of healthy selections.)
- Drink eight to ten glasses of pure, filtered water daily. For every cup with caffeine that you drink, add another glass of water. If you remember from Chapter 2, water makes up 92 percent of our blood, so it is crucial to keep blood volume at a healthy level. When blood volume is low, the body adjusts by narrowing or shutting down capillaries to prevent gases.

- See Cholesterol.
- See "Cardiovascular Corruption," page 17.

Other Recommendations

- Stop smoking and reduce caffeine consumption. An occasional glass of red wine may be beneficial, but more than one alcoholic drink per day should be avoided.
- Losing extra pounds can help reduce stress on the heart. Exercising for 30 minutes three times a week can do wonders for lowering blood pressure and can reduce your risk of stroke and heart attack by over 25 percent.
- It is important to get enough sleep and relaxation, but you may also want to practice relaxation techniques such as visualization, deep breathing, or biofeedback to concentrate on lowering blood pressure specifically and healing the damage that stress has caused (see "Stress-Busting Tips," page 130).
- Dining out can be overwhelming when you are trying to follow a heart-smart diet. Look for dishes that are broiled, poached, roasted, and grilled, and ask that dressings, gravies, and sauces be brought to you on the side so you can control how much you consume.

HIV (HUMAN IMMUNODEFICIENCY VIRUS)

Since the discovery of the acquired immunodeficiency syndrome (AIDS), billions of dollars have gone into the search for an effective way to eradicate this serious threat to humanity. Human immunodeficiency virus (HIV) is thought to be the main causative agent in the development of AIDS. HIV is a retrovirus, a virus that stores its genes as RNA instead of DNA.

Unlike other viruses, HIV reproduces itself inside the cells of the immune system. When HIV gets into our T-cells, it transforms its viral RNA (by using an enzyme reverse transcriptase) into viral DNA and then it is incorporated into the cells of the immune system. Because HIV hijacks our T-helper cells, the generals for the immune system that command all other cells, our immune system does not recognize and destroy the virus. HIV is smart because it has subverted our internal army and uses the commanding cell to thrive and survive.

HIV is able to mutate or change its nature, making it very difficult to destroy with an effective vaccine. The flu virus is similar in its ability to mutate quickly, hence the reason for different vaccines for the many and ever-changing flu strains each year.

Healthy individuals normally have T-helper-cell counts between 800–1200 per cubic millimeter. AIDS is diagnosed when this count drops to approximately 200 or less, and is accompanied by opportunistic infections such as pneumocystis carinii pneumonia, Kaposi's sarcoma, dementia, lymph disorders, and other diseases. Many people live HIV-positive for decades without ever developing AIDS.

According to the Elizabeth Glaser Pediatric AIDS Foundation in the U.S., 1800 children are infected with HIV each day in the world; two American adolescents are infected with HIV every hour; and over 6 million people worldwide are infected each year.

Symptoms

Upon infection, the immune system mounts a serious assault. It is believed that some individuals may have a strong enough immune system to destroy the virus before it has a chance to infect, but in most people by the time the B-cells produce antibodies against the virus, infection is complete and permanent. HIV infection usually begins with acute flu-like symptoms: fever, skin rashes, weakness, muscle aches, and swollen lymph glands under the arms and in the neck and groin. The spleen and liver may also enlarge. The symptoms can last a couple of weeks, just like a bad case of the flu, and then go away. During this time it is easy to infect others who are in intimate contact.

It can take up to a year for a person to test positive for HIV antibodies and during that time the person may have no idea that he or she is infected. After the initial infection, there are no symptoms of HIV. In some cases HIV-infected people with healthy lifestyles have avoided the opportunistic infections and cancers for at least 15 years. If the immune system weakens, however, opportunistic infections will begin to appear; they include pneumonia, Kaposi's sarcoma, systemic candida, herpes, and other conditions.

Causes

HIV is transmitted through blood and body fluids, including semen, blood, saliva, tears, urine, vaginal secretions, and breast milk. The most common routes of transmission are blood-to-blood contact, such as sharing needles or from transfusions prior to the introduction of blood screening; unprotected vaginal, oral, or anal sex; and from an HIV-positive mother to child at any time from gestation to breast-feeding. Opinions on the cause of AIDS vary, but HIV infection is currently believed to be the source of the disease.

HIV and the Balance Between Th-1 and Th-2 Cells

HIV infection causes a decline in the ability of Th-1 cells to produce protective interleukin-2. In the early 1990s it was proposed that the immune dysfunction caused by HIV may be due to an imbalance of Th-1 to Th-2 cells. Researchers have discovered that people just infected with

HIV are predominantly Th-1, but in as little as a few years this changes to a Th-2 dominance. It is believed that those HIV-infected individuals who remain symptom-free after infection have higher numbers of Th-1 cells. In *Basic and Clinical Immunology* by Mark Peakman and Diego Vergani, they stated that "the search is on for therapies that may selectively enhance TH1 and dampen TH2 responses." Synthetic interleukin-2 has been tried and failed as a method to selectively promote Th-1.

Moducare Is Effective at Halting T-4 Cell Decline: Moducare selectively enhances Th-1 and the production of interleukin-2. Patrick Bouic, Ph.D., and his team at Stellenbosch University, Cape Town, South Africa, confirmed this theory in an open-labeled study with a control group and a total of 323 HIV-infected people. The study began in 1993 and the patients, who were diagnosed HIV-positive, were followed for more than five years. Blood parameters—including T-4 cell determination, the degree of apoptosis (programmed cell death), serum cytokine (measurement of the pro-inflammatory interleukin 6, which was shown to activate viral replication in infected cells), and plasma RNA viral load (meaning the total number of cells infected)—were determined.

The trial comprised of two groups of subjects; one group received Moducare and the second was a control group. All were monitored at Tygerberg Hospital's Infectious Disease clinic. Results from this study showed that T-helper cells did not drop in the Moducare treatment group compared to the control group. At the six-month point in the trial, members of the control group were offered the Moducare treatment because their T-helper cells were dropping at the expected rate in HIV infection and there was a risk of death. Researchers felt it was unethical to allow the control subjects to die knowing that the Moducare group did not exhibit the same downward spiral of T-helper cell decline.

As well in the moducare group, apoptosis or programmed cell death, which is proposed as a reason for the excessive T-helper cell loss in HIV-infected individuals, did not show a statistically significant decline; the degree of cell death in the blood of the subjects taking Moducare showed a slight decline. As well, interleukin-6, the pro-inflammatory cytokine that is implicated in the virus's ability to replicate, decreased significantly in the Moducare group.

Sterols and sterolins were not found to have antiviral activity in humans, but it is thought that long-term use may change this. Unfortunately, viral loads were not conducted on all patients since commercial tests were not available until late in the study. Nevertheless, Bouic's team felt confident that Moducare would eventually lead to a decrease in viral load, indirectly via the function of the immune system, but this decrease would not be as dramatic as that induced by current anti-retrovirals. To date, Bouic's research indicates that T-4 cell counts are stabilized with a decrease in serum pro-inflammatory interleukin-6. The importance of Moducare as an auxiliary treatment for HIV/AIDS should not be overlooked. It should be the basis that all other adjuncts are added to. HIV/AIDS persons in North America who combine the anti-retrovirals along with Moducare have significant decline in viral load and an increase in CD-4 counts.

Prescription for Health

AIDS/HIV is a highly complex disease, and in no way do I wish to deny that. The following suggestions are to be used in conjunction with your physician's advice. The goal is to live long term with the virus, reducing viral load and increasing CD-4 cell counts without opportunistic infections.

NUTRIENT	DOSAGE	ACTION
Vitamin A, Micel A	100,000 IU micellized vitamin A for one week, then 5000 IU daily thereafter	Needed because it is deficient in those with HIV/AIDS and is associated with T-helper cell decline
Multivitamin with minerals	Two or three capsules daily or as directed	Assures adequate nutrient status
Moducare sterols and sterolins	Two capsules three times daily for one week, then one capsule three times daily thereafter	See pages 269 and 270 for action
High-potency B-complex and B_{12}	Two or three capsules daily 1000 mcg of B_{12} daily sublingual	Protects against neuropathy and myelopathy
Vitamin C, mineral ascorbates	50 g intravenous infusions daily for two weeks in the acute stage, then 1000–3000 mg in oral form daily thereafter	Inhibits reverse transcriptase
Vitamin E	400–800 IU daily	A potent antioxidant
Selenium	200 mcg selenomethionine daily	A potent antioxidant and immunity booster
Zinc citrate	60 mg daily	Increases the number of T-helper cells
CoQ10	100–200 mg twice daily	Controls opportunistic infections
Reduced L-glutathione or NAC	150 mg twice daily	Reduces TNF and IL-6, is potent antioxidant
Alpha lipoic acid	150 mg three times daily	May slow HIV progression by reducing the activity of reverse transcriptase
Essential fatty acids, Udo's Choice Oil or Omega Essential Balance	2 Tbsp (30 mL) daily	Modulates immune function, may destroy viruses
Curcumin	400 mg three times daily	Inhibits replication of HIV, increases T-helper cells
Garlic (Kyolic)	Two or three capsules daily	Improves digestion and is beneficial for candidiasis
Bromelain	1800 mcu (milk-clotting units) on an empty stomach	Acts as a natural protease inhibitor without the side effects

NUTRIENT	DOSAGE	ACTION
Wobenzym, proteolytic enzyme	Six capsules daily	Acts as a natural protease inhibitor without the side effects, supports immune function, eliminates circulating virus
Women's Whey or proteins+ protein powder	One to two scoops daily	Ensures amino acids for cell repair
Licorice (Glycyrrhizin)	1–2 g of powdered root daily; increase potassium-rich foods such as bananas to ensure adequate potassium	Can inhibit HIV-1; do not take if high blood pressure is present

Health Tips to Enhance Healing

- Follow the nutrition recommendations in Chapter 4. It is essential that those with HIV maintain proper immune function and prevent malnutrition to avoid opportunistic infections. Emphasis must be placed on nutritious food, an aggressive supplementation program, regular exercise, fresh air, positive thinking, and stress reduction. There must also be an avoidance of any substance, activity, or behavior that suppresses the immune system and prevents it from acting at full capacity. (See "The Immune System and Stress," page 45.)
- Eat green foods like blue-green algae, spirulina, wheatgrass, and barley grass, which are rich in plant nutrients.
- Eliminate allergies. See the introduction to this chapter.

Other Recommendations

- Avoid salt, caffeine, sugar, alcohol, soft drinks (diet or otherwise), and cigarettes as they only contribute to the toxic burden on the body and force the digestive, cardiovascular, and excretory systems to work harder in eliminating them.
- Seek out a professional who can provide you with other beneficial therapies such as acupuncture, chiropractic, visualization, hydrotherapy, homeopathy, hyperbaric oxygen therapy, and tradition Chinese medicine.
- If you are sexually active, always use a latex condom to decrease the risk of spreading infection. While there has been success in extending and improving the lives of people with HIV and AIDS, there is no cure and the infection increases vulnerability to other infections, such as pneumonia, which can be fatal.
- Ensure that your primary health-care giver is experienced with HIV, willing to research answers to questions you may have, and is up-to-date on recent studies, breakthroughs, and trends. You must also

educate yourself as to the different types of therapies that are available and participate in the development of your treatment plan.

HYPOGLYCEMIA

Hypoglycemia occurs when the blood sugar (glucose) levels are abnormally low. The diabetic associations believe that hypoglycemia is seen only in those with diabetes, yet due to our diet and lifestyle, hypoglycemia is a very common problem. Blood sugar level is measured in milligrams of glucose per deciliter of blood. The normal range is 60–120 mg/dL depending on how long it has been since the last meal. A fasting blood sugar level can be between 50 and 60 mg/dL. Anything below 45 mg/dL is considered abnormally low.

Symptoms

When the blood sugar levels fall too low, a person may feel weak, shaky, dizzy, tired, nauseous, irritable, lightheaded, anxious, and hungry. There may be swollen feet, sweating, tightness in the chest, blurred vision, lack of concentration, confusion, hunger, insomnia, and heart palpitations. Hypoglycemics may become angry or aggressive with huge mood swings.

The symptoms range from mild to severe depending on the amount of time between meals and the type of food eaten. Hypoglycemia is associated with other ailments, including adrenal deficiency, liver and kidney disease, angina, migraines, and PMS. Typical hypoglycemia is called reactive hypoglycemia because symptoms appear within four hours of a meal, especially if it was high in sugar and fats.

Causes

Diabetes is a common cause of hypoglycemia. Type I diabetics and some Type II diabetics are required to take insulin to lower their blood sugar levels, and if they take too much, skip a meal, drink too much alcohol, or exercise too much, they may induce hypoglycemia.

In non-diabetics, the factors that can induce hypoglycemia are prolonged fasting, long bouts of strenuous exercise (especially if taking beta-blocker medication), pregnancy, and in children, aspirin. It can also arise due to problems with the adrenals, kidneys, thyroid, and immune system.

Hypoglycemia is becoming more common in people following a typical North American diet that is poor in nutrients, low in fiber and complex carbohydrates, and high in sugar and simple carbohydrates. Smoking, stress, alcohol, and caffeine compound the problem.

See recommendations for Allergies, Diabetes, and Hypothyroidism to help control and regulate blood sugar and subsequently insulin.

Prescription for Health

NUTRIENT	DOSAGE	ACTION
Vitamin B-complex	Two or three capsules daily	Important for digestion, metabolism, and nerve function
Multimune containing vitamines A, B_6, C, E, selenium, zinc, magnesium, coenzyme Q10, lipoic acid, reduced L-glutathione	Three capsules daily with food	Supports immune function, contains vitamin A, B_6, C, E, selenium, zinc, lipoic acid, reduced L-glutathione, coenzyme Q10, magnesium; magnesium helps control blood sugar
Vitamin C (buffered with mineral ascorbates, i.e., calcium ascorbate)	2000–3000 mg daily in divided doses	Prevents vitamin C deficiency and protects against the damaging effects of fluctuating blood sugar
Chromium picolinate	200 mcg twice daily	Regulates blood sugar levels
Multimineral without iron	One or two capsules daily	Supports nutrient absorption and repairs deficiency
Women's Whey or proteins+ protein powder	One to two scoops	Small protein-based meals help keep blood sugar stable.
Alpha lipoic acid	300 mg twice daily	Converts glucose to energy, protects against free radical damage, improves insulin sensitivity, recycles vitamin C, and stops neuropathies
Moducare sterols and sterolins	One capsule three times daily	Increases DHEA, inhibits inflammation by IL-6, and decreases the B-cell antibody production against pancreatic tissues
Omega-3 fatty acid	One capsule of fish oil (EPA/DHA) three times daily	Lowers blood pressure, increases levels of good cholesterol, reduces the level of bad cholesterol, and lowers the levels of fibrinogen, a protein that makes blood thicker and stickier; is also necessary for the formation of prostaglandins
Evening primrose oil	1000 mg capsule three times daily with meals	Improves diabetes-related peripheral nerve dysfunction and increases the enzyme activity on omega-6 that is inhibited by abnormal blood glucose and insulin levels
5-HTP	50 mg three times daily	A precursor to tryptophan and to serotonin. Serotonin deficiency predisposes us to hypoglycemia.
Bitter melon	Either fresh, unripened bitter melon or in capsules asrecommended	Normalizes blood glucose

Health Tips to Enhance Healing

- Change your diet to one that is high in fiber and low in sugar and refined carbohydrates. Do not eat any white foods (white sugar, white flour, white pasta, white rice, white potatoes, etc.). Eat brightly colored fruits and vegetables because they are high in vitamins and minerals. Good fruits and vegetables that help stabilize blood sugar are avocado, blueberries, cranberries, grapefruits, kiwi, apples, lemons, turnips, parsley, mustard greens, green pepper, kale, cabbage, bok choy, beets, and spinach. Avoid sweet fruits as they can induce hypoglycemia.

- Use stevia as a sweetener. Avoid refined sugar, syrups, commercial desserts, and most condiments. Read the labels; it may not taste like it, but the sugar content is high in items such as salad dressings, mustard, barbecue sauce, mayonnaise, and ketchup. Don't fall for fat-free or low-fat labeling; the fat content is replaced by sugar. Opt for healthier snacks such as nuts, yogurt, or a protein-rich sports bar that is low in carbohydrates.
- Avoid alcohol, especially if your consumption is excessive or appears to trigger attacks.
- In addition to avoiding the white foods, pay attention to the level of dietary fiber. The ideal type of dietary fiber to consume is water-soluble plant fiber because it prevents rapid rises in blood sugar and improves tissue sensitivity to insulin. Good examples of water-soluble fiber include beans, most vegetables, and fruits such as apples.
- Increase your intake of EPA and DHA by adding regular servings of fish to your diet such as salmon, herring, or mackerel. Other healthy oils come from nuts and seeds such as flaxseed, pumpkin seed, and Udo's Choice oil.
- Eat five or six smaller meals throughout the day instead of three large meals.

Other Recommendations

- Helpful herbs for hypoglycemia are licorice root, garlic, buchu, dandelion root, gotu kola, and alfalfa.
- Spirulina and reishi mushrooms also do well in stabilizing blood sugar.
- Avoid salt, caffeine, sugar, and cigarettes as they can only aggravate the condition.
- If you suspect that allergies are the source of your problem, see the introduction to this chapter.
- Have your physician check you for hypothyroidism.
- If you suspect that you are hypoglycemic, you can have a physician test you. However, some tests may read normal, so follow the diet and supplement program and see if your symptoms abate.

Health Fact

One study found that 75 percent of those with functional hypoglycemia had food sensitivities.

IDIOPATHIC THROMBOCYTOPENIA PURPURA

Idiopathic thrombocytopenia purpura (ITP) is a disease whereby the number of platelets in the body is drastically low, causing abnormal bleeding. Idiopathic means the cause is unknown. In autoimmune idiopathic thrombocytopenia purpura the immune system produces autoantibodies against the platelets, thus destroying them. Platelets are tiny disks in the blood that allow the blood to clot. Platelets are formed in the bone marrow and sit in the spleen for 36 hours before being released into the bloodstream. Platelets must be continually replaced by new platelets because they have limited longevity. In ITP the platelets are damaged or destroyed prematurely, leading to seriously low platelet levels even though the bone marrow may be producing more and more to keep up with demand.

Secondary thrombocytopenia can coincide with other autoimmune disorders such as lupus, inflammatory bowel disease (including Crohn's and colitis), Graves' disease and Hashimoto thyroiditis, rheumatoid arthritis, and scleroderma. There is an increase of ITP being associated with infectious diseases such HIV, herpes, mononucleosis, pneumonia, cytomegalovirus, and Lyme disease.

ITP has acute and chronic variations. Chronic ITP occurs in adults and affects 14,000 to 16,000 new people every year in North America. It is insidious, affects three times as many women compared to men, and remission is rare. Acute ITP appears equally in children of either sex, usually between the ages of two and four, and is often brought on by a viral infection. It comes on suddenly, lasts about six months, and then disappears as quickly as it came. In a small percentage of children, ITP will become chronic and require more aggressive treatment.

Symptoms

Symptoms of ITP are gingival bleeding, easy bruising, and, in women, menorraghia, the excessive loss of menstrual blood. Petechiae are tiny red or purple spots filled with blood that show up in the mucous membranes or skin, particularly around the ankles and lower legs. The petechiae aggregate to become purpura, heavy bruising that appears as patches of purple discoloration on the skin.

As the disease progresses, there can be gastrointestinal bleeding, blood in the urine; skin lesions; nosebleeds; bleeding from the mouth, throat, and other mucous membranes; or in extreme situations, bleeding in the cerebrum. Depression is common with ITP as there are up days and down days, which can make coping with responsibilities of work or family very difficult.

Causes

Macrophages in the spleen and, to a lesser degree, the liver eat the platelets that are coated in IgG autoantibodies. Helper T-cells are increased, suppressor T-cells decrease, and NK cell activity is lower. The macrophage activity stimulates greater macrophage activity, and in serious cases the spleen must be removed to slow down the rate of platelet destruction. However, splenectomies do not guarantee a resolution of the problem and often the disease remains with activity continuing in the liver.

Story of Hope from One ITP Sufferer

I often receive letters from readers who have used some of the products mentioned in the *Healthy Immunity Newsletter*. The following is one of those letters.

> I have been taking Moducare for about three months. I have an autoimmune disease called idiopathic thrombocytopenia purpura (ITP). It is a condition where my immune system attacks my platelets and therefore my blood cannot clot properly. I have had my spleen removed (this means that I am very susceptible to infections). I have taken prednisone and other strong medications that helped for only a brief period. Since taking Moducare, I have had only two viral infections and no sign of platelet drop—this is the first time in 15 years. It has been great! I want to thank you for making such an amazing product available.
>
> —L.V., Pennsylvania

Prescription for Health

Standard medical treatment employs prednisone to stop the immune system from attacking the platelets and high doses of immune globulin are given intravenously to prevent life-threatening bleeding and to keep platelet counts up in children. The following recommendations are focused on halting autoantibody production, correcting the imbalance in the immune system, and reducing bruising and bleeding.

NUTRIENTS	DOSAGE	ACTION
Moducare sterols and sterolins	Two capsules three times daily for one week, then one capsule three times daily as a maintenance dose. Birth to five years of age should take one capsule daily; five to twelve years of age should take two capsules daily; twelve years and older should take the adult dose.	Essential for regulating immune function and controlling autoantibody reactions, is anti-inflammatory

NUTRIENTS	DOSAGE	ACTION
High-potency B-complex	Two capsules daily with meals	Required for metabolism and proper immune function
Multimune containing vitamins A, B₆, C, E, selenium, zinc, magnesium, coenzyme Q10, lipoic acid, and reduced L-glutathione	Three capsules daily with meals	Supports the proper functioning of the immune system, is anti-inflammatory and potent antioxidant
Vitamin C with bioflavonoid	1000 mg of vitamin C twice a day, 500 mg of bioflavonoid daily	Regulates immunity and combats stress, protects platelets from destruction
Vitamin E	100 IU per day	In several studies those with autoimmune diseases had a significant reduction in symptoms.
Spleen extracts	50 mg containing active proteins splenopentin and tuftsin daily	Enhances natural killer cells to protect against infections
Evening primrose oil	1 g three times daily	Is essential for recurring and relapsing autoimmune disease, ensures proper function of suppressor T-cells, is anti-inflammatory

Health Tips to Enhance Healing

- Do not take immune boosters of any type. They can enhance the cytokines responsible for antibody production, thus worsening ITP. The German Commission E does not recommend that those with autoimmune disorders take echinacea.
- Avoid saturated fats from red meats, pork, deep-fried foods, and lard. Research has shown that diets high in saturated fats exacerbated autoimmune disease and increased the number of flare-ups and recurrences.
- Eat plenty of fresh fruits and vegetables, legumes, whole grains, nuts and seeds, healthy oils, fresh fish, free-range poultry, and soy products. Choose organic whenever possible to minimize toxic burden to the system.
- Detoxification and elimination of waste is very important. Eat liver-friendly foods such as kale, carrots, beets, artichokes, lemons, onions, garlic, leeks, and members of the cabbage family (broccoli, cauliflower, Brussels sprouts).

Other Recommendations

- Exercise regularly to improve circulation and to help the detoxification and elimination process.

- Reduce stress. Rest and relax when you can and practice stress reduction techniques (see "Stress-Busting Tips," page 130).
- See autoimmune disease in Chapter 3.

Health Fact

Although ITP can appear subsequent to HIV infection, it should not be interpreted as an increased propensity for developing AIDS. In fact, most HIV-positive people with ITP do not require therapeutics and half of the cases will have a spontaneous resolution within four years.

INFLUENZA

Every year flu season hits and a large percentage of our population suffers its effects. Most people endure a couple of weeks of illness and fully recover, but for some influenza can be serious. Those who are immune compromised, the elderly, asthmatics, and others with chronic lung problems may suffer complications as a result of the flu. Influenza is a viral infection of the upper respiratory tract that is highly contagious. Infections may reside in the ears, nose, throat, bronchial tubes, and lungs. The virus is spread by coughing and sneezing, and enters the body via the mucous membranes of the eyes, nose, and mouth.

The flu vaccine is promoted as the best way to prevent the flu, yet contrary to what we have been told, there are problems with the effectiveness of the vaccine. Most seniors and those that are immune compromised are not protected by their annual flu vaccine. Vaccines work by stimulating B-cells to produce antibodies to the foreign substance—in this case the flu virus. In order for our immune system to do its work, it must operate efficiently. We know the elderly and people with compromised immune systems, such as those with HIV and hepatitis C, do not produce enough antibodies. As a result, those who need the vaccine most are unprotected.

The second problem with the vaccine is that the flu virus keeps mutating, so in order to be protected, the virus in the vaccine has to be the same virus that you are exposed to in the environment. If the virus has mutated and is different from the one in the vaccine, even just slightly, the vaccine is ineffective. Thirdly, the flu vaccine contains a preservative called thimersol, a mercury derivative. Mercury is a neurotoxin (toxic to the brain) and a kidney toxin. Health officials tell us that the little amount of mercury in the vaccine is safe, but no one has studied the effects of years of flu vaccinations. Mercury builds up in the body and is very difficult to remove.

Symptoms

Flu symptoms are similar to that of a cold: fatigue, fever, sore throat, headache, nausea, vomiting, body aches, aching around the eyes, cough, chills, and sweats. The symptoms come suddenly, unlike a cold that may take days for you to feel its full effects. A person may be left so weak and in such discomfort that he or she can't do anything, not even eat.

Fever, which often accompanies the flu, is not an illness but the sign of the immune system fighting off infectious agents such as viruses, bacteria, parasites, and other microbes. Fever of 100–102°F (38–39°C) prevents these agents from multiplying so that the infection dies out, and can also help to rid the body of toxins. Fevers above 102°F (39°C) in adults (or 103°F/40°C in children) must be carefully monitored by a doctor as it is a sign that the condition is worsening. Fevers can be problematic for people with heart conditions because it forces the heart to work harder, and if a fever remains too high for too long, it can induce delirium or seizures, causing dehydration and injury to the brain. Homeopathic treatments such as belladonna, aconite, *Natrum muriaticum*, and *Ferrum phosphoricum* can be quite effective at rapidly reducing fever. For children, Dr. Ronald Reichert, a naturopath practicing in Vancouver and author of *Kava Kava*, recommends Viburcol suppositories by Heel to quickly reduce high fever.

Causes

Strains of the flu virus have been classified as A, B, and C, and pandemics are thought to belong to class A. The genetic material of the flu virus is a single strand of RNA. The virus changes while it copies itself, thus creating slight variations of itself.

Viruses can set up residence in the body when the immune system is weak from fatigue, stress, allergies, and nutritional deficiencies or poor diet, and when we are dehydrated. The mucous membranes around the eyes, nose, and mouth are very rich in immune factors that fight viruses. When we become dehydrated these fluids shrink, reducing the effectiveness of the immune factors. The cheapest virus fighter is plenty of water every day.

Prescription for Health

NUTRIENT	DOSAGE	ACTION
Multimune containing vitamins A, B_6, C, E, selenium, zinc, reduced L-glutathione, coenzyme Q10, lipoic acid, and magnesium	Three capsules with food daily	Boosts immunity, fights viruses, is a potent antioxidant, helps detoxify, contains glutathione, which helps decongest the upper respiratory tract

NUTRIENT	DOSAGE	ACTION
Echinacea	20 drops of tincture several times daily or 1000 mg capsule daily	Boosts immune system and acts as an antibiotic. Do not take longer than four weeks; is contraindicated in autoimmune disease and HIV.
Goldenseal	100 mg three times daily	High in berberine and hydrastine, both potent immune boosters
Astragalus	200 mg three times daily	Boosts immunity and reduces frequency of infection
Garlic	Three capsules daily (Kyolic)	Antiviral in nature, expels mucous, and stimulates NK cell activity
Moducare sterols and sterolins	One capsule three times daily	Enhances immune system, increases gamma-interferon and NK cells
Vitamin A (Micel A)	One dropper of 100,000 units daily for five days	This is my favorite for fighting all kinds of infections. Drop in the back of the throat and let it sit for a few seconds before swallowing. Gets rid of sore throats fast.

Health Tips to Enhance Healing

- Do not eat sugar of any type because it causes your infection-fighting natural killer cells to become inactive, allowing viruses to take hold. No fruit juice.
- Drink herbal teas such as slippery elm, ginger, catnip, and rosehip. Make your own ginger tea by grinding 1 in (2.5 cm) of fresh ginger (which is rich in zinc), add some squeezed lemon and boiling water, and top off with some cinnamon or a sprinkle of cayenne pepper.
- Reduce stress and get plenty of sleep and rest. If at all possible, stay home from work to recuperate fully and not spread the contagion to your coworkers. (See stress and the common cold, page 38.)
- Eat small amounts of solid food. Fresh vegetable juices and flavorful broth will provide the essential nutrients. Eat foods such as radish, daikon, mustard, and turnip greens and those high in vitamins A and C, especially cranberry and blueberry. Use flu-fighters marjoram, cayenne (a decongestant that also reduces fever), and garlic to flavor vegetable dishes. Research has shown that children who eat plain yogurt regularly are better at resisting flu bugs.

Other Recommendations

- Eucalyptus and menthol rubbed on the chest can ease congestion and coughing. Avoid if pregnant.
- Wash hands thoroughly and often, and avoid touching the face, mouth, nose, and eyes.

- Chicken soup actually lives up to its reputation. A study published in *Chest* in 1978 found that chicken soup was more beneficial than warm water. The soup increased mucous production to ease congestion and reduced inflammation. Make sure it is homemade so it doesn't come with unwanted food additives and flavorings.
- Do not give children aspirin (see Fever.) Children with fever should not take any product that contains salicylic acid (aspirin) as the risk of acquiring Reye's syndrome will be significantly increased. Reye's syndrome affects children between the ages of four and 15 and is life-threatening. It usually develops after a bout of cold or flu when aspirin was given as a remedy. Signs to watch for are excessive sleepiness, vomiting, and confusion.

Health Fact

Every year, influenza kills over 20,000 North Americans and hospitalizes another 100,000. The Spanish flu epidemic of 1918 killed almost 30 million people worldwide.

LEAKY GUT SYNDROME
(AND MALABSORPTION SYNDROME)

Leaky gut syndrome (LGS) is caused by years of food allergies, bacterial overgrowth, candidiasis, and stress. These and other factors can cause inflammation of our gut lining, eventually damaging the delicate tissues and allowing openings or gaps for substances to leak into the bloodstream, hence the name "leaky" gut. When waste, bacteria, and partially digested food are allowed to pass into the bloodstream from a damaged or leaky gut, the immune system mounts an assault against these foreign invaders. A leaky gut must be healed quickly, not only to stop the leakage of foreign substances into the bloodstream, but also to quell aggressive immune responses that promote an overproduction of antibodies, which would that lead to further food allergies, cramps, diarrhea, bloating, heartburn, and autoimmune and other chronic disorders.

The antibodies that are produced in response to leaky gut go marauding around the body and may attack other tissues and organs. For example, antibodies that travel to the lungs may promote asthma, and antibodies to the joints will promote arthritis-like symptoms. Leaky gut is implicated in several autoimmune disorders from rheumatoid arthritis to lupus. Toxins are also allowed to access areas of the body that they normally would not have entry to through a leaky gut. These toxins then overload the body's organs, especially the liver.

Breaches and inflammation in the intestinal wall also makes absorption of nutrients very difficult, which is known as malabsorption, thus inducing further stress on the body because of deficiencies.

Malabsorption syndrome, a separate but related condition, occurs when food is not broken down properly or inflammation to the small intestine is so severe that nutrients cannot be absorbed. Once malabsorption sets in, eating the most wholesome diet in the world will not prevent nutritional deficiencies, so extra supplementation must be provided. Even then nutrients taken orally may not be absorbed and injectable nutrients may have to be used. This is especially true for those with celiac disease, Crohn's, or severe candidiasis, or those with autoimmune disorders affecting the gut lining. Those with leaky gut generally have serious vitamin and mineral deficiencies as well.

Although every nutrient is important for the optimal functioning of the body, some nutrient deficiencies promote serious harm. Magnesium is required for hundreds of enzymatic actions, so its deficiency can affect any part of the body. Some researchers suspect that up to 80 percent of the population could be deficient in magnesium, especially because the recommended dietary allowance is too low. Minerals require carrier proteins to help them across the intestine and into the bloodstream. In those with leaky gut, the carrier proteins are often damaged and minerals fail to be absorbed at the optimal rate.

Leaky gut and malabsorption syndrome can affect anyone, but if children are afflicted correction should be taken immediately because they are still developing and their musculoskeletal growth may be permanently affected. According to Dr. Michael Lyon, director of research at the Oceanside Functional Medicine Research Institute, leaky gut syndrome is present in 75 percent of children who have attention deficit disorder.

Symptoms

The symptoms of leaky gut and malabsorption cause intestinal distress: pain, diarrhea, constipation, bloating, gas, irritable bowel syndrome, belching, poor concentration, allergies, fatigue, and weakness. There can also be pale, shiny, greasy stools; problems with vision; muscle cramps; PMS; slow growth rate in children; dry skin and lackluster hair and nails; bruising; and unexplained weight loss. Weight gain can also be a symptom—the appetite may increase because the body is not getting the nutrients it needs. Anemia can arise from an iron or vitamin B_{12} deficiency. If the tongue feels like it is burning, it indicates a B_5 deficiency. Chemical and environmental sensitivities or allergies result from leaky gut. Parasites, virus, and candida overgrowth are common symptoms. Autoimmune disease, especially of the gut lining, and increased autoantibody production and reduced secretory IgA are also seen.

The similarity of leaky gut and malabsorption to other diseases, and the fact that we all experience gastric difficulties at some time or another, make it easy for them to be overlooked as the causal factor for the problem.

SOME SIGNS OF DEFICIENCY OF COMMON NUTRIENTS

Calcium	Bone loss, brittle fingernails, periodontal disease, depression
Folic acid	Anemia, restless legs, digestive problems
Iron	Anemia, cold sensitivity, digestive disturbances
Protein	Peeling nails, grooves and ridges on nails, edema
Selenium	Dry skin, poor immune function, high cholesterol
Thiamin, vitamin B_1	A feeling of pins and needles in the feet and/or hands, anorexia, constipation, pain sensitivity
Vitamin B_2	Sore tongue, cracks at the sides of the mouth
Vitamin B_{12}	No moons on the fingernails (the white part at the bottom that is in the shape of a moon), not including the thumbnails; anemia; pins and needles in feet; palpitations
Vitamin D	Bone loss, hypothyroidism, burning mouth and throat, diarrhea
Zinc	Acne, baldness, brittle nails, white spots on nails

Causes

Long-term antibiotic therapy can also start the process, as can NSAIDs and other prescription drugs that injure the gut lining. Chemotherapy and radiation treatments also cause leaky gut. It is a vicious cycle as some of the causes of leaky gut and malabsorption syndrome (like allergies and candida) are also the end result of leaky gut.

Constipation is clearly implicated. When the bowel becomes blocked with feces, cellular waste, and foreign matter such as bacteria, fungus, parasites, and viruses, the excess toxins inflame the intestinal lining. The inflammation interferes with the processes of digestion and elimination. If this situation is continuous, the accumulation of harmful gases and foreign pathogens endanger the body. If the intestinal lining becomes too weak, spaces open up between the cells, giving easy access to larger molecules of toxins and food that were once prevented from entering the bloodstream.

Any type of digestive problem can lead to malabsorption syndrome if it is allowed to go on for too long. Colitis, celiac disease, Crohn's disease, even chronic diarrhea (to name a few) can injure the intestinal membranes and prevent them from absorbing nutrients. Allergies (particularly to lactose), excessive use of laxatives, alcohol, or other drugs can also adversely affect digestion and absorption. A poor diet low in fiber and nutrients but high in fats and refined carbohydrates will exacerbate any digestive disorder, as will low stomach acid or insufficient digestive enzymes.

Prescription for Health

Go easy on the nutrients because we want to heal the gut so you can then absorb the vitamins and minerals you need. The following, along with the recommendations in Chapter 1, are designed to help heal the gut.

NUTRIENT	DOSAGE	ACTION
Multivitamin with minerals	Use as directed	Prevents deficiency
Moducare sterols and sterolins	One capsule three times daily	Halts inflammatory gut reactions, regulates cortisol, enhances DHEA naturally, regulates immune function. See Prof. Bouic's study on page 109.
P-5-P (the active form of vitamin B_6)	50 mg daily	Heals mucosal lining
Probiotics, a combination of *Lactobacillus acidophilus*, FOS, and *Bifidum bacterium*	1 tsp (5 mL) of 1–2 billion live organisms daily	Restores good bacteria in the gut, stops diarrhea, restores proper elimination
L-glutamine (Jarrow Formulas)	Start with 1 g twice daily and increase over one week to 5 g twice daily on an empty stomach	Heals the gut, which is important for those with radiation-induced diarrhea. Those with leaky gut will notice improvement in four to six weeks.
Omega's Hi-Lignan Flax Seed	1 tsp (5 mL) daily; drink two glasses of water for every tsp of flax powder	Improves transit time, heals mucosal lining of the gut
Digestive enzymes (Prevail)	One or two capsules with each meal	Aids proper digestion
Essential fatty acids, Omega Essential Balance, or Udo's Choice oil, or flaxseed oil	1 Tbsp (15 mL) twice daily	Heals mucous membranes, is anti-inflammatory

Health Tips to Enhance Healing

- Discover the cause by reading Chapter 1 on digestion, and practice the tips for taming tummy troubles. See Bowel Disease, Candidiasis, and Constipation.
- Rule out H. pylori, parasites, or other infections.
- Eliminate food allergies. See the introduction to this chapter for information on testing.
- Once you have healed your gut lining, take a multivitamin with minerals, a high-potency B-complex, and Multimune Antioxidant formula to prevent deficiency and ensure adequate immune function.
- The leaky gut test (intestinal permeability) can be performed to determine if you have leaky gut syndrome. Contact Great Smokies Laboratory (1-800-455-4762) 63 Zillicoa Street, Asheville, NC, 28801-1074. They also offer a plethora of tests to determine candida, fatty acids, vitamin panel, H. pylori antibodies, food allergies, amino acids, and more.

- Do not use NSAIDs (see "Serious Side Effects from NSAIDs," page 13.)
- Use antibiotics only when absolutely necessary (see "Vaccination and Autoimmunity," page 50).

Other Recommendations

- Eliminate all soft drinks, especially diet pops. They often contain aspartame, a substance that contains known toxins. Other artificial sweeteners such as Sorbitol and Sucralose can create gas, bloating, and increased diarrhea, and white sugar depresses immunity. Try using the herbal sweetener stevia instead. It comes in liquid drops and powder form.
- Chiropractic, acupuncture, homeopathy, and reflexology are all beneficial therapies that may be able to provide some relief. Consult a qualified practitioner.

MENOPAUSE

Menopause is the cessation of menses, when hormones of the fertility cycle wind down, the ovaries stop releasing eggs, and pregnancy is no longer possible. For some it can be a greatly anticipated event and for others the time is difficult and tumultuous. The average age of menopause is 51, with perimenopause (the period leading into menopause) starting several years earlier. Menopause is achieved after one year has passed since the last menses, but some women experience symptoms for years before menstruation totally stops and have symptoms up to a decade after. Menopause can be induced at any age by radiation, surgery, and medication. It is not a disease but a normal life process for women.

Symptoms

Menopause is different for every woman. Women consuming the standard North American diet tend to have more menopausal symptoms than women eating traditional diets. Common menopausal symptoms reported include hot flashes, irregular uterine bleeding, weight gain, night sweats, vaginal dryness and thinning, decreased libido, depression, fatigue, nausea, headaches, mood swings, sleep disturbance, changes in cognitive function, bone loss, skin changes, losing hair on the head, hair growth on the body, acne, heart palpitations, urinary tract infections, joint pains, and an increased risk of osteoporosis and heart disease.

Causes

Menopause is a natural event in a woman's life. Every women eventually achieves menopause, but there is some speculation about how menopause begins. Does the brain stop signaling the hormones to stimulate the follicle, or does the follicle stop listening to the brain's signals? Dr. John Lee, author of *What Your Doctor Might Not Tell You About Premenopause*, believes that it is both, and that they are influenced by genetic predisposition and environmental factors such as activity levels, childbearing, exposure to xenohormones, poor diet, low-calorie diets, and severe emotional stress.

Other causes of menopause are premature menopause, oophorectomy (removal of the ovaries), and hysterectomy (removal of the uterus). Premature menopause, between the ages of 15 and 40, will happen to one out of 100 women. Only one-third of those cases will have a traceable cause such as immune dysfunction, infection, metabolic or systemic disease, smoking, reduced blood supply to the ovaries, chemotherapy, surgery, or radiation. The removal of the ovaries and uterus may be done at the same time or separately and is referred to as surgical menopause. An oophorectomy (removal of the ovaries) brings on menopause immediately and the symptoms can be overwhelming due to the sudden decline in hormone production. A hysterectomy in which at least one ovary remains induces a more natural, albeit earlier, menopause.

Prescription for Health

The recommendations below are to help women go through menopause symptom-free, with plenty of energy and a healthy libido, and without the worry of an increased risk of heart disease and osteoporosis. Standard hormone replacement therapy (HRT) is not advised due to the potential cancer-causing risks involved. Scientists are still debating the increased risks of cancer due to HRT. Until we have a clear-cut answer, there are natural alternatives. European studies have shown an increased risk of breast cancer in over 30 percent of women using HRT. As well, the Nurses' Health Study involving 23,000 women found that those taking HRT had double the asthma as women not on HRT. If you do decide to take HRT, make sure you use natural estrogens (Tri-Est containing estriol, estrone, and estradiol) under the guidance of your naturopathic physician. Many laboratories offer complete hormone panels to help determine natural hormone replacement requirements.

NUTRIENT	DOSAGE	ACTION
Vitamin C with bioflavonoids	1000 mg of vitamin C twice daily 500 mg of bioflavonoids twice daily	Decreases the number of hot flashes

NUTRIENT	DOSAGE	ACTION
Vitamin B_6 with a B-complex	50 mg of vitamin B_6 daily Two capsules of B-complex daily	Supports nervous system, is required for metabolism and immune function, reduces PMS symptoms
Vitamin E	400 IU daily	Reduces hot flashes and improves mood. Use vaginal lubricants containing vitamin E.
Calcium with magnesium	1000 mg of each daily	Reduces leg cramps, prevents osteoporosis
DIM	Two capsules daily	Eliminates excess estrogens
Ginkgo biloba standardized to 24 percent	Two capsules daily	Supports cognitive function, improves circulation to hands and feet
Chaste tree (Vitex)	175 mg (or 30–60 drops) daily or 30–40 mg per capsule	Supports proper hormone secretion, reduces PMS symptoms, controls hot flashes
Evening primrose oil	500 mg three times daily	Relieves breast pain, and may alleviate hot flashes
Natural progesterone (I use Life-Flo because it has a metered pump and no messy measuring)	Use as directed. Dosage depends on if you are peri- or postmenopausal	Relieves breast tenderness, hot flashes, irregular breakthrough bleeding, protects against osteoporosis, controls PMS
Dong quai	1 tsp (5 mL) of tincture 1 g of powdered root	Balances estrogen activity; relieves hot flashes and vaginal dryness
Black cohosh, Remifemin	2 mg of 27-deoxyacteine twice daily as found in Remifemin	Reduces depression, insomnia, vaginal dryness, and hot flashes
Moducare sterols and sterolins	One capsule three times daily	Normalizes cortisol, modulates immune function, stops calcium loss due to inflammatory immune factors, enhances DHEA naturally
Gamma oryzamol	100 mg three times daily	Relieves hot flashes
St. John's wort	100 mg twice daily	Alleviates depression. Do not take with antidepressant medications without first consulting your doctor.

Health Tips to Enhance Healing

- Follow a predominantly vegetarian diet and increase your intake of soy and fiber. Fiber carries excess estrogens out of the body. Phytoestrogens, like those found in certain vegetables, legumes, and soy, take up sites in the body that estrogen would like to occupy but because they are already filled, the estrogen is excreted. Several studies have shown that postmenopausal women who eat 200–300 mg of isoflavones from soy foods have a significant reduction in breast cancer, hot flashes, and vaginal dryness. Soy foods are also important for the reduction in cholesterol and heart disease (see "Cardiovascular Corruption," page 17).
- Read about the blood test for breast cancer on page 179.
- See estrogen dominance on page 226.

- Have your thyroid checked for hypothyrodism. (See thyroid self-test, page 22.)
- Avoid constipation (see Constipation).
- Have a dual energy X ray absorptiometry (DEXA) scan to determine bone density.
- Have sex twice a week to maintain optimal immune function and prevent vaginal atrophy.

Other Recommendations

- Reduce stress, get plenty of sleep, and practice relaxation techniques such as visualization, biofeedback, qigong, yoga, and deep-breathing exercises. Go for regular massages.
- Look at menopause as the dawn of a new era that allows you to take time for yourself and do the things you've dreamed about. With fewer obligations to family and career, new opportunities for growth, education, and travel are yours.
- Stop smoking.
- Acupuncture, homeopathy, traditional Chinese medicine, and glandular treatment may all be beneficial for your symptoms. Consult a qualified practitioner.

MONONUCLEOSIS

Also known as the "Kissing" disease, mononucleosis (or mono) is a highly contagious viral infection caused by the Epstein Barr virus (a herpes virus) that affects several glands and the respiratory and lymphatic systems. It tends to affect young adults and teenagers.

Symptoms

Most symptoms of mono are similar to the flu: sore throat, fever, swollen eyes and lymph glands, fatigue that is almost debilitating, headache, an all-over body ache, and no desire to eat. In rare cases there may be a rash that moves around the body. It is also possible that the liver and spleen may enlarge and symptoms such as pain in the upper left abdominal area, jaundice, and depression may be present. In extreme cases, meningitis or encephalitis could develop.

Mono is very stubborn. Although the initial symptoms are gone in less than four weeks, the fatigue and lethargy can linger for another three weeks to a year or more. Attacks may recur within that year or so, growing milder every time. Mono can be chronic and very serious for people with suppressed immune systems, as in those who have had other viral infections or have undergone a transplant. It can often develop into chronic fatigue syndrome.

Causes

Mono is the result of a herpes infection, usually the Epstein Barr virus. It may take only 10 days for mono to develop in children, but in adults it can take much longer. It is not unusual to have outbreaks in camps, schools, and dormitories where people live in close quarters.

Mono is passed through intimate contact. The exchange of fluids while kissing or having sex is an obvious form of transmission, but it can happen by sharing utensils or eating other people's food as well. As it is an airborne infection like the common cold, coughing and sneezing can spread germs as well.

Prescription for Health

NUTRIENT	DOSAGE	ACTION
Multimune containing vitamins A, B$_6$, C, E, selenium, zinc, reduced L-glutathione, coenzyme Q10, lipoic acid, magnesium, and additional vitamin C	Three capsules with food, additional 1000 mg of vitamin C twice daily	Boosts immunity, fights viruses, is potent antioxidant, helps detoxify, contains glutathione, which helps decongest the upper respiratory tract
Echinacea	20 drops tincture several times per day or 1000 mg capsule daily	Boosts immune system and acts as an antibiotic. Do not take longer than four weeks; is contraindicated in autoimmune disease and HIV
Goldenseal	100 mg three times daily	High in berberine and hydrastine, both potent immune boosters
Astragalus	200 mg three times daily	Boosts immunity and reduces frequency of infection
Garlic	Three capsules daily (Kyolic)	Antiviral in nature, expels mucous, stimulates NK cell activity
Moducare sterols and sterolins	One capsule three times daily	Enhances immune system, increases gamma-interferon and NK cells
Vitamin A (Micel A)	One dropperful (equivalent to 100,000 IU) daily for five days, then one drop, which is equivalent to 5000 IU, daily	This is my favorite for fighting all kinds of infections. Drop in the back of the throat and let it sit for a few seconds before swallowing. Gets rid of sore throats fast.

Health Tips to Enhance Healing

- See health tips for Influenza, page 281.

Mono cannot be eradicated with antibiotics, so do not take them unless there is a secondary infection that calls for antibiotic use such as strep throat or an ear infection. If you must take antibiotics, eat plain yogurt or supplement with probiotics to maintain your intestinal flora.

Health Fact

Children under the age of three who contract viral infections are less likely to get asthma or allergies when they are older because their immune system has already had a jump on promoting Th-1 dominance.

MULTIPLE SCLEROSIS

Multiple sclerosis, or MS, is a chronic degenerative disorder of the central nervous system, whereby the myelin sheath is slowly lost (demyelination) over time. Around 400,000 people in North America are affected—more than a million worldwide—and two-thirds of them are women. The myelin sheath protects and surrounds the nerve fibers and transmits information along the nerve. Multiple sclerosis is an autoimmune disease in which antibodies incite inflammation and destruction of the myelin sheath, leaving scars or plaque. The plaque along the spinal cord, optic nerve, and in the brain interfere with communication, resulting in a loss of neuromotor skills.

Most cases occur between the ages of 20 and 40. Like other autoimmune diseases, women are affected more often than men. The appearance of MS in those under the age of 10 is extremely rare. Interestingly, MS is seen more often in those living in the northern hemisphere and extreme southern hemisphere, Canada, Britain, northern Europe, New Zealand, and the northern United States, and is rare in Japan, Africa, and Asia.

Symptoms

There are three levels of symptoms ranging from mild and moderate to severe. Depression appears in 50 percent of MS cases as a reaction to the illness, and cognitive function is challenged, especially memory. There is pain, malaise, and fatigue; the fatigue is so overwhelming that it is usually the cause for stopping work.

Sometimes there is dizziness, numbness, slurring, tremors, lack of coordination, and visual problems. In more severe cases, there may be problems with sexual function, bone density, breathing, bowel and bladder control, muscle cramps, weakness, and paralysis. Thirty percent of persons with MS generally require a wheelchair or will be bedridden.

Causes

Although the cause of MS is not clear and many factors may interact to promote the disease, there are three main theories. There is evidence that viral infection may initiate MS. Several viruses, including herpes simplex virus, measles, rabies, parainfluenza, and others, have been isolated from persons with MS. Viruses may promote an autoimmune process called molecular mimicry, whereby the immune system initially mounted an assault upon a virus that had a very similar "coat" resembling the myelin sheath, causing the immune system to mount antibodies mistakenly against the myelin sheath.

Diet or environment must play a role or patterns of distribution around the globe would not be so clear. Possibly the amount of sunshine and the type of diet may play a role, yet these have not been determined to date. MS primarily attacks people of northern European descent, is rare in East Asia, and is unknown by Africans. Twenty percent of MS sufferers will have a relative who has it, but there are also environmental elements involved. Triggers that have been associated with MS are stress, food allergies, nutritional deficiencies or poor diet, exposure to environmental toxins, and mercury poisoning.

Vaccinosis

In the February 2000 edition of *The Journal of Autoimmunity*, researchers present data showing that MS-like symptoms were reported in 600 people receiving the recombinant hepatitis B vaccine (HBV). Demyelination was seen on magnetic resonance imaging days to weeks after HBV vaccination, yet a French study showed that those vaccinated had less MS. Many of those who were immunized with HBV and developed MS-like symptoms are seeking compensation. As well, evidence linking MS to the measles vaccine shows that we may be creating a bigger problem by vaccinating our children with the measles vaccine. The measles vaccine does not provide life-long immunity and when older children or adults contract measles, they are at higher risk for developing MS. Measles tend to occur at a very early age in the tropics and other areas that are known to have little MS. There is a belief that contracting measles at a young age may be protective against MS. The vaccine does not provide the same type of benefit as the life-long immunity provided by contracting measles naturally. (See "Vaccination and Autoimmunity," page 50.)

Prescription for Health

The following recommendations are not meant to replace your current prescription medications but to support and control autoantibody reactions.

NUTRIENT	DOSAGE	ACTION
Flaxseed oil	3 Tbsp (45 mL) daily	Helps proper myelin and neuron function, inhibits progression of MS
Multimune containing vitamins A, B_6, C, E, selenium, zinc, coenzyme Q10, reduced L-glutathione, lipoic acid	Three capsules daily with meals	Is antiviral, a potent antioxidant; deficiency of B_6 may predispose MS; selenium deficiency is also seen in MS; vitamins and zinc reduce relapses and support immune function

NUTRIENT	DOSAGE	ACTION
Fish oil rich in EPA/DHA, Eskimo-3 or MaxEPA with evening primrose oil	500 mg three times daily along with 500 mg three times daily of evening primrose oil	Inhibits progression of MS
Vitamin B$_{12}$	1000 mcg sublingual tables	Protects myelin sheath
High-potency B-complex	Two capsules daily	Essential for proper neural transmission, protects against deficiency
Phosphatidylcholine	500 mg twice daily	Protects myelin sheath; increases acetylcholine, which is important for muscle function
Reduced L-glutathione	500 mg daily	Essential for detoxification and immune function
Women's Whey or proteins+ protein powder	One to two scoops daily	Ensures adequate amino acids and protein without eating saturated fats
Wobenzym or pancreatic enzymes, bromelain, papain	Three tablets daily of Wobenzym	Reduces circulating immune complexes, halts inflammatory reactions, reduces flare-ups
5-HTP	50 mg daily	Enhances mood

Health Tips to Enhance Healing

- Read Chapter 3 on Autoimmune Disease.
- Avoid all immune boosters, as they enhance autoantibody production responsible for demyelinating nerve fibers.
- Diet is key. The Swank diet developed by Dr. Roy Swank, professor of neurology, University of Oregon Medical School, in the 1950s has been used to slow the progression of MS with excellent results. The diet has to be strictly followed:
  - Less than 10 g of saturated fat daily, preferably less
  - 40–50 g of essential fatty acid-rich oils (see Chapters 4 and 7)
  - No margarine, shortening, or hydrogenated oils; this must be strictly adhered to
  - Fish oils every day
  - Adequate protein from nonsaturated sources
  - Fish three or more times per week
  - No milk; the more I read about milk, the more dangerous I think this food is to our overall longevity
- Eliminate chocolate, alcohol, sugar, coffee, rye, barley, oats, wheat, spices, and salt, as they may aggravate symptoms.
- Stop smoking.

Other Recommendations

- Have dental amalgams removed. (See Toxic Metal Poisoning for more information.)

- When antigens and antibodies interlock, it is called an immune complex. Proteolytic enzyme therapy may be beneficial by penetrating the coating of the immune complex in the tissues and getting them into the bloodstream for elimination, stimulating the breakup of the immune complex and speeding up the inflammation process to reduce tissue swelling. Due to the increased activity, the condition worsens for a short time before it gets better. Use this therapy with the supervision of a naturopath or physician.
- Allergy identification is important in treating MS. See the introduction to this chapter.
- Regular exercise is beneficial for all autoimmune disorders. However, with MS, elevated body temperature can cause nerve dysfunction and worsen symptoms. Swimming is a great exercise because the water supports the body and keeps it cool. Stretching is good for preventing muscle contraction.
- Massage and physical therapy is very valuable for maintaining muscle tone and preventing the symptoms that are associated with restricted movement.
- Do your homework on MS and find all available resources for support.

MYASTHENIA GRAVIS

Myasthenia gravis is a common autoimmune disease in which the immune system produces antibodies that attack the neuromuscular junction. When nerves signal a muscle at the junction, it will contract. Some nerves receive messages from acetylcholine. In myasthenia gravis these acetylcholine receptor nerves are damaged by the immune system, which develops antibodies against them. It generally affects women, striking them during their twenties or thirties; when it affects men, it is during their sixties and seventies. A wide variety of other autoimmune disorders are also seen in those with myasthenia gravis, including lupus, rheumatoid arthritis, alopecia areata, and more.

Symptoms

The onset of myasthenia gravis is noted when the eyelids droop and vision is doubled. Fifteen percent of myasthenia cases will be limited to eye muscle problems. For the other 85 percent, the skeletal muscles become weak, which increases with repeated activity and decreases with rest. It may be difficult to hold up one's head or to carry things. For those with facial muscle problems, smiling will look like snarling, speech becomes nasal or "mushy," and there may be difficulties when trying to chew and swallow. When the affliction is more extensive, the limbs, neck, and diaphragm muscles are involved. If the situation develops to the point where respirators are required or feeding is a problem, then the person is described as being in "myasthenic crisis." Ten percent of those with myasthenia gravis develop life-threatening weakness of the breathing muscles. In severe cases paralysis can occur.

Causes

Myasthenia gravis is thought to be caused by infection, a tumor on the thymus, genetic predisposition, or developmental problems as a fetus. There is also a form of myasthenia gravis that is drug-induced with D-penicillamine, but once medication is withdrawn, the symptoms abate. Antibodies attack the acetylcholine receptors where the nerves and muscle join together, preventing acetylcholine from facilitating muscle contractions. Fewer receptors become available as time goes on, making movement difficult. Like amyotrophic lateral sclerosis (ALS), it affects the voluntary muscles, not the involuntary ones. The reduction in receptors is not limited to the region affected. People with the mildest form of myasthenia (i.e., who have problems only with the eye muscles) have been shown to have fewer receptors in their limbs.

Prescription for Health

The following recommendations are not meant to replace your current prescription medications but to support and control autoantibody reactions. Acetylcholine enhancement and protection of acetylcholine receptors is the focus of the following.

NUTRIENT	DOSAGE	ACTION
Moducare sterols and sterolins	One capsule three times daily	Modulates immune function and cortisol, controls autoantibody production, and reduces inflammation
Flaxseed oil	3 Tbsp (45 mL) daily	Required for proper neuronal function, improves muscle integrity
Multimune containing vitamins A, B_6, C, E, selenium, zinc, coenzyme Q10, reduced L-glutathione, lipoic acid	Three capsules daily with meals	Is an antiviral and a potent antioxidant; deficiency of B_6 may affect muscles, zinc reduces relapses, supports immune function
Fish oil rich in EPA/DHA, Eskimo-3 or MaxEPA	Three capsules three times daily	Inhibits progression of autoimmune diseases
Vitamin B_{12}	1000 mcg sublingual tables	Protects nerves
High-potency B-complex	Two capsules daily	Essential for proper neural transmission, protects against deficiency

NUTRIENT	DOSAGE	ACTION
Phosphatidyl choline	1500 mg twice daily	Increases acetylcholine, is important for muscle function
Reduced L-glutathione	500 mg daily	Essential for detoxification and immune function
Women's Whey or proteins + protein powder	One to two scoops daily	Ensures adequate amino acids for repair
Wobenzym or pancreatic enzymes, bromelain, papain	Three tablets of Wobenzym daily	Reduces circulating immune complexes, halts inflammatory reactions, reduces flare-ups
5-HTP	50 mg daily	Enhances mood

Health Tips to Enhance Healing

- See "Vaccination and Autoimmunity," page 50.
- Do not take immune boosters as they can exacerbate myasthenia gravis.
- Read the health tips for Systemic Lupus Erythematosus (Lupus).
- Maintain an exercise program. While intermittent and growing weakness can be frustrating, regular exercise is beneficial for all autoimmune disorders.

Other Recommendations

- When antigens and antibodies interlock, it is called an immune complex. Proteolytic enzyme therapy may be beneficial by penetrating the coating of the immune complex in the tissues and getting them into the bloodstream for elimination, stimulating the breakup of the immune complex, and speeding up the inflammation process to reduce tissue swelling. Due to the increased activity, the condition worsens for a short time before it gets better. Use this therapy with the supervision of a naturopath or physician.
- Allergies can make autoimmune symptoms worse. See the introduction to this chapter regarding allergies.
- Have yourself tested for heavy metal toxicity with a hair mineral analysis. Get dental amalgams replaced with safer material. Avoid exposure to pollution and toxins and stop smoking. Tobacco has a high heavy-metal content, including cadmium, lead, and arsenic.
- On days that you are not feeling well, rest and stay positive. When you do feel good, take advantage of that time and really enjoy yourself. Your perception of the illness can influence your experiences for the better.

NAUSEA

Nausea, or that sick, queasy feeling in your stomach that makes you feel like you will vomit, is an indication that there is something else happening in the body, most typically a problem in the gastrointestinal tract or it can be due to pregnancy or chemotherapy. Some nausea is severe enough to cause you to vomit or empty the contents of your stomach.

Symptoms

Technically, there are no symptoms of nausea except for intense queasiness in the stomach. However, there can be associated feelings of overall weakness, greater saliva production, decreased appetite, and vomiting.

Causes

There are hundreds of conditions that cause nausea; even riding in a car can induce nausea. Most often nausea is associated with problems in the gastrointestinal tract: constipation, flu, food poisoning, low stomach acid, a lack of digestive enzymes, and inflammation of the stomach lining. Many women experience nausea, called morning sickness, during the first few months of pregnancy and for some it is so intense as to cause vomiting. Nausea can also be brought on by reactions to prescription medication, sudden shock, extreme pain, dizziness, stress, or a hangover. Other sources could be kidney or liver problems or brain tumors.

Prescription for Health

NUTRIENT	DOSAGE	ACTION
Vitamin B-complex	Two capsules daily	Required for digestion and metabolism and reduces nausea
Vitamin B$_6$, in the form of P-5-P	50 mg daily	Reduces nausea, especially in pregnant women
Vitamin C	500 mg three times daily. For those on chemotherapy, increase to 1000 mg three times daily.	Increases T-cell activity to fight infection and protects intestinal cell membrane
Peppermint (enteric-coated)	One or two capsules daily	Aids digestion, reduces intestinal distress
Magnesium	500 mg daily	Calms nerves, reduces nausea
Artichoke	160–320 mg three times daily with meals, assuming standardized to contain 13–18 percent caffeolquinic acids and calculated aschlorogenic acid	Increases bile formation and flow to digest and absorb fats
Ginger	Four 500 capsules daily. It can also be taken as a tea.	Calms upset stomach, reduces nausea

NUTRIENT	DOSAGE	ACTION
Lactobacillus acidophilus	1 tsp (5 mL) twice daily	Increases friendly bacteria and reduces harmful bacteria
Moducare sterols and sterolins	One capsule three times daily. For nausea, hair loss, and vomiting due to chemotherapy, take double the dose until chemotherapy is finished.	Increases T-cell activity to fight infection and reduces inflammation, halts nausea from chemotherapy very effectively

Health Tips to Enhance Healing

- See Chapter 1 for more information on gut problems.
- Herbal teas can be very effective at soothing nausea. Try singularly or combinations of peppermint, chamomile, lemon balm, or fennel. Ginger is especially effective in reducing or eliminating nausea during pregnancy.
- Take oil of oregano (three drops twice a day) if you feel you may have stomach upset from eating something that may have been spoiled. Oil of Oregano is the best treatment for tropical diarrhea and vomiting due to food contamination.
- Drink at least eight to ten glasses of pure, filtered water every day. For every juice, alcoholic, or caffeinated beverage you drink, add another glass of water.
- If symptoms are aggravated during a fatty meal, your bile production could be underactive; stimulate gastric juices with bitter herb teas such as dandelion, plantain, yarrow, wormwood, or gentian.
- Nibbling on whole-grain crackers, dry toast, or eating small portions of plain steamed rice can neutralize stomach acidity. Do not overdo it with big meals; eat smaller portions frequently throughout the day. Eat foods that you like or ones that have pleasant aromas. Avoid spicy, fatty, salty, or strong-smelling foods.
- If smell or taste of food is too strong, eat it when it is cold or lukewarm.
- Avoid processed, packaged, fried, or junk foods as they are nutritionally void and contain harmful fats and chemicals that stress the body. Choose organic produce, wild fish, or free-range poultry to avoid burdening your body with toxins.
- Consume a diet that emphasizes natural, whole foods such as legumes, fresh fruits and vegetables, fish, healthy fats and oils, and nuts and seeds.

Other Recommendations

- If nausea is related to prescription medication, check with your physician if it can be substituted for one that does not cause nausea.

- Get some rest and reduce stress. Practice deep-breathing exercises, biofeedback, visualization, and other therapies to calm the body.
- Get plenty of fresh air and keep cool with the help of wet compresses or stay in shaded areas.
- Close your eyes and rest in a quiet room, or distract yourself with soft music or low background television.
- During an attack, take deep breaths and relax.
- Remove false teeth or retainers and lie on your side in case there is vomiting. Do not lie flat on your back.
- Reduce triggers for nausea if possible (see Constipation, Gallstones and Gallbladder Disease, Hepatitis, Headache, Influenza, Kidney Inflammation, and Stress).
- Check for allergies to foods if nausea is not related to a specific condition.
- When the bones of the head and neck are out of line, chiropractic treatments can be beneficial. Consult a qualified practitioner.

Health Fact

Acupressure bracelets are available for your wrists. Many pregnant women find relief by wearing them during the first trimester.

OSTEOPOROSIS

Our bones are in a constant state of regeneration where the bone is being broken down and rebuilt. Hormones, our liver, kidneys, and immune system all interplay to ensure that bone is maintained. Osteoporosis, meaning "porous bone," arises when bone is broken down faster than it can be rebuilt. Over time a gradual decrease in bone mass causes the bones to become porous, brittle, and fragile, increasing the risk of fracture. Bones of the hip, spine, wrists, and ribs are the most common fracture sites. Osteoporosis affects almost 30 million people in North America, over 80 percent of whom are women. Hip fracture is a dangerous result of osteoporosis. Over 250,000 hip fractures occur each year and many of those affected require long-term nursing care and some patients will even die as a result of hip fracture.

If you have several of the risk factors mentioned below, have a dual energy absorptiometry (DEXA) scan performed to determine bone status.

Major risk factors for osteoporosis include:
- family history
- low stomach acid
- thyroid disease
- corticosteroid therapy (prednisone)
- high-stress lifestyle or Type A personality

- Northern European or Asian descent
- thin, small build
- early menopause
- sedentary lifestyle
- no pregnancies
- smoking
- high caffeine and sugar intake
- high-protein diet

Symptoms

Bone loss occurs silently and often symptoms are not noted until a fracture occurs. Warning signs include back pain around the bottom of the shoulder blades. The pain is relieved with heat, but aggravated by lying flat on the back. Teeth may become loose. There is a loss of height and a rounding of the upper back, known as dowager's hump. Bones can fracture with little stress, and collapsing vertebrae can pinch nerves, causing sciatica.

Causes

If we believe what the media has been telling us, you would think that calcium loss is the only cause of osteoporosis and simply taking gram doses of calcium would solve the problem. Unfortunately, this is not true—calcium alone will not reverse or halt bone loss in most suffering from osteoporosis. Hormones, our immune system, stress, and nutrition combine to maintain proper bone health.

Those with low stomach acid will have a difficult time absorbing calcium carbonate, the most common calcium used in supplements. Less than 10 percent of calcium carbonate is absorbed in those with low stomach acid. Calcium citrate, aspartate, and orotate are much better absorbed compared to carbonate. Calcium concentration is controlled by several hormones and is influenced by our immune system.

Vitamin D also plays an important role in the formation of bone. Vitamin D interacts with the cells of the immune system by reducing the inflammatory cytokines, specifically interleukin-1 and interleukin-12. Carl Germano, RD, and William Cabot, MD, state in the *Osteoporosis Solution* that "In some research circles, osteoporosis is thought to be a type of autoimmune disease."

The inflammatory cytokines of the immune system, specifically IL-1 and IL-6, can cause calcium to be pulled from bone. When we are under stress (and remember, stress can be many things), our stress hormone cortisol is secreted. Cortisol release signals the T-helper-2 cells to secrete IL-6, and IL-6, among other things, pulls calcium from bone. As well, when cortisol goes up our antiaging and immune-regulating hormone DHEA decreases. The body is designed to deal with short-term stressors, but when they become a regular occurrence, the cortisol/interleukin-6 connection causes a breakdown of bone faster than it can be rebuilt.

Osteoporosis can also be influenced by an overactive immune system. When macrophages eat invaders in the course of their daily surveillance, they release nitric oxide and IL-1. Nitric oxide in small amounts protect against bone loss, but when the immune system is fighting infection, macrophages release nitric oxide in large amounts, promoting the breakdown of bone. Fosamax is designed to reduce nitric oxide, although with some terrible side effects. As mentioned earlier, IL-1 also promotes bone loss, so not only does vitamin D have to be available to control the secretion of IL-1 but our macrophages have to be kept in balance as well. Nitric oxide, like vitamin D, is key to regulating bone.

Estrogen protects the body from excessive secretion of IL-1 and IL-6. Estrogen deficiency as found in postmenopausal women, those who have had hysterectomies, or top-level athletes with suppressed menses, is associated with abnormally high levels of IL-1 (which promotes bone loss as explained earlier) and low levels of gamma-interferon (which prevents bone loss).

Other factors promoting osteoporosis include genetic predisposition, hyperthyroidism, hypothyroidism, excessive alcohol consumption, leanness, never being pregnant, side effects of prescription medication, immobility or lack of exercise, not enough sunlight, and smoking. Asians and Caucasians are in a higher risk group. Regular movement and exercise is required to preserve bone mass and increase bone mineral density. However, excessive exercising can also lead to osteoporosis if menses is suppressed or if the immune system is hyperstimulated. Smoking inactivates estrogen, in effect causing estrogen deficiency.

Prescription for Health

NUTRIENT	DOSAGE	ACTION
Calcium citrate	1000–1500 mg daily	Reduces bone loss, protects against fracture
Moducare sterols and sterolins	One capsule three times daily	Regulates cortisol, controls IL-6, IL-1, is anti-inflammatory, controls autoimmunity, naturally enhances DHEA
Vitamin D	200 IU twice daily	Helps increase calcium absorption and inhibits IL-1 and IL-12
Multimune containing vitamins A, B$_6$, C, E, selenium, zinc, magnesium, coenzyme Q10, lipoic acid, and reduced L-glutathione	Three capsules daily with food	An antioxidant, detoxifies liver, supports proper immune function
Magnesium	500 mg three times daily	Essential for absorption of vitamin D and to prevent deficiency
Boron	3 mg daily	Reduces calcium excretion and mimics estrogen

NUTRIENT	DOSAGE	ACTION
High-potency B-complex	Two capsules daily	Reduces the effects of stress, is important for metabolism and to prevent deficiency
Quercetin	500 mg twice daily	Inhibits inflammatory response of IL-8
Curcumin (Turmeric)	600 mg standardized extract	Inhibits inflammatory IL-1 and IL-6
Omega-3 fatty acids, fish oils, or flaxseed oil	500 mg twice daily or 1–2 Tbsp (15–30 mL) of flaxseed oil	Inhibits inflammatory IL-1, IL-6, and pro-inflammatory prostaglandins
Pycnogenol	200 mg twice daily	Prevents damage from excessive nitric oxide production
Ipriflavone	300 mg twice daily	Improves calcium absorption in bone and slows osteoclast activity due to excessive nitric oxide, natural estrogen-like activity

Health Tips to Enhance Healing

- See Menopause. If you have osteoarthritis as well as osteoporosis, see Arthritis. Read "The Immune System and Stress," page 45.
- Rule out hydrocholoric acid deficiency. Low stomach acid impairs calcium absorption. See the introduction to this chapter.
- Reduce consumption of caffeine (it depletes calcium and magnesium), simple or refined sugars (also depletes calcium and lowers bone density), and alcohol (it can lower vitamin D metabolism).
- Include more soy in the diet—the phytoestrogens in soy mimic human estrogen. Although they are a weaker form of estrogen, they help preserve bone mass.
- Eat plenty of green leafy vegetables. They contain vitamin K, which is needed for proper bone mineralization.
- Eliminate all soft drinks. They lower calcium levels and increase phosphate levels.
- Reduce salt. It increases calcium loss.
- Maintain a balanced daily intake of protein—50 g for women (average body weight of 138 lbs/62.5 kg), 63 g for men (average body weight of 174 lbs/79 kg). Too much protein depletes calcium from the bones; too little prevents collagen formation and associated enzymes. Reduce animal protein by opting for vegetable-based protein such as legumes and soy.
- Develop an adequate exercise program that includes weight-bearing activities such as walking, hiking, stair climbing, dancing, weight training, jogging, skiing, or low-impact aerobics.

Other Recommendations

- Eat calcium-rich foods or take your calcium supplements before bed. The blood's calcium level is lower at night, so the rate of calcium absorption is greater.

- Eat a good fat diet to enhance bone density. High saturated fat diets promote bone loss. Read Chapter 4.
- If your medication increases the risk of osteoporosis, inquire if more natural approaches can be taken, or substitute it for one that does not.
- Quit smoking—nonsmokers can avoid menopause longer than smokers by almost two years.
- Take advantage of sunny days when you can and get at least 15 to 20 minutes of sunshine.
- Avoid antacids. They contain aluminum and inhibit the absorption of calcium. (See the antacid story in Chapter 1, page 9.)

Health Fact

- Over 2 million North American men have osteoporosis—and 3 million more are at risk.
- Women in their twenties and thirties can exhibit early signs of osteoporosis.
- By the age of 80 a vegetarian will experience only an 18 percent loss in bone mass, compared to 35 percent in nonvegetarians.

OVARIAN CYSTS

Ovarian cysts are very common and often exist without symptoms. In a normal cycle every month, several follicles, each containing an egg, develop inside the ovary. A surge of luteinizing hormone and follicle-stimulating hormone help release the egg, thereby causing estrogen levels to peak. A drop in luteinizing hormone and follicle-stimulating hormone occurs, the follicle releases the egg, and progesterone increases. If the egg is not fertilized, the cycle starts all over again. When ovarian cysts develop, several follicles mature and enlarge in the ovary to become fluid-filled sacs or cysts. If, however, no egg is released, then no progesterone is secreted and more estrogen is released, thus maturing the follicles into cysts that will grow larger every month until progesterone is secreted.

Cysts can appear in a very short time and disappear just as quickly. Cysts can be alone or in groups, small or large—even as big as a lemon! When cysts are a few centimeters in diameter, doctors will often recommend surgery. However, if a diet and supplementation program is followed, those cysts will usually reduce and disappear. The risk of cancer is present when those cysts become solid. Ovarian cancer is rare, but it is difficult to diagnose and remission rates with conventional medicine are poor.

Sometimes a follicle is able to grow tissue or skin cells within the cyst. These types of cysts will not dissipate and must be surgically removed.

Polycystic ovary syndrome (Stein-Leventhal syndrome) is a disorder in which many fluid-filled cysts are present and male hormones are excessively high. In this disorder, excess luteinizing hormone increases the production of male hormones that can cause acne and coarse hair growth. It is important to correct the hormone imbalance as high levels of male hormones can convert to estrogens, putting the woman at a higher risk of endometrial cancer and endometriosis.

Symptoms

Often ovarian cysts are not noticed until a woman receives a pelvic examination or an ultrasound scan. For those with symptoms, the most obvious symptom is pain, either tenderness to the touch or a constant sore or burning sensation in the abdomen, located in the lower abdomen off to the right or left. Pain may occur during ovulation or intercourse. If a cyst erupts in the pelvic cavity, blood and fluid will discharge, possibly causing pain.

Those with polycystic ovary syndrome will have ovarian cysts, increased coarse body hair, and high levels of luteinizing and male hormones.

Causes

Ovarian cysts occur when there is a hormonal imbalance. Estrogen dominance brought on by poor elimination of waste by the lymphatic system, colon, liver, and kidneys is a factor. Exposure to xenoestrogens is also a factor (see estrogen dominance on page 226). Emotional or physical trauma, prolonged stress, and even heavy exercise can cause an increase in estrogen. A diet rich in meat and dairy products is also responsible for elevating estrogen. Cysts that occur after menopause should be looked at by a physician as there is a greater risk of them being cancerous. The risk of ovarian cancer is increased with the use of fertility drugs or birth control pills, or if you have never been pregnant.

Prescription for Health

NUTRIENT	DOSAGE	ACTION
Natural progesterone cream	40–60 mg daily for five to 28 (or whenever your normal cycle ends); I use ProgestaCare by Life Flo, which delivers 20 mg in a premeasured pump dose.	Keeps estrogen and luteinizing hormones in check

NUTRIENT	DOSAGE	ACTION
Multimune containing vitamins A, B$_6$, C, E, selenium, magnesium, zinc, coenzyme Q10, lipoic acid, reduced L-glutathione	Three capsules daily with food	Supports immune function, is anti-inflammatory, reduces excess estrogens, controls cortisol, is antioxidant
High-potency B-complex	Three capsules daily	Reduces the effects of stress, eases PMS symptoms, balances hormonal state, elevates mood, and controls fluid retention
Multimineral	One or two capsules daily or as directed	Is required for enzymatic reactions in the body and to prevent deficiency, is essential for proper hormone balance
Vitex (chaste tree berry)	40 drops of tincture twice daily	Normalizes hormones
Moducare sterols and sterolins	One capsule three times daily	Reduces inflammation, modulates cortisol, controls inflammatory cytokines, including IL-1 and IL-6)
Evening primrose oil	500 mg three times daily	Is anti-inflammatory, used to treat female disorders
Black cohosh	40 mg daily	Suppresses luteinizing hormone

Health Tips to Enhance Healing

- See "Environmental Estrogens Linked to an Increased Risk of Cancer"on page 70. Also see Menopause.
- Do not use bleached paper products containing dioxins (estrogen mimickers). This includes toilet paper, sanitary napkins, and especially tampons.
- Do not use plastic containers to store food or water. They contain estrogen mimickers. Do not microwave in plastic as the estrogens leach into the food.
- Castor oil packs are excellent at controlling pain. Take six pieces of flannel soaked in castor oil (damp but not dripping) and put them over the area you want to treat. Place a hot water bottle wrapped in a towel on the lower abdomen for 30 to 45 minutes several times a day. This will not only relieve pain but also improve circulation in the pelvic area.
- Follow a vegetarian diet and increase your intake of soy and fiber. Fiber carries estrogen out of the body. Eat plenty of flaxseeds, citrus fruits, cruciferous vegetables, wheat, and buckwheat to eliminate excess estrogen.
- Avoid dairy and meat products. Your diet should focus on fresh fruits and vegetables, wild fish, whole grains, and legumes. Choose organic foods whenever possible to reduce the burden of toxins in the body.

- Detoxification and elimination of waste is very important. Eat liver-friendly foods such as beets, artichokes, lemons, onions, garlic, leeks, kale, carrots, and members of the cabbage family (broccoli, Brussels sprouts, cauliflower).
- Avoid alcohol, caffeine (including medications), sugar, chocolate, coffee, black tea, and soft drinks. Alcohol interferes with liver function. Caffeine and sugar promote inflammation.
- Drink eight to ten glasses of pure, filtered water a day.
- Avoid constipation (see Constipation).

Other Recommendations

- Exercise regularly to improve circulation and help the detoxification and elimination process, but avoid strenuous exercise that will stop ovulation. Polycystic ovarian syndrome is common in obese women.
- Reduce your exposure to xenohormones. Use natural alternatives for pest control, cleaning supplies, makeup, and so on.
- Ovarian cysts are very sensitive to emotions. Actively reduce stress by getting plenty of sleep and practicing relaxation techniques such as visualization, biofeedback, qigong, yoga and deep-breathing exercises. Indulge in hobbies that make you happy.
- Fertility drugs and birth control pills can increase estrogen levels. Those with polycystic ovary syndrome do well on natural progesterone creams.
- Avoid using body talc in the genital area.
- Cool temperatures in the extremities or lower abdomen can cause internal congestion.

PARASITE INFECTION

Parasites can come in all shapes and sizes, from microscopic to several feet long, and they can kill cells faster than the cells can proliferate. It is estimated that eight out of ten North Americans have a parasitic infection, although most people affected have no symptoms. Parasites leave waste in our body and steal our nutrients to feed themselves. Even if symptoms do not manifest, it does not prevent a person from infecting other people. Children are the most susceptible due to their proximity to the ground, their curious natures, which provoke them into touching everything, and their tendency to put their fingers and other objects in their orifices.

North Americans would like to assume that they are immune to contracting parasites, but international travel (of people and food) has literally created a global village. Parasites once contained in the warmer climates, are found in the produce sold in grocery stores and on restaurant plates, just waiting for new accommodation. They lay their eggs or larvae in food, water, or in breaks and wounds on the skin. Giardia lamblia exists in our river systems and likes to set up shop in our small intestine. Pinworms, ringworms, and tapeworms are other intestinal parasites. Mosquitoes and ticks can cause malaria and Lyme disease.

While parasitic infection can be disruptive to your health, it should also be taken as a signal from your body that something else is wrong. Usually, most parasitic infections go unnoticed because the immune system is working at neutralizing and eliminating them. However, if the immune system is weakened, parasites may flourish, and they do have a connection to cancer. Dr. Otto Warburg, director of the Max Planck Institute and winner of the Nobel Prize, believed that cancer cells were allowed to flourish because the cellular process for respiration of oxygen was being replaced by the fermentation of sugar. Healthy cells require oxygen, but cancer cells flourish without it. The environment that generates cancer is the same environment that allows parasites to thrive. Nipping problem parasites in the bud can also lower your risk of cancer.

The research of French-Canadian biologist Gaston Naessons has led to the discovery of somatids. Using a powerful optic microscope that enables the observation of living organisms in the blood, Naessons found tiny bodies he called "somatids," and as the precursor to DNA, they are able to convert energy into matter. Somatids are harmless and live in a cycle of three stages: somatic, spore, and double spore. However, if the immune system deteriorates because of illness, toxins, stress, and other factors, the somatid cycle is extended to include 13 more stages and they become harmful. The mutated somatids have been linked to several illnesses including lupus, MS, and cancer.

Symptoms

The difficult part in diagnosing parasites is that the symptoms can be a result of so many other causes, and testing for parasitic infection is not always accurate. Sometimes it can take several stool samples before parasites are detected, but often physicians give up after the first negative result. Also, not all parasites can be detected through stool samples. Doctors are not trained to suspect parasitic infection unless there was an obvious trip abroad to an exotic locale in their patient's history and may overlook the signs.

Common symptoms of a parasitic infection include nervousness, problems in sleeping, teeth grinding, drooling during your sleep, diarrhea, constipation, gas, and bloating. Parasites are also associated with allergies, anemia, chronic fatigue, irritable bowel syndrome, skin conditions, joint and muscle pain, and growths on the walls of the colon or rectum. Some parasites can induce malabsorption, specifically of vitamin A in the case of

Diphylobothrium latum (tapeworm) and vitamin B$_{12}$ by *Ascaris lumbricoides* (roundworm). Excessive hunger with weight loss (or at least no weight gain) can indicate a tapeworm infection.

If you have traveled, or if these symptoms reappear after you have treated the symptoms, or if you have experienced these symptoms for a extended period, consult a professional experienced with parasitic infection.

Causes

Parasitic infection occurs when we ingest food or water that has not been properly washed or cooked, or when we have been bitten by an insect. Parasites can also enter the body through the skin while a person is swimming or walking barefoot. Risk of infection is heightened when we travel to warmer climates. Unaccustomed to the climate, food, water, and time zone, our resistance is lowered, increasing the likelihood of infection. An immune system weakened by antibiotics and immunosuppressant medication is more vulnerable to infection. Mothers can pass parasites to their children in utero. Not washing hands after a trip to the toilet, or not washing surfaces where food is being prepared increases the risk of transmitting parasites.

Parasites are allowed to thrive if the digestive system is not in good working order. Diets high in sugar, refined flour, and processed foods provide a banquet for parasites. The constipation that inevitably accompanies a person with such eating habits encourages the presence of parasites that thrive on the waste left to putrefy in the intestines because it is not being moved along fast enough. Good bowel health and enough nutrients to optimize the immune system decrease the likelihood of an infection getting to the symptomatic stage. A vitamin B$_{12}$ deficiency leaves the body vulnerable to parasitic infection, which in turn would induce further B$_{12}$ deficiency.

Prescription for Health

NUTRIENT	DOSAGE	ACTION
Multimune contains vitamins A, B$_6$, C, E, selenium, zinc, magnesium, coenzyme Q10, reduced L-glutathione, lipoic acid	Three capsules daily with food	Supports immune function, is potent antioxidant, detoxifies liver
Vitamin B$_{12}$	1000 mcg	Corrects deficiency that encourages parasite infection
Pancreatic enzymes	1000 mg before meals	Improves digestion, helps eliminate parasites
Oil of oregano	Three drops three times daily	Expels parasites
Goldenseal or Oregon grape, containing standardized berberine	50 mg dry powder standardized berberine three times daily	Berberine is effective against many common parasites. It has been shown to be better than prescription parasite treatments.

NUTRIENT	DOSAGE	ACTION
Grapefruit seed extract	Use as directed	Acts as an antiparasitic and is good as a preventative
Garlic (odorless)	Three capsules three times daily	Fights infection and expels parasites
Lactobacillus acidophilus and bifidus	1 tsp (5 mL) daily supplying 1–2 million active organisms	Improve intestinal flora to fight infection
Moducare sterols and sterolins	One capsule three times daily	Regulates immune function, enhances gamma-interferon, NK cells, and cytotoxic T-cells to destroy parasites

Health Tips to Enhance Healing

- Refrain from consuming food or water with higher risk factors such as sushi and sashimi, steak tartare, unfiltered water, and unwashed fruits and vegetables. To make sushi and sashimi safe for eating, they must be frozen for 15 hours before serving. Pure mountain streams you come across while hiking may not be so pure, and some parasites such as Giardiasis may not be eliminated by chlorination.
- Follow a parasite cleanse program—products should contain some combination of herbs such as wormwood, thyme, black walnut leaves and green hulls, garlic, selfheal, centaury, tansy, cloves, turmeric, pumpkin seed, grapefruit seed, butternut bark, fennel seed, and cayenne.
- Diet is a key factor in preventing and fighting parasites. Avoid processed foods and those high in sugar and white flour. Consume a diet that emphasizes natural, whole foods such as fresh fruits and vegetables (raw cabbage, pomegranates, onions, papaya, and blackberries). Fish or lean meat should be well cooked. Nuts and seeds are also good for expelling parasites; stock up on pumpkin seeds and ground almonds. The diet should be high in water-soluble fiber such as Omega's High Lignan Flax Seed, rice bran, or oat bran. Go easy on soy and legumes (just once or twice a week), as they can compound the problem while you are infected. Avoid dairy altogether (see page 7 on MAP, a bacterium found in pasteurized milk).
- If you suspect you have low stomach acid, see the introduction to this chapter.
- Take digestive enzymes (or HCl if stomach acid is low) before a meal. Do not drink during the meal or you will dilute your enzymes. A well-armed stomach can eliminate most bacteria and parasites, rendering them ineffective before they reach the intestines.

- Drink at least eight to ten glasses of pure, filtered water every day to avoid constipation. For every juice, alcoholic, or caffeinated beverage you drink, add another glass of water.
- Relieve constipation since putrefying waste in the intestines makes you a heavenly host to an intestinal parasite (see Constipation).

Other Recommendations

- Wash your hands before preparing food and after handling pets. Avoid having pets up on the furniture.
- At home, drink only pure filtered water. When traveling, drink only bottled water and do not consume drinks with ice.
- Take extra supplements a week or two prior to traveling overseas to boost your immune system and prevent the likelihood of unwanted hitchhikers.
- Get tested for parasitic infection by a diagnostic laboratory using comprehensive digestive and stool analysis (CDSA).

PARKINSON'S DISEASE

First observed in 1817 and described as "Shaker's Palsy," Parkinson's disease (PD) is a progressive disease of the central nervous system that affects about one in every 250 people over the age of 40 and one in every 100 over the age of 60. It wasn't until the 1960s that the biochemical changes in the brain were identified. In Parkinson's, sufferers' dopamine, a neurotransmitter that transmits signals telling nerves to initiate movements, is reduced. As a result, simple movements become impaired and muscle rigidity is possible.

It is more common in men than women. Parkinson's generally begins after the age of 50, but there are increasing incidences of those under 50 becoming afflicted, most notably actor Michael J. Fox, who was diagnosed at the age of 30. It is expected that because we have longer life expectancy, more people will be afflicted with PD.

Symptoms

The initial signs of PD begin slowly. A slight tremor in one hand while it is at rest is often the first sign. The tremor will often disappear while doing a task and during sleep. The tremor can progress to other parts of the body. The body may feel slow and heavy and becomes stiff and easily fatigued. There is difficulty walking or performing simple tasks, and loss of appetite. Often those with Parkinson's will lean to one side and have difficulty moving their legs forward while walking. The facial expression may become frozen, talking is difficult, stuttering may appear, and drooling is common. Some people with Parkinson's experience dementia and depression.

Causes

The underlying cause in most cases is unknown, but it is believed that the cells in the brain degenerate mostly due to free radical damage or toxins that are not being eliminated from the body. A degeneration of neurons in the brain reduces the amount of dopamine available for the body, which becomes less able to produce it. Dopamine is the neurotransmitter that transports signals between nerve cells. In some patients Parkinson's is related to viral encephalitis, an infection that causes massive brain inflammation. Drugs for schizophrenia have caused a Parkinson's-like syndrome because they block dopamine.

Deficiencies in nutrients such as folic acid and niacin can be responsible for some cases of PD. Occupational exposure or excessive supplementation of manganese can lead to toxicity and an increased risk of Parkinson's disease. Excess manganese depletes dopamine and raises the level of neurotoxins. Metal poisoning from mercury and aluminum are seen in some people with Parkinson's.

Prescription for Health

NUTRIENT	DOSAGE	ACTION
Reduced L-glutathione	Intravenous infusion	Intravenous infusions stop tremors and improve mobility dramatically. Dr. Perlmutter uses 1400 mg mixed with saline given in IV for 10 minutes three times per week. This is an essential treatment that dramatically reduces tremors and other symptoms of PD.
Multivitamin with minerals	Three capsules daily	Prevents deficiency
Vitamin B_2 (thiamin)	1 g daily	Increases neurotransmitters
Niacin	500 mg twice daily	Improves brain function
Vitamin B_{12}	1000 mcg sublingually daily	Deficiency is common in the elderly and those on protein-restricted diets
Vitamin B_6	50 mg daily	Required for dopamine conversion; do not take with L-dopa without consulting your physician
Folic acid	400 mcg	Restores possible deficiencies
High-potency B-complex	Two capsules daily	When supplementing B vitamins separately, complement with all B vitamins
Vitamin C	1000 mg three times daily	Acts as an antioxidant; when taken with vitamin E, vitamin C may delay disease progression; when taken with L-dopa, it enhances its supplementation by preventing nausea
Vitamin E	400–800 IU	Acts as an antioxidant; in combination with vitamin C may delay disease progression
Phosphatidyl choline	1000 mg daily	Enhances acetylcholine

NUTRIENT	DOSAGE	ACTION
Phosphatidylserine	1000 mg three times daily	Provides better nerve function and enhances moods
Omega-6 fatty acids, evening primrose oil	500 mg twice daily	May reduce tremors
Moducare sterols and sterolins	One capsule three times daily	Is anti-inflammatory and naturally enhances DHEA
Ginkgo biloba	60 mg three times daily (standardized to 24 percent)	May prevent dementia associated with PD
CoQ10	100 mg daily	A potent antioxidant and free radical scavenger
Octacosonal from wheat germ oil	2 mg daily	Promotes improvement in daily activities and mood
5-HTP	50–100 mg daily	Increases serotonin to alleviate depression

Health Tips to Enhance Healing

- The results of David Perlmutter, MD, using glutathione intravenously are so impressive that every Parkinson's patient should be on this therapy. Levodopa is often reduced significantly upon using the IV glutathione therapy. Physicians should not mix glutathione with anything other than saline, according to Dr. Perlmutter.
- A low-protein diet is essential. When protein is consumed, it should eaten at the evening meal and be from plant-based sources such as soybeans, lentils, tofu, beans, barley, and plain yogurt. This diet can help control movement and coordination. Research has shown that those eating a low-protein diet had a reduction in tremors and tapping, and an improvement in walking.
- Avoid antacids and antiperspirants that contain aluminum. Do not use baking powder that contains alum and do not cook in aluminum pots and pans. Take magnesium, as it competes with aluminum for absorption. Some vaccines contain aluminum salts as a preservative, so avoid those.
- 5-HTP can enhance serotonin levels. The prescription drug Levodopa competes with tryptophan and can lead to reduced serotonin levels.
- Exercise regularly. Keeping active in whatever manner possible while mobility is still fairly good is essential.
- Eliminate alcohol, caffeine, and sugar.

Other Recommendations

- Remove dental amalgams. (See Toxic Metal Poisoning for more information.)
- Avoid manganese. The risk of PD may increase with high levels of

manganese supplementation or inhalation as it accumulates in the basal ganglia.

- Have your iron checked. If it is in excess, give blood. Some studies have shown that those with PD have higher levels of iron, which may promote the disease. Long-term exposure to iron, manganese, and aluminum in the workplace may also increase risk of Parkinson's disease.

- Have blood and urine tests to determine if your exposure to mercury has been excessive. Presence of mercury has been used as an indicator for risk of PD. Avoid long-term exposure, which may contribute to its onset. Consider chelation therapy to rid yourself of the heavy metals. Consult a qualified practitioner.

Health Fact

According to Dr. Michael Murray, ND, one-third of people with Parkinson's disease will acquire dementia, but this progression may be prevented or delayed with ginkgo biloba supplementation and other antioxidant nutrients.

POLYPS

Polyps are benign growths in the passages and cavities of the body. They may occur in the vocal cords, nose, bladder, cervix, colon, and rectum, the last two areas being the most prevalent. In fact, it is estimated that 30 percent of the population will have intestinal polyps. The initial growths look like teardrops, but gradually grow to resemble grapes on a stem. Some types of polyps are indications of a precancerous situation. Familial polyps, Gardner's syndrome, Turcot's syndrome, and Lynch's syndrome are all found in the large intestine and have an almost 100 percent chance of becoming cancerous. Bladder and cervical polyps also carry a risk, so they should be monitored by a physician. Nasal or vocal polyps rarely become cancerous.

Symptoms

Nosebleeds, nasal speech, loss of smell or difficulty breathing may be signs of nasal polyps. A painless hoarse voice, vocal fatigue, and changes in pitch can signal vocal cord polyps. The presence of colon or rectal polyps will usually go unnoticed until you are having a routine physical exam. However, if they are large enough, they can induce cramps, pain in the abdomen, and rectal bleeding. Blood in the urine can indicate bladder polyps. Polyps in the cervix will cause spotting or a watery vaginal discharge, and there may be mid-month, postmenopausal, or postcoital bleeding.

Causes

Polyps tend to grow when there has been repeated irritation or injury to an area. Nasal polyps can arise subsequent to many bouts of hay fever, asthma, allergies, or excessive use of nasal sprays. Cystic fibrosis and an allergy to aspirin have also been linked to polyps. Vocal cord polyps are a result of neglect and a possible infection. Singing without proper technique, excessive screaming, smoking, and allergies are all contributing factors. Vocal cord polyps are more likely to affect females and male children, possibly because high-pitched voices cause a faster vibration of the cords.

Polyps in the colon are usually a sign of poor diet that is low in fiber and high in bad fats and sugar, or an underlying condition such as colitis. Cervical polyps can be caused by hormonal changes, injury to the cervix, or infection, and the risk increases if diabetes is present.

Prescription for Health

The following is recommended for the prevention and treatment of intestinal polyps, the most common type. Also see Cancer and adopt strategies to prevent intestinal polyps from becoming cancerous. If you have nasal polyps, follow the recommendations for asthma and allergies, as nasal polyps are most often associated with those conditions. Those with cervical polyps should follow the treatment plan for menopause to focus on regulating hormones.

NUTRIENT	DOSAGE	ACTION
Omega Hi-Lignan Nutri-Flax	1–2 tsp (5–10 mL) daily with a high-fiber cereal	Soothes gut lining and promotes good elimination
Omega-3 fatty acids	1–2 Tbsp (15–30 mL) of flaxseed or four 500 mg fish oil capsules daily	Reduces inflammation of the intestinal lining and promotes elimination
Lactobacillus acidophilus	1 tsp (5 mL) containing 1–2 billion active organisms twice daily	Improves intestinal flora and reduces harmful bacteria
Moducare sterols and sterolins	One capsule three times daily	Reduces inflammation of the intestinal tract, improves walls of the venous system, increases T-cell activity to fight infection
Peppermint oil	One or two enteric-coated capsules three times daily between meals (0.2 mL active agent per capsule)	Reduces cramps, relaxes esophageal sphincter (reducing pressure from stomach), increases bile flow
Vitamin C	1–3 g daily	Stops inflammation, promotes healing of intestine, strengthens colon wall

NUTRIENT	DOSAGE	ACTION
Digestive enzymes	Two capsules with every meal	Promotes proper digestion of food
Multimune containing vitamins A, B$_6$, C, E, zinc, magnesium, selenium, coenzyme Q10, reduced L-glutathione, lipoic acid	Three capsules daily	Supports immune function, detoxifies liver, is anticancer and a potent antioxidant
Coenzyme Q10	100 mg daily	Is anticancer, supports immune function

Health Tips to Enhance Healing

- For intestinal polyps, follow the health tips for Bowel Disease, Cancer, and Diverticulitis.
- For nasal polyps, read the conditions for Allergy and Asthma.
- Take digestive enzymes before every meal. Do not drink while eating as it dilutes your enzymes.
- If you suspect you have low stomach acid, read the introduction to this chapter.
- If you experience gas, bloating, or constipation after eating a fatty meal, your bile production could be underactive; stimulate gastric juices with bitter herb teas such as dandelion, plantain, yarrow, wormwood, or gentian.
- Regular exercise will help improve digestion. Yoga and tai chi are great for improving circulation, reducing tension, and promoting healthy digestion and elimination. Stretching exercises in which you must touch your toes or draw your knees up to your chest are also good to get the bowels moving.

Other Recommendations

- For quick relief of constipation, take vitamin C to bowel tolerance (see page 94).
- Stop smoking.
- Nasal polyps may benefit from homeopathy. Consult a homeopathic practitioner.
- Have regular physicals to detect polyp formation in its early stages. Consult your physician if you find blood in your stools or if there is rectal bleeding.

Health Fact

USA Today Magazine reported a study held in Leeds, England, that found drinking beer or spirits and smoking increase the likelihood of polyps becoming cancerous. The study used 3356 volunteers, of which 384 were found to have precancerous polyps. Those with a history of smoking had twice the risk of polyps. Those who consumed more spirits or beer had almost twice the risk as teetotalers.

PROSTATE PROBLEMS

Small in size but grand in problems, the prostate is a small, chestnut-sized gland located just below the bladder and wrapped around the urethra. The urethra is the pathway for seminal fluid and urine and when the gland swells, it can inhibit the normal urinary flow and the ejaculation of semen. When the prostate gland swells due to infection, inflammation, or other causes, many gradually worsening symptoms occur. Prostate problems are broken down into three categories: benign prostatic hyperplasia (also called benign prostatic hypertrophy) or an enlarged prostate; prostatitis or infection of the prostate; or, more seriously, prostate cancer. Prostatitis is effectively treated using antibiotics. Prostatitis and benign prostatic hypertrophy are very common prostate problems. Prostate cancer is the second leading cause of death in North American men over the age of 50.

Benign prostatic hypertrophy (BPH) is an enlarged prostate gland that hinders urination by constricting the urethra. There are 180,000 new cases every year and it affects 60 percent of men between the ages of 40 and 59. BPH is also more common in athletes, particularly those who cycle and as such promote repetitive injury to the gland. Cyclists will get BPH at a much younger age than the general population (in fact 80 percent will have BPH by the age of 45). Although BPH is generally harmless, your doctor should diagnose it to ensure you do not have prostate cancer. If BPH is left untreated, obstruction of the bladder can occur, causing kidney damage. This is a life-threatening condition requiring immediate medical treatment.

A digital rectal exam is the first test to be performed where the doctor inserts a lubricated finger into the rectum to feel the prostate gland for swelling or lumps. Next your doctor may order a blood test called a prostate-specific antigen (PSA) test. However, the validity and efficacy of the test has been called into question as the PSA misses cancer growths 33 percent of the time or elicits false-positives in 60 percent of cases where there is no cancer. The strife and disruption for men, who either live with false reassurance (allowing the disease to progress) or who live in fear of a growth that does not exist, cause anguish. The test is also used as the basis for biopsy recommendations, but biopsies are increasingly being scrutinized for a possible role in spreading cancer by puncturing a self-contained cancerous growth. With all that said, a PSA reading above 10 should be cause for further evaluation. A urologist, a specialist in urinary-tract problems, should be consulted and a rectal ultrasound, among other tests, may be performed.

Symptoms

BPH is marked with a frequent urge to urinate, especially at night. The flow of urine may be reluctant or interrupted, be dribbled with less pressure and calibration, and accompanied by an inability to empty the bladder. There may be pain or discomfort during ejaculation. Prostatitis can occur if infection develops from not emptying the bladder effectively. Chronic constipation and low back pain are also symptoms.

Prostatitis is an infection of the prostate characterized by fever, pain while urinating, and a discharge from the penis. Antibiotic therapy is used to treat prostatitis but the recommendations for urinary tract infections can often work as well as antibiotic treatment.

Causes

One cause of BPH is related the hormone testosterone, which is produced by the testes and adrenal glands. As a man ages, his conversion of testosterone using an enzyme called 5-alpha-reductase to the active form of testosterone, dihydrotestosterone (DHT), increases. With more DHT the tissues of the prostate grow faster and the old tissue is not removed fast enough, causing an enlarged prostate. Athletes tend to have higher testosterone levels, which may account for their higher risk of BPH. Chronic constipation also puts extra pressure on the gland, causing inflammation.

Zinc deficiency appears to be critical in the onset of BPH and prostatitis. Zinc is vital for healthy hormone metabolism and is present in prostatic fluid. Zinc supplementation can reduce the size of the gland and enhance the immune system's ability to deal with prostatitis.

Prescription for Health

If you are diagnosed with prostate cancer, adopt these and the Cancer recommendations as well.

NUTRIENT	DOSAGE	ACTION
Multimune containing vitamins A, B₆, C, E, zinc, magnesium, selenium, coenzyme Q10, reduced L-glutathione, and lipoic acid	Three capsules daily with food	A potent antioxidant and anti-inflammatory, detoxifies liver, prevents deficiency, enhances immune function
Moducare sterols and sterolins	One capsule three times daily	German research has shown it effective in reducing symptoms of BPH, and halting the conversion of testosterone to DHT
Zinc	30–60 mg	Reduces prostate size and symptoms, inhibits conversion of testosterone to DHT

NUTRIENT	DOSAGE	ACTION
proteins+ protein poder	One to two scoops daily	High-protein diets inhibit 5-alpha-reductase, which converts testosterone to DHT
PC SPES for prostate cancer	Use as directed by your alternative health-care practitioner	Increases macrophages and T4 cells and stimulates cell death in cancer cells
Lycopene	Two capsules daily	Reduces risk of prostate disease
Flaxseed oil, Udo's Choice oil or Omega Essential Balance	1–2 Tbsp (15–30 mL) daily	Anti-inflammatory, supports cell membranes, reduces BPH symptoms
Lactobacillus acidophilus	1 tsp (5 mL) containing 1–2 billion active organisms daily	Improves intestinal flora to reduce harmful bacteria; required if antibiotics are being taken for prostatitis
Saw palmetto standardized to 85–95 percent fatty acids and sterols	150 mg twice a daily	Prevents testosterone from converting to dihydrotestosterone, thereby preventing growth of prostate; reduces symptoms
Pygeum africanum standardized to contain triterpenes, sterols, and n-docosanol	50 mg twice daily	Alleviates symptoms
Stinging nettle extract	300 mg daily	Suppresses prostate membrane activity, which may in turn lower inflammation and tissue enlargement and inhibit prostate cell growth
Quercitin	500 mg twice daily	Clears symptoms of prostatitis

Health Tips to Enhance Healing

- See Health Tips and treatments for Cancer and Urinary Tract Problems as well.
- Eat soy products. They keep cholesterol levels normalized and may help control DHT.
- Eat pumpkin seeds every day or use Omega Nutrition's delicious pumpkin spread and pumpkin seed oil.
- Keep cholesterol levels below 200 mg/dL, as a higher cholesterol count increases your risk of BPH.
- Get checked for excess cadmium. Stop smoking cigarettes, as they contain cadmium. Cadmium interferes with zinc absorption and increases the enzyme 5-alpha reductase, promoting the conversion of testosterone to DHT.
- Eliminate alcohol, caffeine, and sugar from the diet to decrease inflammation. Alcohol also interferes with zinc.
- Avoid dairy products. After adjusting for age, body mass index, fitness level, and smoking, a Harvard School of Public Health and Brigham and Women's Hospital joint study suggests that men who consumed a higher quantity of dairy products had a higher risk for prostate cancer.

- Researchers at the Fred Hutchinson Cancer Research Center found that three half-cup servings per week of cabbage, cauliflower, Brussels sprouts, or broccoli decreases the risk of prostate cancer by 41 percent.

Other Recommendations

- Modifications in lifestyle and diet can help tremendously. If your physician is recommending invasive or medication therapies, ask for studies and statistics to support that position, and learn the benefits and risks. Do not be afraid to get a second or third opinion. Good physicians will respect your request.

Health Fact

The Journal of the National Cancer Institute reported that a study conducted with 48,000 male subjects found that the men who consumed the highest amounts of lycopene (compared to other subjects) had a 50 percent reduction in risk for prostate cancer.

The Journal of the American Medical Association published the results of a study in 1997 where 322 men with normal PSA readings were asked to have biopsies. Twenty-two percent of the men were found to have cancer that the PSA test had not detected. Another study published by the *New England Journal of Medicine* in 1991 was conducted on men whose PSA readings suggested a cancer presence. Biopsies were performed and 78 percent of those men did not have cancer, in spite of what the PSA suggested.

PSORIASIS

Psoriasis is a very common skin condition that produces skin cells too rapidly, leading to a congestion of cells on the skin's surface. The normal life cycle of skin cells is 28 days, but cells produced by psoriasis mature up to a thousand times faster than healthy skin. More than 7 million North Americans have psoriasis, with its onset generally occurring in the late twenties. Psoriasis can also be associated with an autoimmune form of arthritis called psoriatic arthritis.

Symptoms

Raised patches of red with white flakes or scales appear on the torso, elbows, knees, legs, back, arms, and scalp. When it is in the scalp, it can promote hair loss. In some the nails may become dull, pitted, or ridged and may separate from the nail bed. Psoriasis fluctuates between periods of inflammation and remission and is categorized as mild, moderate, or severe. If the skin becomes too badly damaged there can be fluid loss, bacterial infection, and temperature dysregulation. Approximately 400 people die every year from psoriasis and another 400 are on disability pension. There are psychological ramifications to psoriasis as well, as people may feel shame, embarrassment, social rejection, and anger due to a lack of understanding on the parts of their peers. This psychological aspect can significantly affect relationships.

Arthritis similar to rheumatoid arthritis, called psoriatic arthritis, is sometimes present in those with psoriasis and it is very difficult to treat. There is pain, morning stiffness, swelling, reduced range of motion, pitting of the nails, tiredness, and redness in the eye (conjunctivitis). In severe cases it can lead to deformity of the joints and spine. Difficult to diagnose in people with subtle symptoms, it is believed that 10 to 30 percent of those with psoriasis will also develop psoriatic arthritis. It usually appears between 30 and 50 years of age.

Causes

The cause of psoriasis is unknown, but two theories have emerged: that it is an autoimmune disorder, or that it is caused by a bacterial "superantigen." Either way, there is a glitch in the immune system that tells the body to produce more skin cells. The immune system is often hyperstimulated, promoting inflammatory cytokines in the skin's cells. It may also be that the immune system, after a viral or bacterial infection, becomes primed to attack the skin.

Common triggers for psoriasis flare-ups are poor diet, incomplete protein digestion, a diet with excessive animal fat, bowel toxemia, impaired liver function, a superantigen, and heavy alcohol consumption. Other triggers are reactions to medication, stress, sunburn, illness, injury, nerves, and surgery.

Prescription for Health

NUTRIENT	DOSAGE	ACTION
Moducare sterols and sterolins	One capsule three times daily	Controls inflammation in the skin and reduces allergic reactions. Halts autoantibodies. A long-term treatment; it may take months to see results.
Omega-3 fatty acids DHA/EPA	1 Tbsp (15 mL) of flaxseed oil daily and three 500 g capsules of Eskimo-3 fish oil twice daily	Is anti-inflammatory, promotes remission of psoriasis symptoms
Multimune containing vitamins A, B₆, C, E, selenium, magnesium, zinc, coenzyme Q10, lipoic acid, reduced L-glutathione	Three capsules daily with food	An anti-inflammatory, potent antioxidant, detoxifies liver, supports skin and immune function

NUTRIENT	DOSAGE	ACTION
Omega Hi-Lignan Nutri-Flax	1-2 tsp (5-10 mL) daily	Improves bowel function and reduces bowel toxicity
Vitamin D active cholecalciferol	Oral or topical	Is available by prescription in high doses. Important for proper function of the skin. Also important for preventing deficiencies created when the skin cannot convert vitamin D due to damage from psoriasis.
Milk thistle	100 mg three times daily	Protects the liver and cleanses the blood
Comfrey or stinging nettle tea	Apply to head as a rinse daily	Loosens scales and heals scalp psoriasis
Capsaicin cream	0.075 cream applied to psoriasis several times daily	Anti-inflammatory
Licorice cream containing glycyrrhetinic acid	Apply to psoriasis several times daily	Anti-inflammatory; when compared to corticosteroid creams, licorice was more effective at reducing psoriasis

Health Tips to Enhance Healing

- See Arthritis for information on treatment for psoriatic arthritis.
- See Bowel Disease.
- Avoid saturated fats, as they promote flare-ups of psoriasis.
- Consume a diet that emphasizes natural, whole foods such as legumes, soy products, fresh fruits and vegetables, fish, healthy fats and oils, and nuts and seeds. Opt for foods high in vitamin E and vitamin C (see Chapter 4). Avoid animal meat and choose cold-water fish such as salmon, halibut, and mackerel instead.
- Stress reduction is paramount. Thirty-nine percent of those with psoriasis report that stress initiates the disease. (See "The Immune System and Stress," page 45.)
- Eliminate caffeine, sugar, and alcohol.
- Improve digestion—read Chapter 1.
- Studies have noted that those with psoriasis have lower levels of hydrochloric acid. If you suspect you have low stomach acid, see the introduction to this chapter.

Other Recommendations

- Get a little sun. Psoriasis seems to abate during the summer months and that is thought to be a result of UV radiation.
- Allergies and food sensitivities are common for those with psoriasis. See the introduction to this chapter.
- Try natural alternatives to corticosteroid creams such as Herbacort, or salves with capsaicin, licorice, chamomile, and evening

primrose oil. Botanical Therapeutics makes a great shampoo and conditioner for those with scalp psoriasis.

* Indulge in a sauna and/or steam bath.

Health Fact

The National Psoriasis Foundation states that 56 million hours of productivity are lost annually in the United States due to psoriasis. Treatment costs US$1.6–$3.2 billion every year.

RAYNAUD'S DISEASE/PHENOMENON

Raynaud's disease affects the circulatory system by constricting the arteries in the fingers and toes, causing them to spasm and the skin to discolor. The ears and nose may also be affected. It is more common in women, striking nine times more often than in men. Raynaud's disease begins in the early teens and becomes increasingly pronounced over the next 30 years. When the cause of the disease is known (causes include autoimmunity, frostbite, and surgical complications), it is called Raynaud's phenomenon.

Symptoms

An attack is provoked by emotional stress or by exposure to cold (even touching something cold, such as a refrigerator door). The extremities tingle and, deprived of oxygen, turn white or blue. The loss of blood to the area for prolonged periods, often seen in scleroderma, can result in skin lesions, nail infections, or tissue damage due to the lack of nutrients, so care must be taken to encourage blood flow. Gangrene is a rare result, but can occur.

Causes

Raynaud's disease is thought to be hereditary. Raynaud's phenomenon can be brought on by low thyroid, emotional stress, smoking, caffeine, nutritional deficiencies, and drug reactions to beta blockers, decongestants, oral contraceptives, and migraine relievers. Occupational environment or hazards such as working outdoors and exposure to chemicals such as vinyl chloride (PVCs) are also triggers. Those who use vibrating tools may find that Raynaud's is irreversible even after they no longer work with those tools. When Raynaud's is associated with lupus, rheumatoid arthritis, scleroderma, or Sjogren's syndrome, the symptoms are much more severe.

Prescription for Health

NUTRIENT	DOSAGE	ACTION
High-potency B-complex	Two capsules daily	Reduces stress, improves metabolism and energy production, prevents deficiency
Inositol hexaniacinate (nonflushing niacin)	1000 mg three times daily	Several human studies have shown fewer attacks after exposure to cold and enhanced circulation to fingers and toes
Vitamin E	400 IU twice daily	Promotes circulation
Moducare sterols and sterolins	One capsule three times daily	Anti-inflammatory, regulates immune function
Magnesium	500 mg twice daily	Studies show reduction in reaction to cold
Omega-6 evening primrose oil	Six 500 g capsules daily in divided dose	Reduces reaction time to cold and reduced flare-ups
Omega-3 fatty acids	Four 500 mg capsules of fish oil daily in divided dose	Reduces flare-up and reaction to cold
Ginkgo biloba	60 mg twice daily	Improves circulation
Horse chestnut, Venestat	Two capsules daily	Improves circulation

Health Tips to Enhance Healing

- It is very important to eliminate caffeine from the diet—it constricts blood vessels.
- Stop smoking and avoid exposure to secondhand smoke. Nicotine constricts the blood vessels.

Other Recommendations

- Always dress warmly and avoid exposure to cold. Take warm foot baths or go to bed with warm leg wraps.
- Use borage or evening primrose oil as topical massage oil for your fingers and toes. Massage nightly for two to three minutes.
- Get plenty of rest and reduce stress. Keep a positive outlook. Practice deep-breathing exercises, biofeedback, visualization, and other therapies to calm the body. See Chapter 6 for more ideas.
- Regular exercise is beneficial for increasing circulation. Incorporate some new activities into your life, swing your arms regularly, or rotate them backwards and forwards.
- It is very important to rule out food sensitivities. See the introduction to this chapter.
- Have your physician test you for hypothyroidism.

Health Fact

An investigative news program called "Trade Secrets: A Moyer's Report" showed that companies that produced vinyl chloride (PVC) knew in 1959 that regular exposure to the chemical would result in the disintegration of the hand bones in their employees. They kept the information confidential, did not stop production, did not warn their employees of the impending dangers, nor provide them with adequate protection. Some workers experienced thickened skin on their fingers, and a numbness that would begin in the hand, extending up the arm and to parts of the face.

REITER'S SYNDROME

Reiter's syndrome, also known as reactive arthritis, is comprised of three conditions: acute conjunctivitis, arthritis, and nonspecific urethritis. Inflammation attacks the eye, the joints, mucous membranes, and the urethra. Men are most often affected.

Symptoms

Symptoms of Reiter's often occur one to two weeks after an infection. Fever or weight loss is not unusual. Urethritis, which causes pain or discomfort during urination and a discharge from the penis, may be seen in men. The prostate gland may also enlarge and become painful.

Small, painful sores in the mouth and penis may be seen in some cases. Yellowing of the nails, thickening of the skin, and rashes may also occur.

When the eyes are involved, inflammation, burning, itching, or excessive tearing may be present. Inflammation of the iris is more indicative of a chronic condition. Up to 40 percent of people with Reiter's syndrome can be afflicted with an inflammation of the iris or other ocular disorders.

The swelling, pain, and stiffness of arthritis tend to situate in the lower half of the body, is not symmetrical, and is often associated with a "sausage" digit (an inflammation of the ligaments and tendons in a toe). Generally, Reiter's syndrome has been considered "self-limiting," and that it will just run its course, so often treatment is not even prescribed, yet some symptoms recur for years (see Health Fact). Spinal and joint deformities are seen in severe cases.

Causes

There are two forms of Reiter's. One type follows a genitourinary infection such as chlamydia. Sexually active men are in a higher risk group of contracting it, but Reiter's syndrome can also follow an intestinal infection of salmonella, shigella, or yersinia (see Health Fact). It is believed that you must have a genetic predisposition to develop Reiter's after infection from the above-mentioned bacteria.

Prescription for Health

See Arthritis for Prescription for Health recommendations for joint and inflammatory symptoms.

See Urinary Tract Problems and Prostate Problems for Prescription for Health recommendations for treatment of urinary symptoms. Read Chapter 1 on digestive disorders and Chapter 3 on the immune system to learn about infections and how to prevent them.

See Diarrhea and Parasites for treatment of infectious agents.

Health Tips to Enhance Healing

- Use Weleda eyedrops and eye compresses to relieve conjunctivitis and other eye symptoms.
- Beware of taking non-steroidal anti-inflammatory drugs (NSAIDs). They have severe side effects, especially when used for prolonged periods. (See "Serious Side Effects from NSAIDs," page 43.)

Health Fact

During a papal visit in Ontario, 1608 police officers acted as security guards. Food consumed by the guards had been tainted with salmonella and one-quarter of the officers developed acute gastroenteritis. Three months later, 27 of the affected group had acute arthritis, although it cleared up in nine of them within four months. Five years later, the other 18 officers expressed recurring symptoms or chronic arthritis upon re-evaluation. Diagnosis: Reiter's syndrome. Although Reiter's syndrome is described as self-limited, this study clearly showed that in some cases this is not completely accurate. Four of those officers had to seek alternative employment because their symptoms prevented them from doing their jobs.

RESTLESS LEG SYNDROME

Just as the name suggests, this syndrome is the involuntary twitching or jerking of the legs and it is most prevalent at night. Moving the legs brings only momentary relief, so the continuous urges to move can become annoying and cause restless sleep.

Symptoms

Apart from the desire to move the legs, sometimes the legs will itch, go numb, feel ticklish, or have a burning sensation. Some people feel the need to get up or go for a walk after sitting or sleeping for only a short time. Fatigue is a secondary condition as a result of not getting enough sleep.

Causes

Both the muscles and the arteries spasm in restless leg syndrome. The main culprits attributed to it are stress, anxiety, caffeine, malabsorption, nutritional deficiencies of magnesium or folic acid, and food allergies. This condition is common during pregnancy and in those who smoke. The main cause is magnesium deficiency. Magnesium is lost when we drink caffeinated beverages and during periods of stress.

Prescription for Health

NUTRIENT	DOSAGE	ACTION
High-potency B-complex	Three capsules daily	Prevents deficiency, is important for nerve and muscle function
Multimune containing vitamins A, B$_6$, C, E, magnesium, selenium, zinc, coenzyme Q10, lipoic acid, and reduced L-glutathione	Three capsules daily with food	A potent antioxidant and anti-inflammatory, detoxifies liver, oxygenates cells, prevents deficiency
Vitamin E	200 IU daily	Alleviates symptoms very effectively
Magnesium, preferably in the form of glycinate	500 mg after every meal. If you have kidney problems consult your physician before taking this dosage of magnesium.	Alleviates symptoms of restless leg syndrome, heart palpitation, and twitching eyelids. If you are a heavy coffee drinker, you need more magnesium (100 mg for every cup of coffee consumed).
Valerian or kava kava	Tincture as directed	Calms and relaxes nerves
Ginkgo biloba, standardized extract	60 mg twice daily	Research has shown ginkgo improves circulation in the legs

Health Tips to Enhance Healing

- Avoid caffeinated beverages (coffee, tea, cola, cocoa). Remember that sodas often contain caffeine, as do some food supplements and pain medications.
- Drink herb teas, especially chamomile.
- Eat magnesium-rich foods. (See Chapter 4.)
- Reduce stress.

Health Fact

Two case reports published in *California Medicine* supported the use of vitamin E. One woman, 78, with a 20-year history of restless legs, took 300 IU daily for two months. The other woman, 37, with a 10-year history, took 300 IU daily for six weeks, then 200 IU for four weeks. Both were completely cured.

ROSACEA

Rosacea is a chronic skin disorder causing acne-like breakouts, broken blood vessels, and redness mostly on the cheeks and nose. It generally strikes people after the age of 30 and affects women three times more often than men, although it is usually more extreme in men. If the problem is not addressed, it can cause permanent damage to the skin. It may rarely affect skin on other areas of the body. Rosacea is more common in those with fair skin.

Symptoms

It usually begins with a flush of the face that comes and goes, and tiny bumps can appear. A network of blood vessels may be seen beneath the surface of the skin; as the disease progresses, the redness gets worse. If the skin swells, it may be tender. The eyes can become red, sore, or swollen, even to the point where vision is affected. The skin may thicken over time causing a red bulbous nose called rhinophyma.

Causes

Although the cause of rosacea is not known, there are a number of triggers specific to each individual that aggravate the condition: smoking, hot liquids, spicy foods, stress, caffeine, excessive use of alcohol, gingko biloba, menopausal flushing, a lack of stomach acid or the digestive enzyme lipase, infection, exposure to sunlight, and food and environmental allergies. Nutritional deficiencies of vitamins A and B_2 are also linked to the development of this condition. Rosacea is also often related to excess sebum production. Rhinophyma is common in alcoholics and those who drink alcoholic beverages daily.

Prescription for Health

Antibiotics have been effectively used to treat rosacea in some cases. If using antibiotics, take probiotic supplements as well.

NUTRIENT	DOSAGE	ACTION
Vitamin A	5000 IU daily	Required for healing skin
High-potency B-complex	Two capsules daily	Reduces stress; deficiency has been seen in those with rosacea
Vitamin B₂ (riboflavin)	50 mg daily	Reduces infection in the skin, which plays a causative role
Vitamin C	500–1000 mg twice daily	Enhances collagen formation
Vitamin E	200–400 IU daily	Important for skin repair
Lactobacillus acidophilus	1 tsp (5 mL) of 1–2 billion active organisms daily	Improves digestion by increasing intestinal flora
Evening primrose oil	500 mg three times daily	Is beneficial to the skin and anti-inflammatory
Moducare sterols and sterolins	One capsule three times daily	Controls inflammation in the skin and regulates immune function
Flaxseed oil, Udo's Choice oil, or Omega Essential Balance	1 Tbsp (15 mL) daily	Beneficial for the skin
Zinc	30 mg daily	Prevents rosacea
Pancreatic enzymes	500 mg before meals	Improves digestion and metabolism of fats

Health Tips to Enhance Healing

- Eliminate sugar, dairy, and hydrogenated fats. This is essential to halting rosacea.
- Alcohol is a very strong trigger for rosacea, so reduce or eliminate alcohol.
- It is very important that you take two capsules of digestive enzymes before every meal.
- If you suspect you have low stomach acid that is hindering your digestion, see the introduction to this chapter.
- Drink at least eight to ten glasses of pure, filtered water daily. Water flushes out toxins and encourages efficient elimination.
- Eat foods that encourage healthy liver function such as artichokes, rhubarb, Chinese white radish, black radish, soy, apples, and rolled oats.
- Do not consume hot food and drinks. Let them cool to room temperature first.
- Allergies are also implicated in Rosacea. See the introduction to this chapter.

Other Recommendations

- Use Hauschka Rythmic Skin Conditioner (Sensitive) every night for three months to reduce the appearance of rosacea. This is a very effective topical remedy.

- If you use makeup, use all-natural products, but avoid using other cosmetics or heavy moisturizers.
- Wash your face with natural soaps or cleansers, and keep hair clean. Wash your pillowcases regularly. Avoid using detergents or shampoos with perfumes, scents, colors, or fragrances. Rinse all bedding twice.
- Flushing is provoked by higher temperatures, so avoid conditions that are too hot or too warm, such as you would find in saunas, hot tubs, and hot baths.

Health Fact

Research studies have found that those with rosacea often have a riboflavin deficiency and/or low stomach acid.

SCLERODERMA

Systemic sclerosis (called scleroderma) is an autoimmune disease characterized by hardening and scarring of the skin. Chronic degeneration of connective tissue can also be seen in different organ systems, including the kidneys, lungs, heart, and gastrointestinal systems. Scleroderma is highly individualistic, ranging from mild to severe to fatal. It is invisible when it affects the organs and very visible when it affects the skin. Four times as many women as men are affected and it usually strikes after the age of 25. Young African American women are at an excessive risk of contracting scleroderma.

CREST syndrome is a mild skin sclerosis that is mainly limited to the fingers. It causes calcium deposits in the skin and throughout the body. Raynaud's phenomenon is common. High blood pressure may also occur.

The immune system is dysfunctional in scleroderma. Autoantibodies and excessive immune activation by inflammatory cytokines, especially interleukin-6 and interleukin-1, are seen in scleroderma. Macrophages are also overactive.

Symptoms

Initially the skin hardens, thickens, and becomes tight, shiny, and increasingly painful. The tissues calcify, the skin on the fingers and toes hardens, and there can be Raynaud's phenomenon (see Raynaud's). It can affect large areas of skin or just the fingers. Difficulty swallowing and heartburn may be present especially when the lower end of the esophagus is involved. The joints become stiff and achy. Fatigue, general weakness, and weight loss are not uncommon due to malabsorption from damage to the intestines. At some point, the skin becomes so hard the process stops and although movement may be somewhat restricted, it is not usually crippling. If, however, the disease affects the heart and kidneys, it can be fatal. Within the first seven years of a diagnosis of severe scleroderma, seven out of ten patients will die.

Causes

Scleroderma results when there are spasms in the arteries and abnormal collagen formation. Environmental factors are key in the development of scleroderma. This is evident by the fact that scleroderma-related antibodies are seen in the spouses of those affected with the disease. Ingestion of contaminated salad oils (rapeseed), as well as exposure to solvents like benzene, chemical compounds such as polyvinyl chloride (PVC), and silicone are primary triggers. Eosinophilia-myalgia syndrome (EMS), caused by ingesting contaminated L-tryptophan, resulted in scleroderma in many of those affected with EMS. Hand-arm vibration injury from using equipment like jackhammers can also cause scleroderma. An overstimulated immune system is also clearly involved in scleroderma.

Prescription for Health

The recommendations below are focused on controlling the autoimmune process, increasing circulation to the skin, and regulating collagen synthesis. Do not stop your medications. If you also have Raynaud's or lupus, see those conditions for more information.

NUTRIENT	DOSAGE	ACTION
PABA (para-amino benzoic acid); form used in studies was the potassium salt of PABA, called Potaba	10 g dosages were used in the research	Softens the skin, increases skin mobility, and increases survival rates. Talk to your physician about this successful treatment. Do not take if you have vitiligo.
Moducare sterols and sterolins	One capsule three times daily	Anti-inflammatory, regulates immune function, and controls interleukin-6 and 1
Multimune containing vitamins A, B₆ (P-5-P), C, E, magnesium, zinc, lipoic acid, selenium, coenzyme Q10, and reduced L-glutathione	Three capsules daily with food	Supports immune function, detoxifies liver, is a potent antioxidant and anti-inflammatory, protects against deficiency
High-potency B-complex	Two capsules daily	Reduces stress, improves metabolism and energy production, prevents deficiency
Inositol hexanicotinate (nonflushing niacin)	1000 mg three times daily	Several human studies have shown fewer attacks after exposure to cold and enhanced circulation to fingers and toes
Vitamin E	400 IU twice daily	Promotes circulation
Magnesium	500 mg daily	Required for hundreds of enzymatic reactions in the body, is anti-inflammatory

NUTRIENT	DOSAGE	ACTION
Omega-6 evening primrose oil	Six 500 mg capsules daily in divided dose	Reduces reaction time to cold and reduces flare-ups
Omega-3 fatty acids	Six, 500 mg capsules fish oil daily in divided dose	Reduces flare-ups and reaction to cold

Health Tips to Enhance Healing

- Eliminate caffeine from the diet. It constricts blood vessels.
- Avoid animal meat and choose fish instead. Eliminate sugar and alcohol from the diet.
- Stop smoking and avoid exposure to secondhand smoke. Nicotine constricts the blood vessels.

Other Recommendations

- Rule out allergies. See the introduction to this chapter.
- Reduce stress. (See "The Immune System and Stress" on page 45)
- Rule out hydrochloric acid deficiency (see page 141) and take digestive enzymes.
- See Raynaud's Disease and if you have any other autoimmune disorder, read "Excessive Stress" under Autoimmunity (on page 48) as well for tips on how to alleviate those symptoms.

Health Fact

A study was conducted to determine the effects of omega-6 fatty acids on four patients who had had systemic sclerosis for anywhere from five to 13 years. After one year of receiving 1 g of omega-6 three times daily, all four felt relief from pain, improvement in skin texture and capillary walls, and healing of ulcers. In their conclusion, researchers suggested that 6 g daily would be more beneficial.

SEASONAL AFFECTIVE DISORDER

Seasonal affective disorder (SAD) is a form of "winter" depression that affects 4 to 6 percent of the population. It coincides with the change in seasons, becoming worse as the days grow shorter and there is less light. This is not just the "winter blues" or the fatigue that is more common at wintertime, as it can become as debilitating as other forms of depression. As the days grow longer the symptoms abate and the feelings of normalcy return. Women are affected by SAD four times more often than men, and the condition becomes more prevalent the farther north you go.

Symptoms

The symptoms of SAD are similar to depression—lost libido, inability to concentrate, heightened perception of social rejection, oversleeping, lethargy, anxiety, weight gain due to an increase in sweets and starch cravings, withdrawal from normal activities—and are generally more marked around the winter holidays. A common analogy is that the person is going into hibernation.

Causes

It is believed that the lack of sunlight disrupts the levels of the hormone melatonin. Melatonin is the hormone that stabilizes our biorhythms, regulating our waking and sleeping patterns. A reduction in melatonin secretion can cause a corresponding increase in our stress hormone cortisol and a reduction in serotonin, which is important for managing mood.

A study released in March 2001 suggests that SAD can be triggered by the inflammatory side of the immune system response (IL-6, IL-6 receptor, and IL-2 receptor). Comparing plasma measurements of the SAD group with a control group, the SAD group demonstrated significantly higher levels of IL-6. As we understand more about the immune system, we are learning that it has a role in almost every disease affecting the body.

Prescription for Health

See Depression and adopt the treatment recommendations along with the following that are specific for SAD.

NUTRIENT	DOSAGE	ACTION
Melatonin	1–3 mg 30 minutes before bed	Increases brain melatonin and suppressed cortisol
Moducare sterols and Sterolin	One capsule three times daily	Regulates cortisol and normalizes interleukin-6 and 1
Full-spectrum light therapy	See below	Is antidepressant for SAD and depression

Health Tips to Enhance Healing

- Exercise regularly, even if it is just a walk around the block, and inhale deeply through the nose. Studies have proven that low-to-moderate physical activity can elevate serotonin levels and offset feelings of anxiety or depression. Spend as much time outside as you can.
- Phototherapy is an effective and essential treatment for SAD in addition to the natural remedies mentioned for depression.

Full-spectrum light therapy reproduces natural sunlight. Special light bulbs or a SAD light box or a visor that can be worn are available. Verilux Full-Spectrum Lighting makes excellent bulbs and therapeutic fixtures. Replace all the bulbs in your home and office with full-spectrum lighting. I have a "happy light box" from Verilux sitting on my desk all winter long. I used to get the blues in January, but thanks to my "happy light," I no longer feel depressed. Tanning beds use harmful UV rays and should not be thought of as a source of light therapy.

- See "The Immune System and Stress," page 45.
- Counseling may be beneficial in addition to other therapies.

SINUSITIS (BACTERIAL)

Sinuses are empty cavities lined with mucous membranes. At the bottom of each is a minute opening that empties mucous into the nasal passage to be expelled. If that opening becomes inflamed during infections, allergies, or fungal growth, it closes up, trapping the mucous in the cavity and providing a nurturing environment for bacteria. There are four pairs of sinuses: above and below the eyes, above the nose, and deep in the skull.

Symptoms

Acute sinusitis is accompanied by fever and chills, frontal headaches, and congested sinus passages, which are difficult to clear of a thick discharge. The face is tender to the touch, red, and swollen. In chronic sinusitis, the symptoms are typically less severe with dry cough, postnasal drip, musty breath, and nasal odor. Other symptoms include difficulty breathing, poor sense of smell, and earaches.

Causes

An acute sinus infection usually begins with a cold that promotes a bacterial infection. A weakened immune system, the one that allowed the cold to take hold, is also a contributing factor. Allergies (allergic rhinitis) or sensitivities to food are common instigators of chronic sinusitis. According to Michael Murray, MD, 25 percent of chronic sinusitis cases are the result of a dental infection. Other culprits are smoking, stress, injury to the nose, irritating fumes, and air travel (due to the sudden and frequent changes in air pressure).

Prescription for Health

Antibiotics, although the most common treatment prescribed, are rarely effective. Allergy is the number one cause of sinusitis (see Allergies for treatment recommendations). Read Chapter 3 on the immune system to understand how to get your immune system to destroy the bacteria, reduce inflammation, and control allergic responses.

NUTRIENT	DOSAGE	ACTION
Moducare sterols and sterolins	Two capsules three times daily during acute phase, then one capsule three times daily thereafter as maintenance	Regulates immune function, has been shown in clinical trials to reduce allergic rhinitis and sinusitis, controls cortisol, is anti-inflammatory and reduces IL-6 and IL-1, enhances bacteria- and viral-fighting ability of the immune system
Vitamin C with bioflavonoids	1000 mg every two hours while awake during acute infection and 3000 mg daily thereafter	Fights infection and strengthens collagen along the bronchi
Multimune containing vitamins A, B_6, C, E, selenium, zinc, magnesium, coenzyme Q10, lipoic acid, and reduced L-glutathione	Three capsules daily with food	Supports immune function, is anti-inflammatory, reduces histamine, controls cortisol, detoxifies liver, is antibacterial and antiviral
Bromelain (1200–1800 mcu)	500 mg between meals	Reduces mucous and upper respiratory infections
Goldenseal standardized to berberine	500 mg twice daily	Enhances immune function
Lactobacillus acidophilus	1 tsp (5 mL) containing 1–2 billion live organisms daily	Improves intestinal flora, which fights bacteria
Astragalus	200 mg three times daily	Enhances immune system and reduces infection
Vitamin A (micellized)	100,000 IU daily for five days during acute infection and 5000 IU daily thereafter for maintenance	Fights infection and heals mucous membranes
Echinacea tincture	20 drops in a glass of water taken three times daily for 10–14 days	Strengthens immune system, helps fight bacterial and viral infections

Health Tips to Enhance Healing

- Use Similisan homeopathic nasal spray. It is an excellent adjunct for the recommendations above.
- See Allergies and Candidiasis.
- Avoid sugar and dairy products, especially fruit juice, because the natural sugar content is high. Sugar depresses the immune system and dairy products promote the formation of mucous.

- Draining the sinuses is very important. Local application of warm packs to the sinus area and steam inhalation can help loosen congested sinuses. Steam inhalations can help break up the mucous, especially when you add rosemary or eucalyptus oil to the infusion. Take a hot shower and while showering lay hot cloths on your sinus to facilitate drainage.
- Regular antibiotic use allows bacteria to build up a resistance. Antibiotics also destroy the good infection-fighting bacteria in your intestinal tract. If you do take antibiotics, eat a half-cup of plain yogurt every day to replace lost intestinal flora, but not at the same time as the antibiotic.
- Particularly good for sinusitis is radish juice, which helps remove mucous. Drink the juice of six radishes, one apple, and one cucumber, or add horseradish to meals and soups.
- Practice deep-breathing exercises to improve oxygen intake.
- Maintaining a regular exercise program when you are not suffering from sinusitis will encourage deep breathing and circulate oxygen. (See Chapter 6.)
- Reduce stress. Too much stress and not enough sleep or relaxation takes its toll on the immune system, making it easier for infections to occur. (See "The Immune System and Stress," page 45.)
- Drink eight to ten glasses of pure, filtered water every day. Water is an antihistamine to prevent allergic reactions.
- Avoid caffeine. Herbal teas made from horehound, red clover, anise, mullein, nettle, rose hips, and olive leaf can be quite beneficial in speeding the healing process. Hot water with lemon juice and cayenne can also help.

Other Recommendations

- Apply ice packs or warm compresses, whichever feels good to you.
- Eliminate allergies (see information in the introduction to this chapter).
- Don't use household cleaning sprays, deodorizers, or insect repellents. Have your home checked for environmental hazards such as lead and asbestos.
- Stop smoking.
- Seek out qualified practitioners of acupuncture and homeopathy. Both can be very beneficial in alleviating symptoms of sinusitis.
- If there is swelling around the eyes, consult your physician.

SJOGREN'S SYNDROME

Sjogren's syndrome is an autoimmune disorder or chronic inflammatory disease that causes excessive dryness to the eyes and mucous membranes of the body. The immune system attacks the moisture-producing glands, causing infection, inflammation, or corneal ulcers. It can appear as a primary condition or in conjunction with other autoimmune disorders such as rheumatoid arthritis, lupus, and myasthenia gravis. Two to 4 million North Americans have Sjogren's syndrome. Nine out of 10 people with Sjogren's syndrome will be female and predominantly aged 40 to 50.

Symptoms

Primary Sjogren's syndrome is characterized by an inability of the eyes to tear. The eyes feel gritty and painful, and are sensitive to light, smoke, and fumes. Other areas that can be affected are the salivary glands, nose, skin, and vagina. Mucous membranes lining the gastrointestinal tract and trachea can dry out and become painful and irritated and prone to infections. Pericarditis, or inflammation of the sac around the heart (the pericardium), can be a serious symptom of Sjogren's.

When Sjogren's syndrome is secondary to autoimmune disorders, dry mouth is significantly less present and symptoms expand to other areas of the body. There can be morning stiffness and pain in the muscles and joints, dry cough or other respiratory tract problems, nausea, indigestion and gastritis, renal disease, inflamed blood vessels, nerve problems (especially to the face), allergies, and non-Hodgkin's lymphoma. Fatigue can be debilitating.

The symptoms can range from mild to so severe that it hinders quality of life. Some people may have a remission, while others remain the same or become worse. Sjogren's can develop from a benign autoimmune disease into a lymphoid malignancy (including non-Hodgkin's lymphoma).

Causes

Sjogren's is an autoimmune disease whereby the immune system destroys the exocrine glands (the fluid-secreting glands) and can advance to a systemic multi-organ attack. The cause is unknown, but heredity may play a part. Female hormones and viral infections are being investigated, in particular the retroviruses and herpes viruses (cytomegalovirus, hepatitis C, Epstein Barr, and herpes Type 6). Triggers for Sjogren's syndrome include injury to the arteries or nerves in the face, food and environmental allergies, nutritional deficiencies, wearing contact lenses, and smoking tobacco or marijuana.

Prescription for Health

Those with autoimmune disorders should not take immune boosters as they can overstimulate B-cell activity, promoting autoantibody production. Immune boosters, when taken over the long term, can enhance macrophage function, promoting inflammatory cytokines. The German Commission E does not recommend echinacea for those with autoimmune disease.

NUTRIENT	DOSAGE	ACTION
Bilberry	100 mg twice daily	Improves circulation to the eyes
Moducare sterols and sterolins	One capsule three times daily as a maintenance dose	Essential for regulating immune function and controlling autoantibody reactions, is anti-inflammatory
High-potency B-complex	Two capsules daily with meals	Required for metabolism and immune function
Multimune containing vitamins A, B6, C, E, selenium, zinc, magnesium, coenzyme Q10, lipoic acid, reduced L-glutathione	Three capsules daily with meals	Supports the proper functioning of the immune system, is anti-inflammatory and a potent antioxidant
Vitamin C	1000 mg twice daily	Regulates immunity and combats stress
Vitamin E	100 IU daily	In several studies those with autoimmune diseases had a significant reduction in symptoms
Omega-3 fish oils	1 g three times daily	A powerful anti-inflammatory and controls T-helper-2 reactions
Evening primrose oil	1 g three times daily	Essential for recurring and relapsing autoimmune disease, ensures proper function of suppressor T-cells, is anti-inflammatory

Health Tips to Enhance Healing

- Read Chapter 3 on autoimmune disease.
- Antihistamines and diuretics should never be taken by someone with Sjogren's syndrome.
- Stop smoking tobacco and marijuana and avoid exposure to secondhand smoke.
- Eliminate alcohol, sugar, salt, and caffeine from the diet. They all contribute to dehydration.
- Suck on flavorful lozenges or chewing gum (sugar-free) to keep mucous membranes of the mouth moist.

Other Recommendations

- Rule out allergies. See the introduction to this chapter.
- Weleda eyedrops (either Euphrasia D3, Gencydo 1 percent, or

Cineraria Maritima D3) eyedrops are exceptional for those with dry eyes.

- See "The Immune System and Stress," page 45.
- Lack of saliva creates a vulnerability to bacterial infections in the mouth. Good personal and oral hygiene and preventative dental care should be practiced to minimize severity of symptoms. Get an electric toothbrush and use it at least twice a day. Use mouthwashes that contain soothing herbs and aloe.
- If vaginal dryness is a problem, use a water-based (not oil-based) lubricant.
- Avoid dry, windy climates, air-conditioning, dust, and smoke. Keep your eyes moist with the help of a humidifier.
- If you have another autoimmune disorder, read that section as well for tips on how to alleviate those symptoms.

SNORING

Until recently, snoring appeared to be more annoying than dangerous, but now research has found that it might lead to a greater risk of hypertension, stroke, or heart disease. Severe cases of snoring result in sleep apnea, a condition where the snoring person stops breathing (apnea) and gasps for air because the airway closes, preventing airflow. A person's ability to breathe may be hindered for seconds to minutes and may cause a decrease in oxygen to the brain. Another condition called hypopnea is where the airway is only partially blocked, preventing the person from taking in a full breath. Hypopneic snoring is characterized as heavy, long, and loud.

If a person cannot breathe in enough oxygen, the heart is forced to work harder to make the blood circulate faster, leading to stress on arteries and high blood pressure or irregular heartbeats. The sleeping partner is usually the one to notice sleep apnea or snoring problems.

Symptoms

It may begin innocently enough as heavy breathing during sleep, but gradually snoring grows more evident as it becomes louder and more disruptive, sometimes enough so as to wake the snorer. The snorer may feel tired the next day, even after a full night's sleep, or does not feel refreshed after napping.

Work performance may be affected by the lack of adequate rest. The tendency to snore may start in childhood, but occurrences increase with advancing age and excessive weight. Other signs of snoring include waking up with a dry or sore throat or morning headache, or having night sweats. Snoring children have also been reported to have, in addition to the previous symptoms, poor hearing, a tendency to breathe through the mouth, and enlarged tonsils. According to a study by the School of Dentistry in Cleveland, Ohio, there are also physical differences between children who snore and those who do not. The snorers have narrower pharynxes and a longer distance between the hyoid and mandibular plane.

Causes

When the airways between the throat and nasal passages are partially obstructed, the snorer inhales quickly to get air. The turbulence caused by the inhalation causes the soft palate and uvula (the dangly bit at the back of your throat) to vibrate and create the snore. Snoring is more likely to occur when you are overweight or pregnant, or if the sinuses are congested due to colds, flus, allergies, infections, or nasal polyps. Smoking and excessive use of some medications or alcohol are also linked.

One study monitoring the frequency of snoring among pregnant women found that 4 percent of the women said they snored before pregnancy, while 23 percent more were found to snore by the end of their pregnancy. They also discovered that babies born to snoring mothers have a greater tendency toward lower birth weight.

Prescription for Health

Follow the recommendations for Allergies, Polyps, and Sinusitis in combination with these suggestions.

NUTRIENT	DOSAGE	ACTION
Vitamin C	3000–5000 mg daily in divided doses	Helps reduce inflammation of airways and acts as an antihistamine
Reduced L-glutathione	500 mg twice daily	Reduces inflammation, is antihistamine and antiallergy
Snore Stop by Baywood	Use as directed	Stops snoring, improves air flow
Sage leaves and lindenflower blossoms	1 cup (250 mL) of tea daily	Reduces inflammation of the membranes

Health Tips to Enhance Healing

- Read other applicable conditions: Allergies, Heart Disease, Polyps, and Sinusitis.
- Go to a sleep disorder clinic where specialists in sleep apnea can assess you and provide breathing devices if necessary.
- Use Snore Control homeopathic spray. Some individuals get excellent results using this and other throat sprays with a combination of homeopathic remedies. Snore Control is manufactured by King Bio Pharmaceuticals.
- It is important to rule out allergies. Those with allergies have

swollen mucous membranes in the nose and throat, promoting snoring. Get rid of feather pillows and quilts and remove all allergens from your bedroom.
- Drink at least eight to ten glasses of pure, filtered water every day as it works as a natural antihistamine.
- If you are overweight, losing even 5 lbs (2 kg) can reduce your snoring.
- Stop smoking or drinking alcohol at least three hours before bedtime.
- Air out the bedroom before going to sleep. Do not let pets sleep with you on the bed.

Other Recommendations

- If snoring is really bad, there are mouthpieces that your dentist can construct to pull the jaw forward and open up the air passages. These devices have shown greater success for people with mild to moderate sleep apnea than for those with severe sleep apnea.
- If you normally sleep on your back, try going to sleep on your side or stomach. Try using a neck roll instead of a pillow.
- Avoid taking sleeping pills or antihistamines. They may relax the throat too much and are dangerous for heavy snorers.

Health Fact

Snorers could be arrested for disturbing the peace. Kent Wilson of the University of Minnesota researches snoring and sleep apnea, and reported that 12 percent of his snorers exceeded 55 decibels, the level determined by the Minnesota Pollution Control Agency to be acceptable for night-time noise.

SORE THROAT

Viral infections are the source of most sore throats. As part of the frontline defense, the throat is a barrier that comes in contact with germs and environmental irritants. Sore throats usually last only a few days and are often accompanied by a cold. Although most sore throats are caused by viruses, the presence of streptococcus infection or strep throat should be determined by your physician and may require antibiotic treatment.

Symptoms

The pain of a sore throat can be described as raw, itchy, burning, stabbing, or tender, and the intensity can vary from mild to excruciating.

Swallowing or coughing can be extremely painful. The lymph glands located under the jaw at the side of the neck usually swell and are tender to the touch. A hoarse voice suggests that the problem is located in the larynx.

Causes

As with fever, a sore throat is an indication that a bacterial or viral infection such as tonsillitis, sinusitis, or mononucleosis is present. The tonsils are an integral part of the immune system and removal is not recommended, as they are a significant component of the body's front-line of defense. Antibiotics will not help a sore throat if the cause is viral and several studies have shown that even when throat infections are bacterial, they are generally self-limiting, and in some studies antibiotics were no better than no treatment at all. Streptococcus bacteria can be discovered only by doing a throat culture and fortunately rapid result cultures are available that can determine if the infection is in need of antibiotic therapy. Physicians are trained to prescribe antibiotics in the presence of strep infection even though research has shown that recovery rates were the same whether people were given the antibiotic or allowed the bacteria to run its course. Antibiotics are essential in the case of those who are immune compromised or who have kidney disease or a history of rheumatic fever.

Exposure to excessive amounts of dust, smoke, dry air, or acid reflux can irritate the throat. Sometimes the throat suffers abrasions from swallowing very hot foods or drinks, or when you have been talking, yelling, singing, or coughing loudly or for long periods of time. Other causes of a sore throat can include allergic reactions and tooth or gum infections.

The throat is fairly resilient against invaders, so when it succumbs to infection, it means that the immune system was too weak and unable to adequately mount a counterattack to destroy the virus or bacteria. If you suffer chronic throat infections, read Chapter 3 on the immune system to learn how to enhance it.

Prescription for Health

For those who are not responding to antibiotic treatment or who have recurring throat infections, the following is designed to support immune function and soothe inflamed throat tissues.

NUTRIENT	DOSAGE	ACTION
Vitamin A (micellized, liquid)	100,000 IU in the back of the throat daily for five days. Allow it to bathe mucous membranes. 5000 IU daily thereafter.	Fights bacterial and viral infections, and often alleviates pain of sore throat immediately

NUTRIENT	DOSAGE	ACTION
Vitamin C with bioflavonoids	1000 mg of vitamin C three times daily; 500 mg of bioflavonoids three times daily. Take Multimune as maintenance after infection abates.	Boosts immune function; is antiviral, antibacterial, antihistamine; speeds up healing of mucous membranes
Zinc lozenges	30 mg per day during infection, then take Multimune as maintenance	Alleviates pain and supports immune system. Do not be tempted to eat all of the throat lozenges in one day. Too much zinc can suppress immune function.
Garlic (Kyolic)	Two or three capsules three times daily	Acts as an antiviral and antibacterial
Moducare sterols and sterolins	One capsule three times daily	Regulates immune function, enhances T-cell and NK cell activity and decreases inflammation, regulates cortisol, prevents infections
Lactobacillus acidophilus	1 tsp (5 mL) containing 1–2 billion active organisms daily	Improves intestinal flora and fights bacteria, is essential while taking antibiotics
Goldenseal, standardized to berberine	500 mg daily	Enhances immune function, is antibacterial. Look for goldenseal throat spray at your health food store.
Echinacea tincture	20–40 drops in water three times daily for 10–14 days	Shortens duration of infection, boosts immune function
Multimune containing vitamins A, B$_6$, C, E, selenium, zinc, magnesium, coenzyme Q10, lipoic acid, reduced L-glutathione	Three capsules daily with food	Supports immune function, is potent antioxidant, detoxifies liver, is antiviral, antibacterial, antihistamine

Health Tips to Enhance Healing

- When you brush your teeth, either brush your tongue or use a tongue scraper to remove the bacteria that are hiding on the surface. Change your toothbrush as soon as you feel better and thereafter change it monthly to avoid the growth of bacteria.
- Drink plenty of herbal tea and unsweetened cranberry juice mixed with water.
- Use garlic frequently and liberally in your meals.
- Throat lozenges containing echinacea, vitamin C, goldenseal, and cherry bark are soothing to inflamed throat tissues. Use as directed.
- Read Chapter 3 on the immune system to learn how to prevent infections.
- If you are taking antibiotics, be sure to eat plain yogurt or supplement with probiotics to restore the "friendly" bacteria that will be destroyed.

- Sugar suppresses the immune system, so eliminate it as much as possible from the diet. Do not drink concentrated fruit juice as it is also high in sugar. Keep honey and maple syrup to a minimum as well.
- Water is the cheapest virus fighter you can use. Drink eight to ten glasses during infection to help wash away infection.

Other Recommendations

- Stop smoking. Tobacco leaves a film of tar on the tongue, teeth, and gums that can make infections worse and delay healing. It can also lead to oral cancer.
- Apply warm throat wraps of big cabbage leaves on an hourly basis. You will be amazed how effective this is.
- Gargle every few hours with water, apple cider vinegar, and 1 tsp (5 mL) of sea salt. You can also gargle with solutions made with herbs such as sage, licorice, and fenugreek.
- If a cough or tickle is constant or recurring, have yourself tested for food allergies and environmental allergies. (See Allergies for more information.)

SYSTEMIC LUPUS ERYTHEMATOSUS

Systemic lupus erythematosus (SLE) is commonly known as lupus. This devastating form of arthritis is an autoimmune disease whereby the immune system attacks the connective tissue, affecting mostly the skin, joints, blood, and kidneys. It may appear suddenly or develop over a number of years and most often strikes children and women under the age of 40. In fact, women are afflicted 10–15 times more often than men.

There are three types of lupus. Discoid lupus affects the skin only. Ten percent of those with discoid will develop systemic lupus, although it is believed that those people probably had systemic lupus with discoid lupus as an initial symptom. Systemic lupus involves the skin, joints, and organs, and is the type of lupus that is usually referred to when discussing lupus. The third type is drug-induced lupus.

Lupus is often a chronic lifelong condition with flare-ups and remission. For others, lupus is life threatening when the lungs, kidneys, or heart are attacked by antibodies.

Symptoms

There are a number of markers for lupus. Symptoms for discoid lupus include a rash on the neck or face and in severe cases, symptoms of SLE may be present. SLE markers are: a butterfly or discoid rash over the nose and cheeks like a mask; arthritis joint and muscle pain; mouth ulcers; sensitivity to light and worsening symptoms upon exposure to light; dry eyes and mouth; extreme fatigue; nervous system impairment; kidney damage detected by an abnormal urinalysis; inflammation in the linings of the heart or lungs; low levels of red blood cells and specific white blood cells; and elevated levels of different antibodies.

People with lupus tend to be sensitive to sunlight, and their symptoms flare up and subside in varying intervals. A butterfly rash that appears across the nose is very common. Signs that a flare-up is going to occur include swollen glands and painful, inflamed joints. There can also be fever, headache, mouth ulcers, interstitial cystitis (see interstitial cystitis in urinary tract infections on page 361), weakness, hives, hair loss, and weight loss. After an episode, scars on the skin may remain.

Causes

The actual cause of lupus is still unknown. However, researchers have discovered a variety of conditions that seem to contribute to it or provoke attacks. Viral or bacterial infections are leading suspects. Because women are the ones predominantly affected, it also suggests that there might be a link to excess estrogen or a deficiency in androgen, both factors that trigger autoimmunity. Connections are being found in studies on ultraviolet radiation and its effect on clinical skin disease in lupus.

Other factors that are also commonly associated with a weak immune system are stress, digestive problems due to weak stomach acid, fatigue, vaccination, food or environmental allergies (including toxic metal poisoning and hair dyes), and inherited predisposition.

Some drugs, including hydralazine, procainamide, and beta-blockers, are responsible for creating what is known as drug-induced lupus (DIL) and the condition will remit upon withdrawal of medication.

Prescription for Health

Steroid medications, such as prednisone, immunosuppressive medications (including methotrexate), and NSAIDs are often used to control SLE. Do not stop your medications. The following recommendations are to be used in conjunction with your medication. After following this program for six weeks, have your physician test your autoantibodies. Your medication may need to be reduced. Autoantibody levels should be checked again three months and six months after for further evaluation.

NUTRIENT	DOSAGE	ACTION
Moducare sterols and sterolins	Two capsules three times per day for one week, then one capsule three times daily thereafter	Foundation treatment for SLE, controls T-helper-2 autoantibody production, regulates cortisol, is anti-inflammatory, enhances DHEA naturally
Multimune containing vitamins A, B$_6$ (P-5-P), C, E, magnesium, zinc, lipoic acid, selenium, coenzyme Q10, reduced L-glutathione	Three capsules daily with food	Supports immune function, detoxifies liver, is potent antioxidant and anti-inflammatory, protects against deficiency
High-potency B-complex containing folic acid	Two capsules daily	Reduces stress, is needed for metabolism, lowers homocysteine levels, thereby decreasing the risk of premature atherosclerosis
DHEA	200 mg daily under the guidance of your physician	One study of females with SLE were given 200 mg of DHEA for six months. All subjects noted improvement in all symptoms. May reduce the need for prednisone.
Lactobacillus acidophilus	1 tsp (5 mL) containing 1–2 billion active organisms	Improves intestinal flora to aid digestion
Omega-3 fatty acid	1 Tbsp (15 mL) of flaxseed oil twice daily; 1000 mg evening primrose oil three times daily; or 500 mg of fish oil three times daily	Reduces or prevents inflammation, has been shown to slow progression of autoimmunity
Proteolytic enzymes	Two or three capsules daily	Acts as a potent anti-inflammatory

Health Tips to Enhance Healing

- Read Chapter 3 for more on autoimmune disease.
- Avoid alfalfa sprouts as they cause lupus flare-ups.
- Avoid the sun.
- Research has shown that a diet low in bad fats and low in calories in general caused a reduction in lupus symptoms, flare-ups, and extended periods of remission.
- In order to maintain a higher quality of life, special attention must be paid to nutrition, supplements, exercise, and positive thinking. Although there is an underlying genetic predisposition, avoiding and eliminating triggers can alleviate the severity and duration of symptoms and perhaps reduce the level of medication. Only 10 percent of those with lupus have a parent or sibling with it; only 5 percent of children born to those with lupus will develop it as well.
- Consume a diet that emphasizes natural, whole foods such as legumes, soy products, fresh fruits and vegetables, fish, healthy fats and oils to increase omega-6 intake, and nuts and seeds. Eat plenty of cold-water fish (halibut, herring, salmon, mackerel). Canned

sardines in olive oil are especially beneficial as they are high in omega-3, which can reduce inflammation.

- Avoid caffeine, alcohol, dairy, and animal products, processed foods containing sugar and additives, and any vegetable in the nightshade family (white potatoes, peppers, eggplant, tomatoes).
- Stop smoking and avoid exposure to secondhand smoke. Nicotine constricts the blood vessels.
- Get plenty of rest and reduce stress. Keeping a positive outlook is essential. The Lupus Foundation of America offers much support in dealing with the illness. Practice deep-breathing exercises, biofeedback, visualization, and other therapies to calm the body.
- Regular exercise is beneficial for increasing circulation. Continue your exercise program if mobility is good, but not to the point where pain and inflammation flare up. Engage in activities (like water aerobics, swimming, cycling, and yoga) that support body weight and cushion the joints from damaging impact.

Other Recommendations

- Have hair tested and analyzed for toxic levels of heavy metals present in the body.
- Get checked for possible allergies. See the introduction to this chapter.
- Consider removing old mercury fillings and having them replaced with safer materials. However, ensure that you are not allergic to those substances before having them put into your mouth. If you choose to replace fillings, do it slowly over time so as not to release too much mercury into the bloodstream at once. (See Toxic Metal Poisoning.)
- When antigens and antibodies interlock, it is called an immune complex. Proteolytic enzyme therapy may be beneficial by penetrating the coating of the immune complex in the tissues and getting them into the bloodstream for elimination stimulating the breakup of the immune complex, and speeding up the inflammation process to reduce tissue swelling. Due to the increased activity, the condition may worsen for a short time before it gets better. Use this therapy with the supervision of a naturopath or physician.
- Avoid taking oral contraceptives, penicillin, hydraline, anticonvulsants, sulfa drugs, and procaineamide. Ask your doctor if they are really necessary or if there are safer alternatives.

THYROID
(HYPOTHYROIDISM, HYPERTHYROIDISM)

The thyroid is a small gland that lies below the Adam's apple in the neck and wraps around the trachea. It secretes thyroid hormones that control many metabolic functions in the body. Thyroid hormones stimulate the production of proteins and increase the use of oxygen by cells in the body. Iodine is required by the thyroid to produce thyroid hormones. A careful recycling process occurs in the thyroid to ensure that adequate thyroid hormones are available to control the body's metabolic rate. Thyroid hormone comes in two forms: thyroxine T4 and triiodothyronine T3. Most T4 is converted in the liver into the active form of thyroid T3. About 80 percent of the T3 is produced via the liver and the other 20 percent is produced directly by the thyroid.

A delicate balance must be maintained to keep a steady metabolic rate in the body. The hypothalamus and pituitary glands work in concert with the proteins of the body, T4, the liver, and other organs to maintain that balance.

When the thyroid produces too much thyroid hormone, hyperthyroidism develops. Autoimmune reactions against the thyroid can cause hyperthyroidism. Graves' disease is one such condition in which the immune system malfunctions, causing an increase in thyroid hormone. The result is a goiter, a greatly enlarged thyroid gland. Thyroiditis, an inflammation of the thyroid gland, can initially cause hyperthyroidism, but eventually the damage to the thyroid caused by the inflammation causes hypothyroidism or low thyroid function.

Hypothyroidism is when the thyroid gland produces too little thyroid hormone. It is estimated that approximately 25 percent of the population is affected by hypothyroidism and women are predominantly affected.

Symptoms

The symptoms of hypothyroidism are varied. Hypothyroidism causes the body's metabolic rate to slow dramatically and often early symptoms are misdiagnosed as depression. Slowed heart rate, hoarse voice, slowed speech, swollen and puffy face, drooping eyelids, intolerance to cold, constipation, and weight gain are hallmark symptoms. The hair often becomes sparse, coarse, and dry, and there is a loss of eyebrow hair. The skin will become dry, scaly, thick, and bumpy and may have raised, thickened areas on the shins. Carpal tunnel syndrome, muscle weakness, confusion, depression, dementia, heart disease with high cholesterol and triglyceride levels, hormone disruptions, shortness of breath, and extreme fatigue may also be present. Women with hypothyroidism may also experience heavy menstrual bleeding, infertility, and when they do become pregnant, they are at increased risk of miscarriages, premature deliveries, and stillbirths.

Have your thyroid function checked by your doctor, but don't be surprised if the results come back normal even though you have a large number of the symptoms above. Many people have subclinical low thyroid and yet are diagnosed with normal thyroid based on the current tests. The Barnes basal temperature test can better help determine thyroid function (see Chapter 2, page 22). Hypothyroidism is a serious health risk for many other conditions. Nutritional therapies do not work as well in those with underactive thyroid, so correction is essential.

Causes

Hashimoto's thyroiditis is the most common cause of hypothyroidism due to the autoimmune process that attacks the thyroid. Eventually the thyroid cannot produce enough thyroid hormone, causing hypothyroidism. The treatment of hyperthyroidism using radioactive iodine and surgery is the second most common cause of hypothyroidism.

Decades ago iodine was added to salt to make iodized salt to treat goiter and subsequent thyroid problems, but many people are no longer eating salt and as a result we are seeing an increase in hypothyroidism. As well, eating foods containing goitrogens, which block iodine uptake, may be associated with an increase in hypothyroidism.

Those living in northern regions such as Canada are not getting enough sunshine to produce vitamin D, a cofactor in thyroid hormone production, so as a result are more prone to hypothyroidism. Trace minerals are also required to make thyroid hormone, and deficiencies in these minerals promote hypothyroidism.

Prescription for Health

You should not stop your thyroid medication. It is essential for providing adequate thyroid hormone. The recommendations below are designed to support thyroid function.

NUTRIENT	DOSAGE	ACTION
Moducare sterols and sterolins	One capsule three times daily as a maintenance dose	Essential for regulating immune function and controlling autoantibody reactions, is anti-inflammatory
High-potency B-complex	Two capsules daily with meals	Required for thyroid, metabolism, and proper immune function
Multimune containing vitamins A, B₆, C, E, selenium, zinc, magnesium, coenzyme Q10, lipoic acid, reduced L-glutathione	Three capsules daily with meals	Supports the proper functioning of the immune system, is anti-inflammatory and a potent antioxidant, provides nutrients to make thyroid hormone
Vitamin C	1000 mg twice daily	Regulates immunity and combats stress

NUTRIENT	DOSAGE	ACTION
Multimineral with trace minerals	Two capsules daily	Minerals are essential precursors to thyroid hormone
Omega-3 fish oils	1 g three times daily	A powerful anti-inflammatory and controls T-helper-2 reactions, improves skin and hair symptoms
Women's Whey protein powder containing amino acids including tyrosine	One scoop (30 g) daily	Tyrosine binds with iodine to make thyroid hormones

Health Tips to Enhance Healing

- See Graves' Disease and Hashimoto's Thyroiditis.
- Reduce the consumption of foods that impede the absorption of iodine (called goitrogens) if you have hypothyroidism. These foods include soy, turnips, cabbage, mustard greens, peanuts, pine nuts, and millet.
- Do not take immune boosters as they can overstimulate the immune system and increase antibody production.
- Armour Thyroid extract should be taken under the guidance of your physician. In many cases it has been used in place of prescription thyroid medication.
- Avoid fluoride toothpaste and fluoridated water as they compete with iodine for absorption.
- It is not advised to supplement the diet with iodine because there is such a delicate balance required by the thyroid to function properly that too much iodine can be damaging. If you are eating too much iodized salt, switch to sea salt or reduce your salt intake.
- Ensure you get adequate sunshine. The thyroid gland requires vitamin D to function properly. Those living in northern regions have higher rates of low thyroid and Hashimoto's.
- Detoxification and elimination of waste is very important. Eat liver-friendly foods such as kale, carrots, beets, artichokes, lemons, onions, garlic, and leeks.
- Stress reduction is essential. See "Excessive Stress," page 48.

TINNITUS

Tinnitus is a common condition that affects almost 36 million North Americans, with a greater prevalence for women and African Americans. Tinnitus is noise originating in the ear instead of from the outside environment. Seven million people are affected to such an extent that they are unable to lead normal lives. Tinnitus is also a symptom of Ménière's disease, a disorder that causes attacks of severe hearing loss, dizziness, or vertigo, causing nausea, vomiting, and tinnitus.

Symptoms

Although tinnitus is referred to as ear ringing, ringing is not the only sound heard. There can be a high-pitched sound or squealing, buzzing, throbbing, ticking, or hissing sounds. The sound may be constant or intermittent or pulsing along with the heartbeat. It can be annoying and distracting, and sometimes painful as well.

Causes

Tinnitus can occur when there is injury or damage to the hearing nerve endings in the inner ear, or if there is stiffening of the middle ear bones (called otosclerosis).

Ear infections, wax buildup, exposure to loud noise, medications (such as aspirin, anti-inflammatories, sedatives, antibiotics, and antidepressants), and nutritional deficiencies can all contribute to the condition. Circulatory disorders, or poor circulation caused by smoking, alcohol/drug use, and caffeine are often a factor. Allergies, thyroid problems, diabetes, autoimmune diseases, Ménière's disease, presence of a tumor, TMJ (temporomandibular joint dysfunction), and injury to the head or neck are other possible sources.

In younger people, tinnitus is generally a result of loud noise, whereas in older people it is associated with hearing nerve impairment. The worse tinnitus is, the more pronounced the associated depression, anxiety, and insomnia.

Prescription for Health

NUTRIENT	DOSAGE	ACTION
Vitamin A	5000 IU daily	Receptor cells of the ear are dependent upon vitamin A for proper function
Moducare sterols and sterolins	One capsule three times daily	Controls cortisol, reducing interleukin-6, thereby improving calcium homeostasis
Vitamin B$_{12}$, sublingual tablet	1000 mg daily	Restores possible deficiency and ensures adequate iron. Iron deficiency is associated with hearing loss.
Vitamin D and calcium	500 IU of vitamin D daily 1000 mg of calcium daily	Essential for maintaining calcium homeostasis. Imbalanced calcium is indicated in hearing loss.
Magnesium	500–1000 mg twice daily. If you have kidney dysfunction consult your physician before taking magnesium.	Magnesium deficiency is linked to the development of tinnitus
Zinc	30–60 mg daily	Zinc is concentrated in sensory tissues of the ear
Coenzyme Q10	100 mg daily	Ensures adequate oxygen to delicate auditory hairs

NUTRIENT	DOSAGE	ACTION
Ginkgo biloba	200 mg (standardized to 24 percent flavoglycosides)	Shown to reduce tinnitus and improve circulation
Omega-3 essential fatty acids, fish oil, or flaxseed oil	1000 mg three times daily of fish oil 1–2 Tbsp (15–30 mL) of flaxseed oil	May reduce sensorineural hearing impairment

Health Tips to Enhance Healing

- Rule out heavy metal toxicity, especially aluminum, lead, and cadmium. (See Toxic Metal Poisoning.)
- Eliminate allergies. One study was of 23 patients with Ménière's disease. They had failed to respond to standard treatments and were tested for food allergies. When foods that promoted ear symptoms were eliminated, all patients showed a reduction in hearing loss and reduction of tinnitus.
- Increase your protein intake by using Women's Whey or proteins+ protein powder.
- Reduce animal fat and cholesterol that may be reducing oxygen and nutrients to the ear by increasing blood platelet stickiness. (See Cholesterol to learn how to maintain cholesterol levels.)
- Drink eight to ten glasses of pure, filtered water a day. Water reduces platelet aggregation.
- Avoid stimulants that cause constriction on the blood vessels such as sugar, caffeine, salt, alcohol, and smoking.

Other Recommendations

- Have your physician check your blood pressure and rule out other disorders such as anemia, hypothyroidism, hypoglycemia, hyperlipo-proteinemia, and inflammation of the inner ear. Confirm that there are no side effects from other possible medications you are taking.
- Protect your ears from loud noise, or wear protective earplugs or ear phones if noise exposure is unavoidable.
- Reduce stress.
- Some people find relief from the tinnitus by masking it with low volume radio static or a ticking clock in the background. There are also tinnitus maskers that can be adapted to hearing aids to provide a more appealing sound that can compete with tinnitus.

Health Fact

Of 120 patients that were found to have hyperlipoproteinemia (high lipoprotein in the blood) and tinnitus (most were also overweight and had related conditions such as diabetes), 83 percent improved their symptoms after five months on a high-protein, low-carbohydrate, calorie-restricted diet.

TOXIC METAL POISONING

Investigative news reporter Bill Moyers opened his March 26, 2001, television special, "Trade Secrets: A Moyers Report," by having a blood sample taken to determine the level of toxins in his body. Mount Sinai Hospital checked his blood for 150 common industrial chemicals. He tested positive for 84 of them. Of that 84, only one would have been present if he lived more than 100 years ago—lead. At the age of 66, Bill Moyers was told he wouldn't have to worry about what those chemicals could do to him, but the doctor was concerned about the effects that level of chemicals would have on a pregnant 21-year-old female and her fetus. We are living at a time of excessive toxic exposure. Our children receive 35 percent of their lifetime toxic load before they are five years old. Many chemicals pass through the placenta to the fetus and through breast milk to our babies. Trace amounts of 17 pesticides were found in the top baby foods sold in the United States.

The Environmental Protection Agency has 80,000 chemicals registered for possible use. Fifteen thousand are manufactured in commercial quantities, and of those 15,000 only 43 percent have been tested for their short-term effect on our health; no long-term studies have been completed. In a report for the major chemical, rubber, and petrochemical companies in response to concerns about the safety of their products, scientists stated that "very little data exists." In other words, the chemical industry cannot prove their chemicals are safe. Commercially grown foods are no better. They contain high levels of toxic heavy metals and xenoestrogens from pesticides and they are lower in selenium, which is an important mineral for detoxification. Farm workers experience pesticide-induced illnesses, cancer, chronic fatigue, and other conditions.

Mercury, lead, cadmium, and aluminum, to name a few, are extremely toxic substances and can be breathed in, ingested, and absorbed through the skin. Once in the body they make their way to the bloodstream. Some of these substances (like lead and cadmium) are so similar to minerals that the body needs (such as zinc and calcium) that the body assimilates them in the same way. Cadmium is stored in the liver and kidneys. Lead goes into the bloodstream and other organs before settling in the bones where it remains until the body undergoes significant physical stress such as pregnancy, illness, or organ failure. Fifty percent of mercury is stored in the kidneys; it is also stored in the brain and central nervous system.

The earth has become a toxic dump and substances have polluted our water, air, and food. We must find some way of dealing with these toxin-loaded necessities of life. Your immune system becomes overloaded when it is assaulted by too many toxins and dysfunction is the result. Alternative medicine researchers and physicians believe that heavy metal poisoning is a major factor in autoimmune disorders, especially multiple sclerosis.

Cadmium, mercury, lead, arsenic, nickel, and aluminum are the main heavy metals that are commonly found in human tissues at unacceptable levels. Heavy metals do most of their damage to our immune systems, rendering them defenseless against pathogens. How do heavy metals find their way into our body? Different heavy metals have different routes of entry into the human system, yet all are devastating to the immune system.

We are exposed to lead through leaded gasoline, canned food with leaded seams, milk and meats from animals fed contaminated food, and leaded paint. These are a few of the sources of this extremely toxic metal.

Mercury, a potent neurotoxin, is found mainly in fish, especially canned tuna fish, and mercury amalgam dental fillings (silver fillings in your teeth). Having your mercury amalgam fillings removed is especially important to those with autoimmune diseases. Although North American dental associations refuse to admit that there is a connection between certain autoimmune diseases such as multiple sclerosis and mercury poisoning, anecdotal cases of remission after removal of amalgams are reason enough to have them replaced.

Cadmium exposure through cigarette smoke is the main reason for toxicity of this metal. Fertilizers, fungicides, rubber, and paint are also common sources. Smoking cigarettes not only increases your chance of lung cancer but also exposes you to over 6000 chemicals, all of which need to be detoxified by the body.

Arsenic, one of the most toxic heavy metals, is found in herbicides and insecticides, paint, and cigarette smoke. Arsenic is also found in the tips of the needles of coniferous trees, and arsenic poisoning has been seen in forestry workers and tree planters as well.

Aluminum is probably one of the most common heavy metals that we are exposed to. Aluminum sulfate is used in the water-purification process to remove impurities from our water. Studies conducted in France have found there is a direct connection between Alzheimer's disease and traces of aluminum in tap water. This neurotoxin is also found in antiperspirants, baking powder, stomach antacids, aluminum household pots, pans, and foil, and it is also prevalent in many laxatives.

Nickel is another heavy metal that is required in the body in minute quantities, but when exposure is too high, nickel toxicity develops. Nickel exposure through dental appliances, including braces, can cause allergic reactions and immune dysfunction. Children who have just had their braces attached have higher incidence of appendicitis than children without braces. The link has yet to be explained.

Chelation Removes Heavy Metals

Protection from exposure is important, but like most of us you have probably been exposed to these common heavy metal sources over your lifetime without even knowing it. High-dose antioxidants, especially vitamin C and reduced L-glutathione, help the body deal with free radicals and increase detoxification via the liver and kidneys. Chelate means to latch onto. In the case of heavy metals, the chelator attaches onto the metal, carries it into the blood, then on to the kidneys to be excreted via the urine.

Intravenous chelation commonly uses EDTA (ethylene-diamine-tetra acetic acid), which is injected directly into a vein. IV chelation is very effective at attaching to the heavy metals mentioned above, along with minerals that have been deposited in the blood and on the walls of arteries and veins. Although chelation will also remove other minerals along with the bad guys, your chelating physician will return these to your bloodstream to ensure adequate levels. Chelation is especially important to help detoxify those with autoimmune disorders so that your total toxic load can be reduced, allowing your immune system to function appropriately without extra burden. Most people feel better after several IV chelation treatments. For those who are having their mercury amalgams removed, chelation therapy can accelerate the mercury detoxification process.

Gasoline attendants, printers, hairdressers, jewelers, dentists, plumbers, painters, and those who work with solvents are at high risk of poisoning from toxins in the workplace.

Toxins are stored in our fat tissue. They disrupt protein metabolism and the function of our kidneys as well as overloading our liver. Certain foods and nutritional supplements can aid the elimination of toxins and heavy metals from our body.

Symptoms

Toxic poisoning can be recognized through symptoms such as dizziness; lack of coordination; numbness; hyperactivity; vomiting; headaches; fatigue; tremors; weakness; infertility; bloody diarrhea; anorexia; emotional problems such as depression, anger, and instability; and loss of hair, memory, vision, smell, hearing, libido, and ambition. It is also associated with having a metallic taste in the mouth, dermatitis, blue gums, gum disease, and loosened teeth. Illnesses linked to toxic metal poisoning include Alzheimer's, Parkinson's, chronic fatigue syndrome, attention deficit disorder, colitis, kidney disease, osteoporosis, nephritis, emphysema, and the autoimmune diseases. The immune system is seriously weakened, the thymus gland shrinks, and fewer T-cells are produced.

Causes

What makes one person susceptible to environmental pollution while another person remains healthy? Certain enzymatic pathways must be available to detoxify the body, but if the body is overloaded with detoxifying other chemicals, then the new arrivals are free to cause damage while they wait their turn. If there are any nutritional deficiencies, then the enzymatic actions that need to take place can't happen. If chemicals and pollutants continue to assault the body, it can break the body's point of tolerance and disease sets in. Also, if the previously mentioned pollutants and toxins have damaged the enzymatic pathways, then the pathways are no longer able to function.

The greatest source of mercury poisoning comes from dental amalgams. Several countries have banned the use of mercury fillings. However, authorities in North America have been dragging their heels even though the evidence is overwhelming. Other sources of toxic metal poisoning are hair dyes, shellfish, ocean fish, refined grains, coffee, tea, printers' and tattoo inks, paints, wood preservatives, floor wax, pesticides, sewage, vehicle exhaust, talcum powder, antiperspirant, jewelry, lead crystal ware, aluminum cookware, glazes, pipes, solder in tin cans, batteries, hemorrhoid suppository preparations, antacids containing aluminum, and cosmetics.

Prescription for Health

NUTRIENT	DOSAGE	ACTION
Sulphoraphane, indole-3-carbinole or DIM	Use as directed	Detoxifies excess estrogens, toxins, and detoxifies the liver
High-potency B-complex	Two or three capsules daily	Essential for metabolism, detoxification of sulpha drugs and antibiotics
Vitamin C with bioflavonoids	1000–2000 mg three times daily	Helps remove heavy metals, enhances glutathione important for detoxification, strengthens the immune system
Calcium citrate and magnesium	1000 mg of calcium citrate daily; 500 mg of magnesium daily	Competes with lead; higher levels of lead can be present if there is calcium deficiency; helps eliminate cadmium
Multimune containing vitamins A, B_6, C, E, selenium, zinc, magnesium, reduced L-glutathione, lipoic acid, coenzyme Q10	Three capsules daily with food	A potent antioxidant; glutathione, zinc, vitamins A, C, and E are essential for detoxifying heavy metals and toxins; coenzyme Q10 and lipoic acid are for energy production; selenium chelates mercury
Lipotropic factors that include choline and methionine	1000 mg each of choline and methionine daily	Promotes the flow of bile and helps detoxify the liver and improve fat metabolism
Alpha lipoic acid	100 mg daily	Detoxifies heavy metals
Milk thistle	100 mg three times daily	Protects the liver from toxins, enhances the activity of glutathione

NUTRIENT	DOSAGE	ACTION
Garlic (Kyolic)	200 mg three times daily	Helps excrete metals out of the body
Moducare sterols and sterolins	One capsule three times daily	Protects and regulates immune function, controls inflammatory cytokines, enhances DHEA naturally, controls cortisol
Omega's Hi-Lignan Flax Seed	1 tsp (5 mL) daily	Improves transit time, helps heal mucous membranes of the digestive tract, eliminates bowel toxins

Health Tips to Enhance Healing

- Take saunas as often as possible. The skin is the largest detoxification organ and saunas help to eliminate toxins through the skin. Dry brushing the skin is another excellent detoxification method. Get a soft, natural bristle brush from the health food store and before your shower or bath (see detoxification bath below), brush your skin from the tips of your toes toward your heart and from the tips of your fingers towards your heart. Then climb into the detoxification bath.

DETOXIFICATION BATH

1 box (2 cups/500 mL) baking soda
2 cups (500 mL) Epsom salts
a few drops of lavender essential oil

Run your bathwater through a showerhead filter. The water should be very warm and you should soak until the water becomes tepid. Get out, dry yourself off, and rub sesame oil on the soles of your feet (optional) and then get into bed. This is wonderful. I have a detoxification bath twice a week.

- Toxins are released by bacteria and candida yeast (see Candidiasis).
- Detoxify your liver with the supplements mentioned above and eat plenty of organically grown Brussels sprouts, asparagus, avocado, garlic, onions, broccoli, cabbage, caraway seeds, dill, peppers, whole grains, and Women's Whey or proteins+ containing amino acids.
- Vitamin C, reduced L-glutathione, selenium, and milk thistle will ensure the liver is better able to detoxify chemicals and toxins.
- Have dental amalgams replaced with safer material. Some insurance companies will cover this cost, but don't rush into having them done all at once. Have fillings replaced one by one to prevent excess mercury vapor from entering the bloodstream. Ask your dentist to use a rubber dam during the procedure—it will act as a barrier when the mercury comes out. Leading researcher and

author of *It's All in Your Head*, Hal Huggins, DDS, recommends you make an early morning appointment. Mercury vapors from other patients' dental work hang around in the air for a while and can be breathed in. Be sure to take supplements to aid in the detoxification process. Supplementation should start two weeks prior to the first amalgam removal and continue for three months after the last one. It can take three to six months for mercury to be eliminated from the body.

- Avoid exposure to pollution and toxins. Stop smoking. Cigarettes have 6000 toxins including cadmium, lead, and arsenic.
- Drinks or acidic fruits and vegetables such as tomatoes that come in cans should be avoided. It was not all that long ago that North American manufacturers stopped using lead to seam tin cans; other countries may not have changed their manufacturing processes for goods that we import.
- Avoid constipation to ensure regular excretion of toxic substances. (See Constipation.)
- Shellfish, if caught close to shore, and ocean fish such as swordfish and shark can contain high levels of industrial waste. Avoid them altogether, or when preparing ocean fish broil them so the fat drips to the bottom of the pan. Toxins are stored mainly in the fat.
- Drink eight to ten glasses of pure, filtered water daily. For every juice, alcoholic, or caffeinated beverage consumed, drink another glass of water. Do not drink from the tap or suspect sources. Lead is still found in older water pipes. Aluminum is used in the water purification process.

Other Recommendations

- Diagnostic laboratories can check for toxic metal levels in the system through hair mineral analysis.
- See information about xenoestrogens in Chapter 4.
- See chelation therapy above. Consult a professionally trained practitioner for therapy.
- Contact the American College for Advancement in Medicine (ACAM). All chelation doctors are certified by this organization and they also have a physician referral service for alternative medical doctors. Call toll-free in the U.S. (1-800-532-3688) or go to www.acam.org or e-mail acam@acam.org.

Health Fact

One of the chemicals found in Bill Moyer's blood was DDT. The doctor pointed out that DDT has been banned in the United States since 1972 (although it may be found on imported goods from countries that still use DDT). According to a public health statement released by the Agency for Toxic Substances and Disease Registry, DDT is stored in the fatty tissue and is slow to leave the body. Levels will remain constant or increase if there is increased exposure, but should decrease as exposure decreases. DDT is excreted through urine and breast milk.

ULCERS (STOMACH AND INTESTINAL)

A healthy gastrointestinal tract has a protective lining of the stomach and upper intestine. If the lining and the tissue underneath becomes damaged, ulceration can develop. If the ulcer is ignored, the sore can erode the stomach wall, causing it to bleed. Peptic ulcer is a term used to describe the most common types of ulcers that occur in the stomach (gastric ulcer) and duodenal (the first part of the small intestine). Duodenal ulcers are more common than gastric ulcers. Esophageal ulcers occur when acid reflux (gastroesophageal reflux disease) from the stomach occurs, ulcerating the esophageal lining.

Gastric and esophageal ulcers can become cancerous. All ulcers are potentially life-threatening and should be treated aggressively.

Symptoms

Those with peptic ulcers may or may not have symptoms, but in those who do, abdominal pain occurs about an hour after eating or during the night. Cramping, burning, and gnawing are some of the adjectives used to describe the pain. Often the symptoms are mistaken for heartburn. Nausea, bleeding, and inflammation are other signs of an ulcer. Relief can often be obtained temporarily by drinking water, vomiting, eating food, or taking an antacid. If your vomit resembles coffee grounds (blood), you have blood in your stool, or you experience extreme abdominal pain, consult your physician immediately.

Causes

Previously it was thought that anxiety or stress induced excess stomach acid that damaged the gastrointestinal lining. Research is now documenting strong links supporting the idea that many ulcers are a result of a *Helicobacter pylori* bacteria infection. *H. pylori* infection can be determined by a blood test. The *H. pylori* take up residence on the gastrointestinal lining and injure the lining and the mucous layer that guards against digestive juices. *H. pylori* infection may be allowed to flourish due to low vitamin C concentration in the stomach acid and low hydrochloric acid. One study published in 2000 demonstrated that smokers have significantly less vitamin C in their gastric juices than nonsmokers, which is interesting because smokers are twice as likely to have ulcers. As well, smokers have an increase in hydrochloric acid output, worsening symptoms. Another study published in March 2001 found that of the diabetics who were experiencing peptic ulcer symptoms, 77 percent had an *H. pylori* infection.

Stress and anxiety still increase the risk for ulcers because they do raise stomach acidity. Eating large meals that overburden the digestive system and following a diet that is low in fiber and high in fat and refined carbohydrates are also to blame. Allergies and some medications, in particular NSAIDs, are other factors that optimize the environment for an ulcer. (See "Serious Side Effects from NSAIDs," page 43.)

See page 9 to read about the myth that those with ulcers and heartburn are secreting too much stomach acid. Those with gastric ulcers often do not secrete enough stomach acid and as a result suffer bloating, gas, leaky gut, and malabsorption.

A new cause of peptic ulcer occurs as a result of aspirin treatments prescribed to reduce heart attacks. Aspirin in dosages over 75 mg per day are associated with an increase in gastrointestinal bleeding. Vitamin E and other nutrients would be a better choice to improve lipid profiles and reduce the risk of heart attack. (See Chapter 2.)

Prescription for Health

All symptoms of ulcer need to be treated by a medical doctor. The following are recommended in addition to your physician's advice. *H. pylori* requires antibiotic treatment or supervised bismuth treatment by your physician.

NUTRIENT	DOSAGE	ACTION
Licorice DGL chewable tablets	380 mg on an empty stomach. Two capsules daily for acute ulcer and one daily for maintenance. Research studies used a dosage of 760 mg three times daily.	Soothes inflammation
Moducare sterols and sterolins	One capsule three times daily	Regulates immune function to fight bacteria, is anti-inflammatory, enhances DHEA, controls cortisol (our stress hormone)
Multimune containing vitamins A, B₆, C, E, selenium, zinc, magnesium, coenzyme Q10, lipoic acid, reduced L-glutathione	Three capsules daily with food	A potent antioxidant, contains vitamin C, which is known to heal ulcers, has antihistamine action, supports immune function, detoxifies liver
L-glutamine	1000 mg twice daily	Known to help heal mucous lining of the intestinal tract
Oregano oil	Three drops twice daily in water	Antifungal, antibacterial, antiviral, anticandidia

NUTRIENT	DOSAGE	ACTION
Omega Hi-Lignan Flax Seed	1 tsp (5 mL) daily	Increases transit time, eliminates bowel toxins
Lactobacillus acidophilus	1 tsp (5 mL) containing 1–2 billion active organisms	Improves intestinal flora to fight bacteria

Health Tips to Enhance Healing

- If you must use an antacid, try Flora Distributors Fruitin, which acts as a protective barrier without the dangerous additives of over-the-counter antacids (some antacids contain aluminum).
- See Chapter 1 to learn how to improve your digestion and tame your tummy troubles.
- See Bowel Disease, Candidiasis, and Constipation.
- Quit smoking. Smoking doubles your chance of developing a peptic ulcer, interferes with healing the ulcer, and encourages its reoccurrence.
- Drinking 32 oz (1 L) of raw cabbage juice per day has been known to be very effective for peptic ulcers. As well, drink aloe vera juice, which heals the intestinal tract, and cranberry juice, which inhibits bacteria.
- Eat cooked rhubarb once a day until your ulcer has healed. Sweeten rhubarb with other sweeter fruit or stevia. Do not use sugar as sugar inhibits your immune system's ability to fight *H. pylori*.
- Eliminate allergies. See the introduction to this chapter.
- Eat foods that are nutritious and easy on the stomach during attacks. The best for bleeding ulcers are avocados, yams, potatoes, steamed carrots, and plain yogurt. Steam the vegetables and mash them, or eat organic baby food.

Health Fact

A study held between April 1998 and July 1999 in Liege, France, on 152 patients found that 72.8 percent of those with gastric ulcers and 78.5 percent of those with duodenal ulcers also had an *H. pylori* infection.

URINARY TRACT PROBLEMS
(BLADDER INFECTIONS, INTERSTITIAL CYSTITIS)

Urinary tract infections, or UTIs, refer to infections of the urethra, bladder, and kidneys that are caused by bacteria, viruses, fungi, and several different parasites. They can occur in both men and women, but adult women experience these infections twice as often as men due to the proximity of the urethra to the vagina and rectum. Treatment must be swift as UTIs can cause permanent damage to the urinary tract, chronic infections, kidney disease, and, in men, worsen prostate problems. In men with enlarged prostates or prostate cancer, urinary tract infections are often a result of the underlying condition.

It is called cystitis when infection is located in the bladder, and urethritis when the urethra is affected. A more serious condition, pyelonephritis or kidney infection is most often the result of bacteria in the bladder traveling to the kidneys. It can also be caused by a weakened immune system that allows infections in the blood to affect the kidneys. Infants, children, and adolescents can also be affected with urinary tract infections; 5 percent of teenaged girls develop a UTI.

Urine tests can determine the presence of infection in most individuals, but many, especially women, will have all the symptoms of UTIs with no bacteria present in their urine.

Interstitial Cystitis

Interstitial cystitis is a chronic inflammation of the urinary bladder lining and the bladder muscle that is not caused by bacteria. While there is no bladder autoantigen that has been identified, it is often coincides with lupus and other autoimmune diseases, leading researchers to believe it may be an autoimmune disorder. The continual inflammation eventually results in a shrunken bladder that cannot hold adequate amounts of urine, causing those afflicted to plan their life around the location of toilets. It is predominantly a female affliction; only 10 percent of interstitial cystitis cases occur in men. In men it will often be undiagnosed because the symptoms are so similar to prostate pain. Although rare, interstitial cystitis has been diagnosed in children. It is estimated that more than 1 million people in North America suffer with interstitial cystitis. Food allergies are thought to be a major factor in initiating and promoting this disease. The symptoms of irritable bowel syndrome may be present with interstitial cystitis, thus compounding the problem.

Symptoms

When urination brings a burning pain and increases in frequency, urinary tract infections are usually suspected. There may also be urination at night, lower abdominal pain, and the urine may smell or be darker in color. The volume of urine excreted may be reduced and fever and a flu-like feeling may also be present. Blood can appear in the urine. If it is a kidney infection, there can be pain in the lower back. Children may experience urinary incontinence during an infection. Urinary tract infections are often overlooked in young children with fever.

The early symptom of interstitial cystitis is frequent urination, day or night. In severe cases it can happen 60 times in a day. Eventually the need to urinate becomes urgent; there may be blood in the urine and pain or spasms of the abdomen, urethra, or vagina. The capacity of the bladder is reduced and the bladder wall bears scars and hemorrhaged punctures. Sexual activity for both men and women may be curtailed because it is too painful. The lifetime implications for one's sex life and the chronic pain can lead to depression, ranging from moderate to severe, and has led to suicide. Other symptoms may be present such as migraines, joint or muscle pain, gastrointestinal problems, or allergies.

Causes

The vast majority of UTIs are caused by bacteria (E. coli), which are commonly found in the vagina and/or intestine and have been introduced through the urethra. The bacteria are transferred from the anus to the urethra. Women are more susceptible to infection than men because their urethra is shorter and situated closer to the anus. Risks that can create a vulnerability to UTIs are blockages in the urethra (due either to past infections or structural abnormalities), antibiotics use, stress, pregnancy, food allergies, sexual contact, oral contraceptives, diaphragms, conditions such as diabetes, a weakened immune system, or hormonal imbalances brought on by menopause. Herpes virus is also a cause of UTIs because during an active outbreak, it may be so painful to urinate that the bladder is not fully emptied, thus allowing for infection.

Candida overgrowth is also a source of fungal infections in the urinary tract. (See Candidiasis.) Parasites, including worms and protozoa, also cause UTIs.

In men UTIs are predominantly caused by enlarged prostate or prostatitis. Treating the underlying condition generally eliminates the UTI (see Prostate Problems). In children, one-third of UTIs are a result of reflux—when urine flows back up the ureters from the bladder to the kidney. The kidneys can become scarred if reflux is not diagnosed and there are repeat infections. Another cause is bladder instability where the bladder attempts to void urine before it is full and it later becomes impossible to hold it in.

The cause for interstitial cystitis is unknown, although some researchers theorize that it may have begun with an initial infection. However, testing for an infectious presence has been inconsistent so no conclusions can be drawn at this time. Interstitial cystitis can appear as a symptom of lupus or endometriosis, and can be aggravated by the environment (i.e., diet and lifestyle). Fortunately, there is now an effective natural treatment containing calcium glycerophosphate called Prelief, available from AkPharma Inc., Pleasantville, NJ 08232, 1-800-994-4711.

Prescription for Health

A three- to 14-day course of antibiotics may be prescribed for the treatment of UTIs, yet some researchers believe that natural treatments should be tried first, and only if fever and pain persist for several days should antibiotic therapy be prescribed. (Read about antibiotic-resistant bacteria, page 55.)

NUTRIENT	DOSAGE	ACTION
Cranberry capsules or cranberry juice (unsweetened and must not contain aspartame or sugar). Mix unsweetened cranberry with other unsweetened juice like apple or pear.	16 oz (500 mL) daily or 500 mg capsules three times daily	Prevents E. coli bacteria from adhering to urinary tract; protects stomach lining from H. pylori
Vitamin C, mineral ascorbates, including calcium, magnesium, potassium ascorbate	1000 mg twice daily	Antibacterial, supports immune function
Lactobacillus acidophilus	1 tsp (5 mL) with 1–2 billion active organisms daily	Improves intestinal flora to fight bacteria, is essential for those taking antibiotics
Goldenseal standardized for berberine content	500 mg daily	Antibacterial, inhibits bacteria from adhering to the bladder wall
Uva ursi tea	1 cup (250 mL) daily	Uva ursi acts as a diuretic, alleviates pain, and fights bacteria (*do not use if pregnant)
Multimune containing vitamins A, B$_6$, C, E, selenium, magnesium, zinc, coenzyme Q10, lipoic acid, reduced L-gluthatione	Three capsules daily	Supports immune function, detoxifies liver, enhances bacteria and virus fighting ability
Moducare sterols and sterolins	One capsule three times daily	Regulates immune function, is anti-inflammatory, anti-bacterial, enhances DHEA naturally, controls cortisol, stops autoimmune reactions

Recommended for Those with Interstitial Cystitis

Prelief (calcium glycerophosphate)	Two tablets whenever you have acidic foods or drinks	Research has shown that 70 percent of those with interstitial cystitis report relief from pain; 61 percent report a decrease in the urgency to urinate
Gota kola (Centella asiatica)	200 mg twice daily	Strengthens bladder wall, reduces the formation of scar tissue
Moducare sterols and sterolins	One capsule three times daily	Halts autoimmune processes, is anti-inflammatory
Horsetail and marshmallow tea	1–2 cups (250–500 mL) daily	Horsetail strengthens bladder wall, marshmallow calms an irritated bladder

Health Tips to Enhance Healing

- See Allergies, Candidiasis, and Prostate Problems to understand and eliminate the underlying cause of your UTIs. Read Chapter 3 to understand how important a proper functioning immune system is in fighting infections.
- Water is the cheapest substance you can take to eliminate and prevent bladder infections. Drink an 8 oz (250 mL) glass of pure, filtered water every hour that you are awake during the day, but do not drink during meals or else you will dilute your digestive enzymes.
- Avoid foods that have been noted for exacerbating symptoms such as spicy and acidic foods, caffeine, citrus fruits, chocolate, and alcohol. Caffeine can cause spasms in the bladder. Reduce or eliminate intake depending on the severity of your symptoms.
- Drink 16 oz (500 mL) of pure, unsweetened cranberry juice daily to inhibit bacterial growth (do not buy the commercial cocktail type you find in supermarkets, which are laden with sugar). Be sure to add natural cleansers and diuretics such as celery, parsley, and watermelon to your diet.
- Eat plenty of plain yogurt or take acidophilus supplements to boost intestinal flora, especially if you are taking antibiotics.
- Castor oil packs or a hot water bottle on the inflamed area may help soothe spasms.
- Smoking has been indicated to aggravate interstitial cystitis.

Other Recommendations

- Eliminate allergies. See the introduction to this chapter.
- If possible, avoid taking antibiotics for urinary tract infections. Excessive use can lead to the creation of "supergerms" that grow increasingly resistant to antibiotics. Antibiotics also destroy the beneficial bacteria in the intestines that help fight infections. For most urinary tract infections, natural treatment and methods of prevention will be enough.
- Go to the bathroom every two to three hours to empty the bladder. Holding it can increase the likelihood of infection and raise the risk of bladder cancer. Also, empty the bladder after sexual intercourse or exercising.
- Wear cotton underwear to keep the area dry and increase the flow of air. After swimming or water skiing, change into dry clothes quickly.
- Practice good daily hygiene and keep the genitals and anus clean. For those with recurring infections, do not use douches, tampons, sanitary pads, bleached toilet paper, or commercial bubble baths.

- Avoid exposure to heavy metal toxins. Aluminum and cadmium may lead to infection.
- Sitting on cold or damp surfaces can aggravate symptoms. Stay warm.
- Support groups can help you to cope with the changes in lifestyle brought on by the illness. Look for one in your area. Check out the Interstitial Cystitis Association's web site for more information at www.ichelp.com, or you may prefer personal counseling. If you feel uncomfortable talking about intimate feelings with members of the opposite sex, don't hesitate to request a counselor with whom you would be more relaxed.

Health Fact

Three-quarters of those living with interstitial cystitis experience clinical depression prompted by painful sex and complaints from partners about the infrequency of intercourse. In a study that was conducted on women with interstitial cystitis, it was found that of the 23 percent who were not in relationships, one-third felt that interstitial cystitis was the mitigating factor for the breakup. Supportive families and partners can be instrumental in maintaining a high quality of life for those dealing with the disease and can strengthen the bonds of the relationship in the process.

VARICOSE VEINS

Varicose veins are lumpy, bulging blue veins in the legs. Women get them four times as often as men, and roughly half of the people over 50 have some type of varicose vein (hemorrhoids are a type of varicosity in the veins of the anus). Veins have little valves on the inner walls of the vessel to prevent blood from flowing backwards. Valves can become dysfunctional due to damage to the vein walls. When this occurs, it prevents proper one-way circulation and blood pools in the veins. The extra fluid causes the veins to stretch and bulge.

Although they are visually unappealing, varicose veins are not harmful if they are small and appear close to the surface of the skin. However, if varicose veins are located deeper within the leg, ulcerations, deep-vein blood clots, or bleeding under the skin can occur. In serious cases, there can be complications such as inflammation of the veins (phlebitis), clots that can relocate in the lungs (pulmonary embolism), and leg ulcerations requiring immediate medical attention.

Symptoms

When the veins get sluggish, the legs can feel tight, heavy, or restless, and there can be aches or leg cramps, pain, and swelling. The veins may itch and sores may develop.

Causes

Veins are fragile and pressure caused by obesity, smoking, pregnancy, and occupational environment (either too much standing, sitting, or heavy lifting) can cause the veins to dilate, leading to damage of the valves. In fact, 10 times the normal pressure is forced on the veins if a person stands for many hours. Other causal factors include heart or liver disease, constipation, tumors in the abdomen, vitamin C deficiency, birth control pills, hormone replacement therapy, and genetic predisposition.

Prescription for Health

Sclerotherapy and surgery to remove large and bulging veins can have excellent results. The following recommendations are effective in eliminating spider veins at the surface. Larger veins will most often not be eliminated but will be reduced in size, and symptoms will be alleviated.

NUTRIENT	DOSAGE	ACTION
Omega's Hi-Lignan Flax Seed	1–2 tsp (5–10 mL) daily	Eliminates constipation and soothes mucous membranes of the entire intestinal tract, softens stool
Horse chestnut seed extract or Venastat	100–150 mg daily containing escin or Venastat as directed	Increases antioxidant activity, inhibits enzymes that destroy venous walls, improves venous tone
Flaxseed oil or Udo's Choice or Omega Essential Balance	1–2 Tbsp (15–30 mL) daily	Soothes intestinal lining and promotes elimination
Moducare sterols and sterolins	One capsule three times daily	Reduces inflammation caused by IL-6 activity, promotes proper immune function
Multimune containing vitamins A, B₆, C, E, selenium, zinc, magnesium, lipoic acid, coenzyme Q10, reduced L-glutathione	Three capsules daily	Supports immune function, is a potent antioxidant, supports vein integrity, detoxifies liver, prevents deficiency, repairs blood vessel walls, prevents blood clotting and bruising, improves circulation
Bromelain	500–1000 mg after every meal	Anti-inflammatory, prevents hard, lumpy skin around bulging varicose veins
Gotu kola (Centella asiatica)	30–60 mg of triterpenic acid content twice daily	Enhances connective tissue integrity and increases blood flow
Flavonoids or cyanidins from bilberry or grape seed extract or pycnogenol	150–500 mg daily	Improves the integrity of capillaries and veins, protects collagen from damage in varicose veins, is a potent antioxidant and antihistamine

Health Tips to Enhance Healing

- See Constipation, Hemorrhoids.
- Reduce weight. Even an extra 10 lbs (4.5 kg) puts added pressure on your venous system.
- Eat foods high in fiber.
- Drink at least eight to ten glasses of pure, filtered water every day. Water maintains a healthy level of blood volume and prevents constipation.
- Apply witch hazel ointment topically twice a day to reduce swelling and tone veins.
- Avoid standing or sitting for long periods. Regular exercise is mandatory for circulation disorders and maintaining weight.
- Stop smoking. Nicotine constricts blood vessels.

Other Recommendations

- When traveling for long periods of time, make sure that you stand up and move around every once in a while to keep circulation going and prevent blood clots from forming in the veins. Wear loose clothing and drink plenty of water.
- Supportive elastic stockings specifically for varicose veins, when used in combination with the above recommendations, can dramatically reduce the appearance of unsightly veins.
- Hydrotherapy can alleviate pain and improve circulation. Fill a bathtub full of cold water and walk on the spot for 20 minutes. An alternative is to spray cold water on the legs, front and back, for 10 seconds every morning in the shower.
- When sitting or lying down, raise the legs above the heart for 20 minutes every day.
- Shift your weight and stand on your toes periodically if you must stand for long periods of time. If you sit at a desk, wiggle your toes and flex your leg muscles to keep blood flowing. Do not cross your legs and avoid putting pressure on your legs.
- Do not scratch veins if they are itchy, or you may cause further damage.

Health Fact

Foods that are especially rich in vitamin C and bioflavonoids (and therefore good for alleviating or preventing varicose veins) will aid venous circulation. Eat green leafy vegetables, avocados, radishes, turnips, mustard and turnip greens, garlic, onions, green peas, green peppers, broccoli, currents, cantaloupes, red or black grapes, lemons, blackberries, blueberries, cherries and the spices cayenne and ginger.

VASCULITIS

Vasculitis is a complicated autoimmune disease with inflammation and destruction of the blood vessel walls. It may be acute or chronic and it is often a secondary disease in many autoimmune conditions, including rheumatoid arthritis, Wegener's granulomatosis, Sjorgren's, and lupus. Vasculitis can affect any blood vessel in the body attacking and damaging various organs or tissue leading to fibrosis (interstitial fibrous tissue), necrosis (tissue death), or thrombosis (blood clots).

Symptoms

Symptoms are varied depending on the type of vasculitis. Most individuals feel run-down, experience pain in the joints and muscles, and may have fever and night sweats. Signs of vasculitis include bleeding of the mucous membranes, patches of hard purple patches in the skin (purpura), and bleeding in the lungs and kidneys. When it affects the aorta and major branches, it can cause loss of pulse, gangrene, and hypertension in the kidneys. If blood vessels are damaged to the point that circulation is obstructed, tissue death may occur. Pain, headaches, and blindness result when inflammation of the arteries in the head occur. In giant cell arteritis, one form of vasculitis, there can be pain with eating, facial pain, and throbbing headaches.

Causes

Although in most cases the cause of vasculitis is unknown, certain triggers and underlying conditions have been observed. Studies have shown that those with vasculitis have a serious deficiency of the enzyme glutathione peroxidase as a result of low levels of selenium and vitamins E and C. Sensitivities and allergy to certain chemicals and food are implicated. It can appear as a secondary process with other autoimmune disorders. Vasculitis is associated with hepatitis virus infection and it is thought that inflammation starts when the immune system mistakenly attacks blood vessels thinking they are the virus (molecular mimicry, see Chapter 3). The immune system is voracious and will attack these vessels, damaging the vessel and disrupting the tissues, organs, and nerves and cutting off blood supply to those areas. Some researchers believe that several viruses are involved in initiating vasculitis. Drugs have also been shown to promote vasculitis.

Prescription for Health

Those with autoimmune disease should avoid immune boosters that enhance macrophage function as the increase in interleukin-1 that macrophages release promotes increased inflammatory factors known to exacerbate autoimmune disease. Continue to take any medications prescribed by your physician, including corticosteroids. Once you have been on the following treatment for six weeks, have your physician test your autoantibodies. If autoantibodies are reduced, your physician will adjust your medication accordingly. Retest again at three and six months

NUTRIENT	DOSAGE	ACTION
Moducare sterols and sterolins	One capsule three times daily as a maintenance dose	Essential for regulating immune function and controlling autoantibody reactions, is anti-inflammatory
High-potency B-complex	Two capsules daily with meals	Required for thyroid and immune function
Multimune containing vitamins A, B_6, C, E, selenium, zinc, magnesium, coenzyme Q10, lipoic acid, reduced L-glutathione	Three capsules daily with meals	Enhances intracellular glutathione seen in those with vasculitis, supports the proper functioning of the immune system, is anti-inflammatory and a potent antioxidant, helps fight viruses
Vitamin C	1000 mg twice daily	Regulates immunity and combats stress
Vitamin E	100 IU daily	Reduces flare-ups of vasculitis
Omega-3 fish oils	1 g three times daily	A powerful anti-inflammatory and controls immune-mediated reactions
Evening primrose oil	1 g three times daily	Essential for recurring and relapsing autoimmune disease, ensures proper function of suppressor T-cells, is a potent anti-inflammatory

Health Tips to Enhance Healing

- Read Chapter 3 on autoimmune diseases for tips on how to alleviate symptoms. See Lupus, Multiple Sclerosis, Scleroderma, Sjorgren's, etc., if you have one of those autoimmune diseases as well.
- Rule out allergies; see the introduction to this chapter. Several case studies and small research studies have shown that the elimination of food allergies and environmental allergens resulted in the elimination of purpuras (bluish-purple bruises). When allergy-causing foods were reintroduced, vasculitis symptoms returned.
- Eliminate caffeine from the diet. It constricts blood vessels.
- Avoid animal meat and choose fish instead. Eliminate sugar and alcohol from the diet.

- Stop smoking and avoid exposure to secondhand smoke. Nicotine constricts the blood vessels.

Other Recommendations

- Reduce stress. (See "Excessive Stress," page 48.)
- Rule out hydrochloric acid deficiency (get an HCl test) and take digestive enzymes. See the introduction to this chapter.

VITILIGO

Vitiligo is a depletion of melanocytes, the cells that produce the pigment melanin that gives the color to our skin, eyes, hair, and genitals. Due to the destruction of the pigment-producing cells, those with vitiligo will develop white patches of skin on the affected area. Hair growing from the depigmented area (beards, eyebrows, eyelashes) will also be white. It strikes up to 5 million people in North America. Of those affected most will develop a loss of pigmentation before the age of 40. Both genders are affected equally. It may stay localized or spread to the entire body and it may happen quickly or gradually over decades.

Often vitiligo is found along with other autoimmune diseases including Addison's, alopecia areata, pernicious anemia, and others. It also has a hereditary component as children born to parents with vitiligo have a higher risk of developing it.

Vitiligo is not life threatening, but it is emotionally and psychologically damaging. Children and adolescents can be devastated by their appearance and focus should be on maintaining self-esteem. Support groups may offer the emotional support required to deal with this disfiguring disorder.

Symptoms

Depigmentation of skin color is generally the first symptom. There may be a few patches that are small or many patches that cover the body or it may only affect one side of the body. The depigmented skin is more common in sun-exposed areas—the face, hands, and lips. People with darkly colored skin may lose pigment inside their mouth.

Causes

The cause is not clear, but half of vitiligo cases have a genetic history. It is often present with other autoimmune disorders, such as alopecia areata, Type I diabetes, Addison's disease, or pernicious anemia. Antibodies that destroy tyrosinase (an enzyme needed to convert tyrosine to make melanin, as well as antibodies to melanocytes) have been detected in 80 percent of cases. These antibodies destroy and damage the cells that make melanin.

Heavy metal toxicity has also been associated with vitiligo. Drug-induced vitiligo usually corrects itself once the offending drug has been eliminated. Thyroid disease, nutritional deficiencies, or injury to the skin brought on by disinfectants or chemicals can stimulate the condition. Stress, either emotional or physical, can also provoke more patches to appear.

Depigmented areas can occur after a wound or lesion on the skin has healed. Fungal infections, eczema, and psoriasis often leave lightened areas in the skin folds of the elbow, knees, and other areas once healed.

Prescription for Health

The following recommendations can aid skin repigmentation. Corticosteroid treatments should never be stopped without your physician's advice. It can take up to two years to repigment skin.

NUTRIENT	DOSAGE	ACTION
Copper (those taking over 15 mg of zinc daily may be deficient in copper as zinc inhibits absorption of copper)	2–3 mg daily. Doses higher than this should be determined by your health-care professional.	Activates tyrosinase, the enzyme required to make melanin. A deficiency of copper results in tyrosine not being converted to tyrosinase, thus causing albinism and vitiligo.
Women's Whey or proteins+ protein powder	One to two scoops daily	Ensures adequate amino acid intake containing tyrosine
Moducare sterols and sterolins	One capsule three times daily	Stops autoimmune reactions, controls cortisol, enhances DHEA naturally, is anti-inflammatory
L-phenylalanine and a 10 percent phenylalanine cream applied topically to depigmented areas	50 mg/kg daily. In Canada, the cream must be prescribed by your doctor, and a compounding pharmacy can supply it.	Helps to repigment areas; the body needs phenylalanine as a precursor to tyrosine
Essential fatty acids, Omega Essential Balance, or Udo's Choice oil	1–2 Tbsp (15–30 mL) daily	Improves skin integrity, is essential to proper hormone function; those with autoimmune disorders have experienced a decrease in symptoms
Khella, Khellin extract	100 mg daily	Research using Khellin extract, plus UVA therapy, has shown it stimulates melanin production and repigmentation in a large percentage of those with vitiligo without the side effects associated with standard synthetic prescription psoralen plus UVA therapy.

NUTRIENT	DOSAGE	ACTION
High-potency B-complex	Two or three capsules daily	Essential for metabolism, the digestion of foods, protects against the effects of stress

Health Tips to Enhance Healing

- See Chapter 3 on the immune system and autoimmune disease.
- See Addison's disease, Anemia, and Scleroderma if vitiligo is a secondary process to another autoimmune disease.
- Heavy metal poisoning, especially arsenic and nickel, is associated with vitiligo. Constant exposure to nickel may cause depigmentation. Nickel-containing dental braces and eyeglass frames have been documented to promote vitiligo in those skin areas exposed over the long term. See Toxic Metal Poisoning.
- Low stomach acid is also related to developing vitiligo and other autoimmune conditions. If you suspect you have low stomach acid, see the introduction to this chapter for information on how to correct the problem.
- Take digestive enzymes before a meal, but do not drink fluids while eating as they will dilute digestive enzymes.

Other Recommendations

- Exposing affected skin to the sun may stimulate pigmentation, but be cautious. Use sunscreen with maximum UV protection, do not overdo it, and avoid sunning yourself between 10 a.m. and 2 p.m. when the sun is the hottest. Affected areas have no protection against UV rays, so do not skimp on the sunscreen.
- If you know you will be coming into contact with chemicals or cleansers, wear protective clothing so as not harm affected areas. Wash gently and moisturize well.
- Topical creams with antioxidants may be beneficial. Look for products that contain carotenes, vitamin C, and green tea. Ask your dermatologist about phenylalanine-containing cream, as one research study showed excellent repigmentation in those taking both oral and topical phenylalanine.
- Vitiligo can be especially hard on the self-esteem of children and adolescents. Building self-esteem by encouraging activities and hobbies that they enjoy and can excel at is paramount. If coping is difficult, and friends and family might not be enough, try talking to a counselor or to a support group about it.

Health Fact

Dr. Melvyn Werbach reported in his book *Nutritional Influences on Illness* that as early as 1945, a connection was made between the severity of vitiligo and low stomach acid. Of the 29 patients evaluated, only 10 percent had normal HCl levels, and 35 percent had no HCl at all. Those with the most severe vitiligo had the worst HCl levels and also had B vitamin deficiency. When a B-complex and HCl were supplemented, vitiligo symptoms improved.

WARTS (CERVICAL DYSPLASIA, HPV)

Warts are a viral skin infection caused by any one of almost 60 human papilloma viruses (HPV) and they affect a large percentage of the population. Plantar warts are located on the soles of the feet and are difficult to eliminate. Warts commonly appear on the hands, feet, nails, and face, but can appear anywhere on the body. Most warts are painless, yet others can put pressure on nerves, especially plantar warts.

Venereal warts (condylomata acuminata) are found on the genitalia of both men and women and they are very contagious and transmitted sexually. When warts appear on the cervix, it is critical they be treated aggressively because HPV infection (as well as herpes simplex Type 2) is the main cause of cervical dysplasia, a precancerous condition (although not all HPV infections result in cervical dysplasia). Today we have an epidemic of cervical cancer caused by the human papilloma virus Type 16 and 18. Over 90 percent of cervical cancers are related these two types of HPV. HPV-16 and 18 do not cause external genital warts. Penile warts rarely become cancerous, but there is a risk. Genital warts are a sign of a weakened immune system and can also cause cancer of the vagina, mouth, throat, or esophagus.

Warts can also infect the mouth if a person sucks a wart growing on a finger. They can also be transmitted through oral sex.

Symptoms

Plantar warts are usually confined to the feet. They look like calluses in that they are white but different in that their center is hard and the area can be tender and may bleed from the pressure of the body's weight. Common warts come in all shapes, sizes, and colors. They can be dark, gray, yellowish, or skin-tone, with a rough surface and most often not more than half an inch across. Flat warts, which are most often seen in children, are smooth, scaly, and yellowish-brown in color.

Genital warts are red or pink, flat or tall, and can surface in groups or individually. Women with genital warts must have regular PAP smears to rule out cervical cancer. Standard medical treatments to remove genital warts are less than satisfactory and most often the warts return frequently.

Causes

The human papilloma virus and a weakened immune system are the cause. Warts often spread to other parts of the body in those affected, but transmission from person to person is less common. Genital warts, on the other hand, are very contagious and are transmitted sexually, but may not manifest for at least three months after infection, which means they can be passed on without the carrier's knowledge. A pregnant mother may pass genital warts to her child during birth.

A healthy immune system can help to fight off the HPV virus most of the time. The recurrence of warts suggests that the immune system is suppressed or weakened either by illness or immunosuppressant drugs. This is especially the case with genital warts. The risk of cervical dysplasia is higher when the HPV infection is associated with smoking, intercourse before the age of 18, HIV, and engaging in sex without using condoms.

Stress reduction is important to keep cortisol levels in check. Cortisol is implicated in increasing our risk of viral infections. (See "The Immune System and Stress," page 45.)

Prescription for Health

The following recommendations seek to enhance the immune system, destroy the virus, and prevent recurrences. Those with HPV-induced cervical dysplasia should adopt the recommendations for cancer.

NUTRIENT	DOSAGE	ACTION
Moducare sterols and sterolins	One capsule three times daily	Regulates immune function, enhances virus-fighting activity, controls cortisol, enhances NK cell and T-helper-1 cell activity. In a pilot study women with HPV CIN-III lesions had their lesions return to normal.
High-potency B-complex	Two or three capsules daily	Important for immune function, metabolism and digestion, hormone balance, and to prevent deficiency in women taking birth control pills
Folic acid	1–10 mg daily; 5–10 mg dosages should be monitored by a physician	Deficiency can promote cervical dysplasia and increase the risk of cervical cancer
Beta glucans, PSP, reishi, maitaki, cordyceps, shiitake mushroom extract	600 mg twice daily	Enhances immune function, NK cells, gamma-interferon and macrophage function

NUTRIENT	DOSAGE	ACTION
Multimune containing vitamins A, B$_6$, C, E, selenium, zinc, magnesium, coenzyme Q10, lipoic acid, glutathione	One capsule three times daily	Supports immune function; glutathione detoxifies liver, enhances NK cells; vitamins A, B$_6$, C, E, selenium, and zinc have been shown to reverse or reduce dysplasia, are potent antioxidants
Lactobacillus acidophilus	1 tsp (5 mL) daily containing 1–2 billion active organisms or 1 cup (250 mL) of acidophilus-rich yogurt	Enhances immune function and intestinal flora and aids digestion
Omega-3 fatty acids from flax or Eskimo-3 fish oils from Tyler	1–2 Tbsp (15–30 mL) of flaxseed oil or six 500 mg capsules of fish oil	May delay onset of malignancy
Oil of oregano	Three drops twice daily in water and apply topically on common and plantar warts	Antiviral, antibacterial
Garlic (Kyolic)	Two capsules daily and plenty of fresh garlic in foods	Boosts immunity, helps fight viruses (see below for topical treatment)
Wobenzym	Three to five tablets daily	Disables viruses

Health Tips to Enhance Healing

- See Cancer if you have genital warts and read Chapter 3 on how to enhance your immune function.
- Stop smoking. The incidence rate of cervical dysplasia is two to three times higher in smokers.
- Do not put fingers that have warts on them in your mouth to prevent transmission to your mouth.
- If you are on birth control pills and continue to have genital warts, choose another form of birth control. Birth control pills deplete the body of vitamins B$_6$, B$_{12}$, and C, folic acid, zinc, and riboflavin.
- Take plant sterols and sterolins. Over 65,000 cases of cervical cancer are diagnosed each year in North America and over 10,000 women will die as a result. The fear of cervical cancer sends most women to their doctor for an annual Pap smear. Often women are told that their Pap smear is abnormal, showing cell changes called cervical dysplasia. As mentioned earlier, many have HPV-induced cervical dysplasia. A small pilot study using Moducare sterols and sterolins was undertaken to see if HPV-induced cervical dysplasia could be reduced or reversed by enhancing immune function.
- Thirteen women with CIN III (cervical intraepithelial neoplasia, low-grade squamous epithelial lesion) cervical lesions were divided into two groups. Seven were given Moducare and six were given a placebo (a fake pill). The results of the study showed that all six in the placebo group had no improvement of disease. In the

treatment group receiving Moducare, the lesions were completely eliminated in three patients, with the other four showing no further progression of the lesions. Although this was a small sample, it provides enough encouragement that further research should be performed.

Other Recommendations

- Place a piece of raw peeled garlic on common warts without it touching the healthy skin, and cover with a bandage. Leave it for 24 hours. There will probably be blisters and in a week's time the wart will fall off.
- Never have unprotected sex. Condoms are very effective at preventing the transmission of HPV. Reduce exposure to the virus by not having sex with people who have genital warts or who have come into contact with genital warts. Do not assume that a person is not infected because there are no visible warts.
- Clean genital area gently but well and air dry. Do not aggravate the skin. Wear cotton underwear and abstain from intercourse until the warts are gone.
- Have Pap smears every year to detect early changes in the cervix. If you have genital warts, seek attention from a physician or naturopath. While natural therapies can be effective at reversing cervical dysplasia, the condition should be supervised and evaluated for changes in the cervix.
- Quite often common and plantar warts will resolve themselves without treatment. Do not try to remove warts by yourself. Consult a qualified practitioner if your warts bother you or cause pain.

Health Fact

Researchers investigated whether plantar warts were more common in adolescents who used locker rooms as opposed to shower rooms. One hundred forty-six students (ranging in age from 10 to 18) from a swim club and a public school were interviewed and had their feet examined. Twenty-seven percent of those who used communal shower rooms had plantar warts, compared to 1.25 percent of those who only used locker rooms, suggesting that the infection is increased in those who expose their feet to infected, moist surfaces.

CHAPTER 8

RECIPES FOR A HEALTHY IMMUNE SYSTEM

We know that frying foods and barbecuing or blackening foods promotes trans fatty acids, cancer, and heart disease. You learned in Chapter 4 that extra-virgin olive oil is the only "supermarket" oil safe for human consumption. You have thrown away all the bad oils and margarines and have purchased some of the organic, cold-pressed nut and seed oils and spreads from the health food store and you are ready to start cooking. The following tips and recipes will show you how easy it is to make healthy fats a part of your diet and how to adapt current recipes to this new way of using fats and oils.

HEALTHY COOKING

To low-heat sauté, use several tablespoons of water or vegetable stock instead of oil. Cover the bottom of the pan with the ingredients you wish to sauté and slowly add more until cooked to the desired consistency. Place your large sauté pan on low heat. Add more liquid as required to prevent sticking and stir often. Sautéing in this manner will keep the temperature inside the pan at a safe level of 212°F (100°C).

- Coconut oil or ghee (which is clarified butter) are the only oils that can be heated to 375°F (190°C). Certain oils, such as flaxseed, walnut, borage, soy, canola, hemp, Omega Essential Balance, and Udo's Choice, must be added at the end of cooking once the food has been removed from heat. The goal is to use as little oil as possible during the cooking process. Add oils after cooking is finished to give the satisfying flavor and texture that we crave.
- With the exception of extra-virgin olive oil, supermarket oils should never be consumed, especially processed corn and canola oil, as they are genetically modified. Supermarket salad dressings

often contain these oils, so be sure to purchase your salad dressings from the health food store or, better yet, make some of the recipes I recommend.

- Never *fry* with any of the oils I recommend (other than coconut oil or ghee), since these oils are very sensitive to heat, which will destroy their healing ingredients and make them toxic. See the chart provided on page 380 to determine cooking methods for different oils. Always add the health-giving, no-heat oils after cooking, once the pot has been removed from the heat. Fats and oils add a wonderful creamy texture and full body to foods.
- Low-heat sauté foods in water, chicken or vegetable broth, and wine. Adopt this method mentioned above.
- Steam vegetables or fish. Boiling vegetables leaches the important phytonutrients, especially the sterols and sterolins, into the water, which is then tossed down the drain.
- Poach or simmer foods, especially fish.
- Soups and stews are a safe cooking method as foods are cooked over low heat.

Low-heat oven roasting up to 250°F (120°C) is excellent for garlic, chicken, meats, fish, and vegetables.

When baking breads and muffins at temperatures around 325°F (165°C), the moisture keeps the inside temperature under 212°F (100°C).

For full flavor of nut oils, add after cooking.

The best addition to any kitchen is a food processor. Choose a heavy-duty appliance, such as a Cuisinart or Braun, that has several blades and attachments. It is invaluable when preparing vegetables, spreads, desserts, salad dressings, and much more. A food processor is used in the preparation of several recipes; it is not a requirement, just a time-saving process. If you do not own a food processor, then a good knife or a blender, coffee grinder, or hand-held blender may provide similar results.

Some of my recipes recommend Omega Hi-Lignan Nutri-Flax. It is certified organic, finely ground, and contains 4.8 mg/gm of lignans and is great to add to many baked goods. High-lignan flax can be added to any of your favorite baking recipes. Just substitute the fibrous ingredients, i.e., ¼ cup (60 mL) of wheat germ can be replaced with ¼ cup (60 mL) of high-lignan flax. I recommend that you not add more than ½ cup (125 mL) of this high-lignan flax to your baking recipes or the result may be a muffin, bread, or pastry that is just too heavy.

Several different seed and nut oils are recommended in the following recipes. Their essential fatty acid content is important as well, as this determines the temperatures they can withstand in cooking. Each oil is chosen not only for its culinary delights but also for its essential fatty acid (EFA) content and ability to be heated (or not). Although I am recommending

More Healthful Hints

- Do you have gas or feel bloated? Do you belch or have a big belly? Plant-based enzymes aid the digestive system. Look for a well-rounded formula in your local natural health food store.
- Lactic acid in natural yogurt and sauerkraut helps enzyme production. Countries where these foods are consumed regularly (such as Russia, Bulgaria, and Romania) have lower cancer rates per capita and have the highest number of centenarians.
- Garlic is antiviral and antifungal, reduces cholesterol, and is rich in selenium. It also increases white cell production.
- Jalapeño and cayenne peppers contain capsicum, which is a powerful antioxidant. They also rev up your fat-burning furnace and aid weight loss.
- Tomatoes are rich in the phytonutrient lycopene, a powerful cancer-protective agent. Tomatoes should be eaten with oil to increase the absorption of lycopene.
- Dark vegetables are rich in carotenoids and chlorophyll, both of which have powerful anticancer properties.
- Sesame oil is the most stable oil for low-heat sautéing.

Omega Nutrition's and Udo's Choice oils because those are the ones I use, you can purchase any brand-name organic, cold-pressed nut and seed oils.

ESSENTIAL FATTY ACID PROFILE OF DIFFERENT OILS

Oil	Omega-6	Omega-9	Other
Coconut	—	7%	Saturated fat 91%
Garlic-chili flaxseed	15%	21%	Omega-3 54%
Hazelnut	14%	77%	
Olive	15%	63%	
Pistachio	30%	54%	
Pumpkin	55%	25%	
Safflower	78%	12%	
Sesame	45%	40%	
Sunflower	71%	16%	
Hi-oleic sunflower	15%	75%	

TEMPERATURE CHART

No Heat (120°F/49°C) Superpolyunsaturates (condiments, salad dressings)	Low Heat (212°F/100°C) Polyunsaturates (sauces, baking)	Medium Heat (325°F/165°C) Monounsaturates (light sautéing) For optimal flavor add after cooking	High Heat (375°F/190°C) Saturates (high-heat sautéing)
Flaxseed oil Omega Essential Balance oil Udo's Choice oil Borage oil Canola oil Hemp seed oil Soy oil Walnut oil	Safflower oil Sunflower oil Pumpkin oil	Almond oil Hazelnut oil Olive oil Pistachio oil Sesame oil	Coconut oil Ghee (clarified butter used in Indian cooking methods)

THE TRUTH ABOUT COCONUT OIL

Nearly four decades ago, data gathered from experimental diets mistakenly concluded that coconut oil raised blood cholesterol levels. Scientists now know that coconut oil was not the villain. Health problems were caused by the omission of essential fatty acids in experimental diets, not by the inclusion of coconut oil in them. Diets that include any hydrogenated products always result in high serum cholesterol levels because these products contain harmful trans fatty acids and lack heart-healthy EFAs.

In the late 1980s consumer activists, including the Center for Science in the Public Interest, reinitiated the war against coconut oil and attempted to stamp out newly discovered scientifically proven benefits. As a result of this misinformation, food giants have been replacing this healthy, naturally saturated oil with hydrogenated, refined oils full of harmful trans fatty acids.

Researchers noted that the Polynesians and Bicolanos (of the Philippines) include coconut oil in their daily diets and have low serum cholesterol levels and little coronary heart disease. When nonhydrogenated, saturated fats are part of an essential fatty acid-rich diet, and little or no change is seen in serum cholesterol levels. For years we were told not to eat eggs because they would raise our cholesterol, and then researchers discovered that eggs were not a problem. It is the oxidized cholesterol and trans fatty acids in processed foods that are raising our cholesterol.

Current research shows that not all saturated fatty acids raise cholesterol. There are two groups of saturated fats—medium chain and long chain—and each acts differently in the body. Long-chain saturates store as fats and are associated with LDL, the bad cholesterol. Medium-chain saturates found in coconut oil do not clog arteries, nor do they cause heart disease. Instead, medium-chain saturates are easily digested and are also a source of fuel and energy.

Because coconut oil is naturally saturated, it does not need to be hydrogenated. The hydrogenation process causes fat to change from liquid to solid at room temperature and is used in the manufacturing of most margarines and shortening. The result of hydrogenation is a poisonous molecular distortion of the fatty acids, turning them into harmful trans fatty acids. Researchers have pointed out that these warped fatty acids raise LDL (the bad cholesterol) and lower HDL (the good cholesterol).

Not only is coconut oil slightly lower in calories than most other fats and oils, less coconut oil is required when cooking or baking. It is also a source of medium-chain triglycerides (MCTs), which are especially valuable to people who have trouble digesting fat. MCTs enable the body to metabolize fat efficiently and convert it into energy rather than storing it as fat. Dieters, weight lifters, and athletes find coconut oil beneficial for this reason.

Coconut Oil for Immune Dysfunction

Coconut oil is ideal for immune-suppressed individuals too. Why? Almost 50 percent of its fatty acid content is lauric acid, a disease-fighting fatty acid. Lauric acid, also found naturally in human breast milk, protects infants from being infected by many viruses and some bacteria. Besides human milk, coconut oil is one of the few significant sources of lauric acid.

Coconut oil, one of the most stable oils, is naturally solid at room temperature (below 76°F/24°C). It is nondairy and has no trans fatty acids. It is great for baking. It whips up easily and makes batter the perfect consistency. Use three-quarters the amount of coconut oil as a substitute for butter, shortening, or lard in your family recipes, or simply use coconut oil instead of butter or margarine on toast, crackers, and more.

In the following recipes, I recommend using Omega Coconut Butter. It is certified organic, and no solvents are used during processing. It is nonhydrogenated and free of trans fatty acids. The piecrust recipe is excellent.

Any favorite recipe in your cookbooks can be altered to include the new cooking methods that use a minimum of oils for frying. Use any of the several oils mentioned, combined with chives, dill, and garlic to top cooked potatoes, drizzle on fresh vegetables, and combine with your favorite herbs and vinegars for an excellent salad dressing and more. Your options are as limitless as your imagination.

RECIPES

The following recipes are quick, delicious, and rich in essential fatty acids, phytonutrients, and fiber.

Breakfast

APPLE OATMEAL

1 cup	old-fashioned oats (thick-cut are the best)	250 mL
1 cup	water	250 mL
1 cup	apple juice	250 mL
3	medium-size apples, grated	3
1 handful	raisins, rinsed (optional)	1 handful
dash	cinnamon	dash
3 Tbsp	flaxseed oil or Udo's Choice or Omega Essential Balance	45 mL
2 Tbsp	Omega Hi-Lignan Nutri-Flax	30 mL

Place first six ingredients in a heavy saucepan. Cover and cook over low heat for 20 minutes. Stir occasionally. Remove from heat and stir in oil. Spoon oatmeal into individual serving dishes and sprinkle with Omega Hi-Lignan Nutri-Flax.

Makes 2 servings.

APPLESAUCE SURPRISE

1 cup	organic applesauce	250 mL
dash	cinnamon	dash
2 Tbsp	Omega Hi-Lignan Nutri-Flax or Udo's Choice Wholesome Fast Food Blend	30 mL
½ cup	plain or vanilla yogurt	125 mL

Mix all ingredients and serve immediately.

Makes 1–2 servings.

FLAX PUDDING

This pudding tastes so good your family won't believe it is healthy.

6 Tbsp	flaxseeds (or 5 Tbsp/75 mL or Omega Hi-Lignan Flax Seed)	90 mL
2 cups	milk, soymilk, or Rice Dream	500 mL
2 Tbsp	ground hazelnuts, almonds, or pistachios	30 mL

1	large banana, mashed	1
1 Tbsp	honey (optional)	15 mL
	juice of one orange	
1	apple, peeled, cored, and grated	1
	whipped cream as desired	
	strawberries or fresh fruit for garnish	

Pulse the flaxseeds in a coffee grinder for a few seconds. Bring milk to a boil in a double-boiler and stir in ground flaxseeds with a whisk to prevent lumps (add all of the ground flaxseed or Omega Hi-Lignan Nutri-Flax at once); boil for 30 seconds, remove from heat, and pour into a bowl. Let cool. It will have the consistency of pudding. Mix ground nuts, banana, honey, and orange juice into the flax pudding mixture. Gently mix in grated apple and spoon into parfait dishes layered alternately with fresh fruit and real whipped cream. Top with a strawberry and a dab of whipped cream.

Makes 4 servings.

MOM'S BEST RICE PUDDING

When I am making any other rice dish, I make extra rice for this wonderful dessert or breakfast treat.

3 cups	cooked brown rice, prepared according to instructions on package	750 mL
6	eggs, well-beaten	6
1½ cups	milk (soy or rice milk can be substituted)	375 mL
½ cup	maple syrup	125 mL
1 tsp	vanilla	5 mL
1 tsp	cinnamon	5 mL
1	apple, grated (optional)	1
¼ cup	Omega Hi-Lignan Nutri-Flax or Udo's Choice Wholesome Fast Food Blend (optional)	60 mL
2 Tbsp	Omega Essential Balance or flaxseed oil or Udo's Choice Ultimate Oil Blend (optional)	30 mL
1 cup	yogurt (optional)	250 mL

Mix together first six ingredients (and the grated apple if you are using it) and pour into a buttered casserole dish. Bake in a preheated 350°F (180°C) oven for 30–40 minutes or until firm. The pudding should be thick, not runny. Once cooled, stir in flax, oil, or yogurt if desired.

This can be served hot or cold for breakfast. Applesauce or whipped cream can top this great treat.

Makes 4 servings.

YOGURT SHAKE

1 cup	plain acidophilus yogurt	250 mL
2 Tbsp	Omega Hi-Lignan Nutri-Flax or Udo's Choice Wholesome Fast Food Blend	30 mL
1 Tbsp	Omega Essential Balance or Udo's Choice Ultimate Oil Blend	15 mL
½ cup	fresh fruit	125 mL
1 cup	organic fresh apple juice or juice of choice	250 mL
3	ice cubes	3
1 scoop	Women's Whey Protein Powder	1 scoop

In a blender combine all ingredients and blend until smooth. Drink immediately.
Makes 1–2 servings.

YOGURT VARIATIONS

1 cup	plain acidophilus yogurt	250 mL
2 Tbsp	Omega Hi-Lignan Nutri-Flax or Udo's Choice Wholesome Fast Food Blend	30 mL
¼ cup	granola	60 mL
1 Tbsp	Omega Essential Balance, or flaxseed oil, or Udo's Choice Ultimate Oil Blend fruit of your choice (bananas, strawberries, mango, blueberries, and papaya are excellent)	15 mL

Mix all ingredients and enjoy.
Makes 1 serving.

Appetizers, Dips, and Snacks

BLACK BEAN SALSA

2	ripe tomatoes, chopped	2
¼–½ cup	chopped cilantro	60–125 mL
⅓ cup	finely chopped onion	80 mL
½–3	serrano chili peppers salt to taste	½–3
1	can (15 oz/425 g) of organic Eden black beans, drained and rinsed juice of two limes	1
¼ cup	Omega Garlic-Chili Flax Seed Oil	60 mL

Place tomatoes in a medium bowl. Add the cilantro and onion to the tomatoes. Cut open the chilies, remove all the seeds, and dice very fine. Add chilies, salt, and beans to the tomato mixture. Pour lime juice and Omega Garlic-Chili Flax Seed Oil over all ingredients. Mix, cover, and refrigerate for one hour.

Makes 3–4 cups (750 mL–1 L).

FALAFELS

One cup (250 mL) of dry beans equals 2–2½ cups (500–625 mL) cooked. You can soak and cook your own beans and then put them in individual freezer bags for future use. This is not only economical but makes for quick meals. Freezing soaked and cooked beans also makes them easier to digest and causes less gas and bloating

4 cups	cooked garbanzo beans (they should be very soft)	1 L
6	cloves garlic, minced	6
½ cup	finely chopped fresh parsley	125 mL
½ cup	finely minced onion	125 mL
1 tsp	cumin powder	5 mL
dash	cayenne pepper	dash
2	eggs, beaten	2
2 Tbsp	tahini (page 402)	30 mL
4 Tbsp	Omega High-Lignan Nutri-Flax or Udo's Choice Wholesome Fast Food Blend	60 mL
2 Tbsp	flour	30 mL
6	pita bread	
	tahini sauce, tsatziki, grated cheese, lettuce, tomato, onions, cucumber, and sprouts for garnish	

Using the food processor, mash garbanzo beans into a soft paste. Combine all ingredients except flour until well mixed. Refrigerate for at least one hour. Lightly roll into balls, then roll in the flour and bake on a cookie sheet at 400°F (200°C) for 20–25 minutes or until crispy on the outside. Place 3 or 4 falafels in a pita bread with tahini sauce (page 402) and tzatziki (page 403), grated cheese, lettuce, tomato, onions, cucumber, and sprouts.

Makes 20–24 falafels.

GUACAMOLE

3	ripe avocados, mashed	3
	juice of one small lemon	
3	garlic cloves, pressed	3

½ cup	chopped tomatoes	125 mL
2 Tbsp	finely minced green onion	30 mL
2 Tbsp	sour cream	30 mL
3 Tbsp	Omega Essential Balance or Udo's Choice Ultimate Oil Blend	45 mL

Mix avocados with lemon juice and add garlic. Mix thoroughly. Add chopped tomatoes and green onion. Stir in sour cream and Omega Essential Balance. Serve as a condiment to fajitas or bean tortillas, with nachos, or as a layer in the Seven-Layer Mexican Party Dip (page 387).

For a quick version, use ½ cup (125 mL) salsa in place of tomatoes and minced onion.

Makes 4 servings.

HUMMUS

2 cups	cooked chickpeas (garbanzo beans) or 1 can (16 oz/500 mL), drained (save liquid)	500 mL
4	garlic cloves, minced	4
3 Tbsp	tahini (optional)	45 mL
3 Tbsp	olive or flaxseed oil	45 mL
⅓ cup	freshly squeezed lemon juice	80 mL
⅓ cup	reserved liquid from chickpeas	80 mL
1 tsp	cumin	5 mL
	salt to taste	

Add all ingredients to food processor and blend until smooth. If the hummus is too thick, add 2 Tbsp (30 mL) of Udo's Choice Ultimate Oil Blend and add more lemon juice.

Serve as a dip for vegetables or spread for crackers or warm pita bread.

Makes 2 cups (500 mL).

DELICIOUS ARTICHOKE DIP

2	cans (14 oz/400 mL) water-packed artichokes, drained	2
6–8	garlic cloves	6–8
1 cup	homemade mayonnaise (page 408)	250 mL
1 cup	freshly grated Parmesan cheese	250 mL
1 cup	grated Emmenthal or sharp Swiss cheese	250 mL
2 Tbsp	freshly squeezed lemon juice	30 mL
½–1 cup	grated Asiago cheese	

Preheat oven to 375°F (190°C). Combine all ingredients except Asiago cheese in a food processor and blend until well mixed. Pour into an ovenproof casserole dish. Sprinkle with grated Asiago cheese. Bake until hot and bubbly, approximately 25 minutes. Remove from oven. Serve with bread, crackers, or vegetables.

Makes 3 cups (750 mL).

SEVEN-LAYER MEXICAN PARTY DIP

Cilantro is one herb known to help chelate (pull) mercury out of the human body. With our daily exposure to mercury, we should be eating plenty of cilantro.

2 cups	refried beans (page 398)	500 mL
1 cup	grated Monterey Jack cheese	250 mL
2 cups	guacamole (page 385)	500 mL
2 Tbsp	finely chopped parsley	30 mL
2 Tbsp	finely chopped cilantro	30 mL
1 cup	sour cream	250 mL
2	tomatoes, chopped	2
4 or 5	green onions, finely minced	4 or 5
1 bag	organic blue or yellow corn tortilla chips	1 bag

Preheat oven to 350°F (180°C). In a 9 in × 12 in (23 cm × 30 cm) glass baking dish, evenly spread the refried beans and cover with half of the grated cheese. Next, spread the guacamole, then sprinkle on the parsley and cilantro. Next, spread a layer of sour cream and green onions and then the chopped tomatoes. For the last layer, add the remaining grated cheese and sprinkle with parsley.

Bake until the cheese melts and the dip is hot throughout. Serve at once with tortilla chips.

Makes 6–8 servings.

SPANAKOPITA

FILLING:

6	eggs	6
2 cups	crumbled feta cheese	500 mL
3 Tbsp	extra-virgin olive oil	45 mL
1 cup	ricotta, or cottage, or quark cheese	250 mL
1 cup	finely chopped onion	250 mL
¼ cup	finely chopped parsley	60 mL

1 large handful	chopped fresh basil, stems removed	1 large handful
1 tsp	ground fennel seeds (grind them yourself for better flavor, using a clean coffee grinder)	5 mL
2 Tbsp	flour	30 mL
2 lb	fresh spinach, thoroughly washed and dried and chopped into 1 in (2.5 cm) pieces,	1 kg

PASTRY:

| 1 lb | package filo pastry dough, thawed | 0.5 kg |
| 1 cup | melted better butter (page 407) made with olive, hazelnut, or almond oil | 250 mL |

Combine all ingredients for the filling and mix thoroughly. Set aside.

Preheat oven to 325°F (165°C). Use a wide pastry brush or a 2 in (5 cm) natural bristle paint brush (not one you have used for painting). Brush the bottom and sides of a 10 in × 13 in (25 cm × 33 cm) baking dish with melted better butter. Place one sheet of filo in the dish, then brush the top with melted butter. Place another sheet of filo over it and brush again with better butter. Continue until you have 8–10 layers of filo. Spread the filling onto the filo sheets. Then cover with 8–10 sheets of filo, again brushing each sheet with better butter. The secret to spanokopita is in the filo pastry. Remember that each sheet of filo should be spread with better butter or oil to ensure a flaky, light dish when baked.

Bake uncovered for one hour. Serve with warm pita bread, tsatziki sauce (page 403), and Greek salad.

Makes 6 servings.

Salads

MARINATED BROCCOLI, BEAN SPROUT, AND CHERRY TOMATO SALAD

Broccoli is very high in sulphoraphane, a powerful anticancer phytonutrient. Chew each bite fully to ensure that you absorb the maximum amount of sulphoraphane. Recipe should be made several hours before serving to allow the dressing to flavor the vegetables and soften the broccoli.

Researchers at the Fred Hutchinson Cancer Research Center noted that it took only three half-cup servings per week of broccoli, Brussels sprouts, and cauliflower to decrease the risk of prostate cancer by 41 percent.

2 cups	bean sprouts	500 mL
1	medium red pepper, sliced	1
3 cups	chopped broccoli, cut into bite-size pieces	750 mL

1	small red onion, thinly sliced	1
1 cup	halved cherry tomatoes	250 mL
½–¾ cup	pistachio nut oil, or Omega Essential Balance Oil, or Udo's Choice Ultimate Oil Blend, or extra-virgin olive oil	125–180 mL
2 Tbsp	Omega Apple Cider Vinegar (or to taste)	30 mL
6 Tbsp	organic and wheat-free tamari	90 mL
2	garlic cloves, pressed	2
¼ cup	black sesame seeds	60 mL

Combine sprouts, red pepper, broccoli, onion, and cherry tomatoes in a large serving bowl.

Combine the oil, vinegar, tamari, and garlic in a container and shake well.

Pour dressing over salad and toss well. Garnish with black sesame seeds. Cover and refrigerate until serving, tossing occasionally.

Makes 6 servings.

SHRIMP AND SUGAR SNAP PEA SALAD

SHRIMP MIXTURE:

36	large shrimp, deveined, shelled, and lightly steamed until cooked	36
½ lb	sugar snap peas or snow peas with ends removed	250 g
1	English cucumber, thinly sliced	1
¼ cup	finely chopped parsley	60 mL
2	thinly sliced celery stalks	2

DRESSING:

5 Tbsp	Omega Essential Balance Oil or hazelnut oil	75 mL
¼ cup	Omega Apple Cider Vinegar	60 mL
1 Tbsp	toasted sesame oil	15 mL
4 Tbsp	organic and wheat-free tamari	60 mL
1 Tbsp	Dijon mustard	15 mL
1 Tbsp	liquid honey	15 mL
	coarsely ground black pepper	
	sea salt to taste	

SALAD BED:

| 3½–4 cups | cooked whole wheat couscous (or if you are wheat allergic, use 1½ cups/ 375 mL of rice noodles cooked according to package directions, or use fresh wild greens) | 875 mL–1 L |

In a large bowl combine shrimp, peas, cucumber, parsley, and celery. Mix dressing ingredients and pour over shrimp mixture. Refrigerate for two hours. Place couscous on a serving dish and arrange shrimp on top.

Makes 6–8 servings.

TABOULI SALAD

This is an excellent summertime salad, as it is very refreshing. It is also a great side dish to serve with falafels.

1 cup	dry bulgar wheat (found in the bulk food section of your grocery or health food store)	250 mL
1½ cup	boiling water	375 mL
⅓ cup	freshly squeezed lemon juice	80 mL
4	garlic cloves, minced	4
½ cup	finely minced green onions	125 mL
1 cup	finely chopped parsley	250 mL
2	large tomatoes, chopped	2
1 cup	finely chopped red pepper	250 mL
½ cup	oil of your choice (pistachio or hazelnut oil work very well) freshly ground pepper to taste	125 mL

Soak the bulgar in the boiling water for at least 30 minutes until soft. Combine remaining ingredients and add to the presoaked bulgar. Refrigerate for several hours.

This recipe can also be made with couscous instead of bulgar, which gives it a much lighter texture. Cook 2 cups (500 mL) of couscous as directed on package. Fluff with a fork to prevent clumping while cooling. Once cooled, add all the other ingredients.

Makes 4 servings.

Soups

BLACK BEAN SOUP

This soup is delicious and easy to prepare.

2 cups	chopped onion	500 mL
6	garlic cloves, minced	6
2 tsp	cumin	10 mL
2 tsp	coriander	10 mL
4 Tbsp	olive oil	60 mL
2	cans (14 oz/400 g) black beans	2

	(or 2 cups/500 mL of dry beans soaked and cooked in 4 cups/1 L of water)	
2 cups	vegetable stock or puréed tomatoes	500 mL
½ cup	chopped red pepper	125 mL
½ cup	finely chopped parsley	125 mL
½ cup	chopped cilantro	125 mL
⅛ tsp	cayenne pepper	0.5 mL
	juice of medium freshly squeezed lemon	
½ cup	Omega Essential Balance Oil or Udo's Choice Ultimate Oil Blend chopped green onions, cilantro, sour cream, or yogurt for garnish	125 mL

In a large, heavy-bottomed pot, sauté onions, garlic, cumin, and coriander in olive oil until onions are soft. Add beans, vegetable stock or puréed tomatoes, red pepper, parsley, and cilantro. Simmer over medium heat for 30 minutes. Purée soup in blender or use a hand-held blender in the soup pot. (A hand-held blender is the greatest gadget—you will never have to transfer hot soup to a blender again.) If the soup is too thick, add a little more stock. Add cayenne pepper. Remove from heat and stir in freshly squeezed lemon juice and Omega Essential Balance Oil.

Serve garnished with chopped green onions, cilantro, and a dollop of sour cream or yogurt. This soup can be frozen without the garnishes.

Makes 6 servings.

LENTIL CARROT SOUP

When my children were small and not too impressed with vegetables, I would purée the entire pot. They loved this soup with a dollop of yogurt or sour cream and big slices of whole grain bread.

6 cups	vegetable stock	1.5 L
1	bay leaf	1
2½ cups	raw lentils	625 mL
2 cups	chopped carrots	500 mL
1½ cups	chopped onions	375 mL
1 cup	chopped celery	250 mL
6	garlic cloves, crushed	6
1 cup	diced potato or yams	250 mL
1 tsp	cumin	5 mL
½ tsp	oregano	2 mL
	black pepper to taste	
2 cups	diced fresh tomatoes	500 mL
¼ cup	red wine	60 mL

¼ cup	Omega Essential Balance Oil or	125 mL
	Udo's Choice Ultimate Oil Blend	
½ cup	chopped parsley	125 mL
½ cup	minced green onions and parsley	125 mL
	for garnish	

Simmer vegetable stock, bay leaf, and lentils for four to five hours. In a separate pan sauté carrots, onions, celery, garlic, potato, and herbs and spices. Add to lentil mixture and simmer for 15 minutes. Add tomatoes and red wine and simmer until vegetables are cooked to desired tenderness. Remove bay leaf before serving. The longer this soup simmers, the better. Remove from heat and stir in Omega Essential Blend Oil. Garnish with chopped parsley and green onions.
Makes 6 servings.

MINESTRONE SOUP

This is a rich soup and makes a hearty meal when served with warm buns or bread topped with better butter. I always try to use fresh herbs when in season. Home-soaked and cooked beans can be used in place of canned. My reason for recommending canned is simply to save time.

6	garlic cloves, crushed	6
2 cups	chopped onion	500 mL
1 cup	sliced celery	250 mL
4 Tbsp	olive oil	60 mL
2 cups	sliced carrots	500 mL
1 cup	chopped red pepper	250 mL
	sea salt or mineralized salt to taste	
¼ cup	finely chopped cilantro	60 mL
2	bay leaves	2
2 tsp	fresh oregano	10 mL
2 tsp	fresh basil	10 mL
4 cups	soup stock (use nonhydrolized vegetable bouillon cubes)	1 L
1	can (14 oz/400 g) garbanzo beans or pinto beans, drained and rinsed	1
2 cups	tomato purée	500 mL
1½ cups	chopped fresh tomatoes	375 mL
¼ cup	dry red wine	60 mL
½ cup	dry pasta cooked firm and set aside	125 mL
½ cup	Omega Essential Balance Oil or Udo's Choice Ultimate Oil Blend	125 mL

	freshly grated Parmesan cheese, for garnish	
	freshly ground coarse black pepper, for garnish	
1 cup	finely chopped parsley	250 mL

Frizzle garlic, onions, and celery in olive oil in a large, heavy-bottomed soup pot. Add carrots, red peppers, salt, and fresh herbs. Cover and simmer for 5 minutes. Add stock, beans, tomato purée, tomatoes, and red wine. Cover and simmer on low heat for 20 minutes. Remove bay leaves. Add pasta. Cook until tender. Remove from heat, stir in Omega Essential Balance Oil, and top with freshly grated Parmesan cheese, black pepper, and parsley.

Makes 8 servings.

Vegetables

GINGERED ASPARAGUS OR GREEN BEANS

This is a fabulous recipe that brings out the best of these vegetables.

¾ cup	Omega Apple Cider Vinegar	180 mL
1½ Tbsp	freshly grated gingerroot	25 mL
2 Tbsp	maple syrup	30 mL
1 lb	fresh asparagus or green beans	500 g
2	garlic cloves, minced	2
3–4 Tbsp	sesame oil	45–60 mL
½ tsp	sea salt	2 mL
1 tsp	low-salt soy sauce or organic and wheat-free tamari	5 mL

Combine vinegar, grated gingerroot, and maple syrup and bring to a boil. Cook uncovered over medium heat for 10–15 minutes to make a deep ginger tasting sauce and set aside.

Cut off ½ in (1.5 cm) from base of asparagus, or clip off ends of green beans. Steam vegetable until tender, about 5–8 minutes. Remove from heat and rinse with cold water to stop the cooking.

Combine garlic, oil, sea salt, and soy or tamari with vinegar mixture. Arrange asparagus or green beans on a plate. Cover with marinade and refrigerate for one to two hours before serving.

Makes 4 servings.

OIL-LESS VEGETABLE STIR-FRIZZLE

Any combination of your favorite vegetables will work in this recipe. I have just chosen the ones my family likes.

1 cup	vegetable stock	250 mL
3–4 Tbsp	organic and wheat-free tamari or low-salt soy sauce	45–60 mL
3	garlic cloves, pressed	3
1 Tbsp	peeled and finely sliced fresh ginger	15 mL
1 tsp	sesame oil (for flavor only)	5 mL
1	large coarsely chopped onion	1
1	medium head of broccoli, cut into bite-size pieces	1
2	carrots, sliced diagonally	2
1	red pepper, coarsely chopped	1
½ cup	pistachio oil, or Omega Essential Balance Oil, or hazelnut oil, or Udo's Choice Ultimate Oil Blend	125 mL

In a wok or very large pot, combine stock, tamari, garlic, ginger, and sesame oil. Heat liquid and then add all the vegetables except the red pepper. Cook until veggies are tender-firm, then add the red pepper. Cover and cook to the desired tenderness. Remove from heat and stir in the oil you chose. Serve with rice and Excellent Ginger Sauce (page 401).

Makes 2–4 servings.

Main Dishes

CAULIFLOWER CURRY

CURRY SAUCE:

1 tsp	coriander	5 mL
1 tsp	cumin	5 mL
¼ tsp	ground cloves	1 mL
4	garlic cloves, peeled	4
1 tsp	peeled and grated fresh gingerroot	5 mL
½ tsp	turmeric	2 mL
⅛–¼ tsp	cayenne pepper	0.5–1 mL
½ cup	water	125 mL

CAULIFLOWER MIXTURE:

2 cups	coarsely chopped onion	500 mL
1	large cauliflower, cut into bite-size pieces (sliced yams and cubed potatoes can be added for variation)	1
	juice of 1 lemon	
3 Tbsp	pistachio nut oil	45 mL

Mix sauce ingredients in blender or food processor, or with a whisk, until well blended. Set aside.

Low heat saute onions in olive oil and 2 Tbsp (30 mL) of water until soft. Add cauliflower or other vegetables. Add sauce mixture and cook covered, on low heat, until cauliflower or other vegetables are tender but not soft. Once cooked, remove from heat. Stir in lemon juice and pistachio nut oil.

Serve with brown rice, veggies, and plain yogurt. Sprinkle with toasted sesame seeds.

Makes 4 servings.

GREEK SPINACH FETA CASSEROLE

This dish is a favorite for those with hectic schedules. Even my children, who hate cooked spinach, enjoy its taste when it is baked.

4 cups	brown rice, cooked (3 cups brown rice, 1 cup wild rice can be mixed for a festive touch and increased nutritional value) (2 cups raw brown rice cooked in 4 cups water or 1½ cups raw brown rice with ½ cup raw wild rice cooked in 4 cups of water)	1L
1 cup	finely chopped onion	250 mL
1	medium red pepper, finely chopped	1
1	small yellow pepper, finely chopped	1
4	garlic cloves, minced	4
5	eggs, beaten	5
1 cup	skim milk (soy or rice milk can be substituted)	250 mL
1½ cups	crumbled feta cheese	375 mL
½ cup	pitted calamata olives (optional)	125 mL
3 Tbsp	organic and wheat-free tamari or low-salt soy sauce	45 mL
6 Tbsp	extra-virgin olive oil or pistachio nut oil	90 mL
1 Tbsp	crushed fennel seeds	15 mL
½ cup	chopped parsley	125 mL
2 lbs	raw spinach, chopped, or 1 large bag (washed and dried well)	1 kg
1½ cups	grated cheddar cheese	375 mL

Preheat oven to 375°F (190°C). Mix all ingredients except the cheese together, adding each in the order listed. Spread mixture into a buttered casserole dish 9 in × 12 in (22 cm × 30 cm) and sprinkle the top with the grated cheese. Bake for one hour until bubbling hot and the cheese is melted.

Serve with Greek salad, pita, and hummus dip for a Greek treat.

Makes 6 large servings.

CHICKEN FAJITAS

2 Tbsp	extra-virgin olive oil	30 mL
2 Tbsp	water, chicken stock, or vegetable stock	30 mL
2 cups	chicken tenders with tendon removed	500 mL
1 cup	thinly sliced onion	250 mL
1 cup	thinly sliced red pepper	250 mL
⅛ tsp	cayenne pepper	0.5 mL
¼ tsp	cumin	1 mL
¼ tsp	coriander	1 mL
¼ cup	salsa (choose mild or hot)	60 mL
⅛ cup	Omega Essential Balance or Udo's Choice Ultimate Oil Blend	30 mL
1 package	soft tortilla shells	1 package

CONDIMENTS:

Sour cream, salsa, avocado, grated cheese, lettuce, tomato

Place olive oil, water, and chicken tenders in a deep skillet. Sauté on very low heat until chicken is almost cooked. Add onions, red peppers, spices, and salsa. Cook until onions and red peppers are hot and chicken is thoroughly cooked. Remove from heat and stir in Omega Essential Balance Oil or Udo's Choice Ultimate Oil Blend. Heat both sides of the tortilla shells on a hot skillet. Spoon chicken mixture and condiments onto tortilla shell and roll.

Makes 4 servings.

DR. RON'S VEGETARIAN CHILI

This vegetarian chili is quick and easy if you use a food processor to prepare the vegetables and canned beans.

2	large onions, finely chopped	2
8	garlic cloves, minced	8
3 tsp	chili powder (more if you like it very hot)	15 mL
2 tsp	cumin powder	10 mL
2 tsp	coriander powder	10 mL
	salt and pepper to taste	
¼ tsp	cayenne pepper	1 mL
1 cup	finely chopped celery	250 mL
¼ cup	olive oil	60 mL
2–4 tbsp	water	
2 cups	grated carrots	500 mL
2 cups	grated zucchini	500 mL

1	large red pepper, chopped	1
1	large green pepper, chopped	1
2 cups	chopped fresh tomatoes	500 mL
1	can (16 oz/500 g) stewed tomatoes	1
1	can (16 oz/500 g) tomato sauce	1
1	can (8 oz/250 g) tomato paste	1
1	can (14 oz/400 g) kidney beans, drained and rinsed	1
1	can (14 oz/400 g) of pinto beans, drained and rinsed	1
½ cup	Omega Essential Balance or Udo's Choice Ultimate Oil Blend	125 mL
1	small jalapeño pepper, finely chopped (optional)	1

In a very deep, heavy-bottomed pot, sauté (over low to medium heat) the onions, garlic, jalapeno pepper, spices, and celery in the olive oil and water until soft. Add carrots, zucchini, and chopped red and green peppers. Frizzle for 5–10 minutes, stirring occasionally. Add more water if needed to keep veggies from sticking. Add the fresh and stewed tomatoes, sauce, and paste. Add beans. Turn heat down to minimum and let simmer for several hours. Remove from heat and add Omega Essential Balance Oil just before serving. It is great when served with warm, hearty buns and a dollop of sour cream or grated sharp cheese.

Makes 6 servings.

GINGER TOFU

1 lb	firm tofu	0.5 kg
2 tsp	peeled and freshly grated gingerroot	10 mL
2 tsp	sesame seed oil	10 mL
2	garlic cloves, pressed	2
4 Tbsp	organic and wheat-free tamari	60 mL
½ cup	water	125 mL
1 tsp	cornstarch	5 mL
⅛ cup	Omega Essential Balance Oil or Udo's Choice Ultimate Oil Blend	30 mL

Rinse and drain tofu and slice into ½ in (1.5 cm) thick rectangles. Place them in a shallow marinating dish. In a separate bowl, combine gingerroot, sesame oil, garlic, tamari, and water. Pour over tofu pieces. Marinate overnight.

Preheat oven to 325°F (190°C). Drain marinade from tofu and pour into a saucepan. Place tofu on a well-oiled (or nonstick) baking sheet and bake at for 30 minutes.

Mix cornstarch into remaining marinade in saucepan and cook over medium heat, stirring constantly until thick. Remove from heat and stir in Omega Essential Balance Oil before serving. Pour over baked tofu. Serve with rice and Oil-less Vegetable Stir-Frizzle (page 393).

Makes 4 servings.

RATATOUILLE

1	large onion, coarsely chopped	1
6	garlic cloves, minced	6
2 Tbsp	water	30 mL
4 Tbsp	olive oil	60 mL
1	small eggplant, cubed	1
1 cup	tomato sauce	250 mL
1	bay leaf	1
1 tsp	fresh basil	5 mL
1 tsp	oregano	5 mL
⅛ tsp	finely chopped rosemary	0.5 mL
1	large zucchini, cubed	1
1	medium red pepper, cubed (seeds removed)	1
1	medium green pepper, cubed (seeds removed)	1
3	large tomatoes, coarsely chopped	3
3 Tbsp	tomato paste	45 mL
½ cup	Omega Essential Balance Oil or Udo's Choice Ultimate Oil Blend	125 mL
½ cup	chopped parsley	125 mL

In a large, deep pot, frizzle onion and garlic in water and olive oil until onion turns translucent. Add eggplant, tomato sauce, bay leaf, basil, oregano, and rosemary. Mix ingredients, cover, and simmer on low heat for 20 minutes. Stir in zucchini and red and green peppers and simmer for another 5 minutes. Stir in tomatoes and tomato paste. Mix thoroughly. Simmer until vegetables are cooked to desired tenderness. Turn off the heat and stir in Omega Essential Balance Oil or Udo's Choice Oil and chopped parsley.

Add some good hearty bread and a side dish of brown basmati rice and you'll have the full meal deal.

Makes 6 servings.

REFRIED BEANS (FRIJOLES REFRITOS)

This recipe can be used as the filling for enchiladas, tortillas, seven-layer dip, or as a main course with salad.

2	cans (16 oz/454g) black beans or pinto beans (or 2 cups/500 mL raw or 3–4 cups/750 mL–1 L cooked)	2
1	large onion, finely chopped	1
3 Tbsp	olive oil	45 mL
4	garlic cloves, minced	4
1 tsp	coriander	5 mL
1 tsp	cumin	5 mL
½ cup	salsa	125 mL
¼ cup	chopped fresh cilantro	60 mL
⅛ cup	Omega Essential Balance or Udo's Choice Ultimate Oil Blend	30 mL
1 cup	grated Monterey Jack or sharp cheddar cheese	250 mL

Drain the cans of beans, reserving the liquid from one can. Set aside. (If you get gas from eating beans, then discard all the liquid and rinse the beans.)

In a deep skillet, frizzle onion with olive oil, garlic, coriander, and cumin until onion is soft. Slowly add beans, ½ cup (125 mL) at a time. Mash the beans with a potato masher. Add salsa and chopped cilantro. Heat thoroughly. Remove from heat and stir in Omega Essential Balance Oil and Udo's Choice Ultimate Oil Blend. Top with grated cheese.

Refried beans can also be placed in soft tortilla shells with guacamole, sour cream, lettuce, sprouts, tomatoes, salsa, and cheese.

Makes 6 servings.

SOUTHWESTERN CHICKEN AND BLACK BEAN PASTA

¼ cup	olive oil	60 mL
4	garlic cloves, minced	4
2 lbs	chicken tenders (tendon removed)	1 kg
1	medium onion, chopped	1
1	red pepper, diced	1
½ cup	chopped fresh cilantro	125 mL
½ cup	chopped fresh parsley	125 mL
⅛ tsp	cayenne pepper	0.5 mL
1	can (16 oz/500 g) black beans, drained and rinsed	1
1	can tomato paste	1
1	can (16 oz/500 g) stewed tomatoes or 8 large fresh tomatoes, chopped with stems removed	1
6 Tbsp	Omega Garlic-Chili Flax Seed Oil	90 mL
16 oz	cooked whole grain pasta	500 g

freshly grated Parmesan cheese, for garnish
freshly ground pepper, for garnish

In a deep pan, slowly saute olive oil, garlic, chicken, and onions on low heat until thoroughly cooked. Add red pepper, cilantro, parsley, cayenne, and black beans. Cook until heated.

After the chicken, vegetables, and bean mixture has been cooked, add the tomato paste and stewed tomatoes. Simmer for 5 minutes. Remove from heat and add Omega Garlic-Chili Flax Seed Oil. Stir thoroughly, then serve with cooked, drained pasta. Serve hot and garnished with Parmesan cheese and organic freshly ground pepper.

Makes 6 servings.

SPINACH QUICHE

1 cup	grated Swiss cheese or Emmenthal cheese	250 mL
1	prepared piecrust (page 405)	1
6	eggs	6
2	garlic cloves, pressed	2
1 cup	finely crumbled feta cheese	250 mL
½ cup	finely minced onion	125 mL
½ cup	finely chopped mushrooms	125 mL
⅓ cup	finely minced parsley	80 mL
¼ cup	chopped fresh basil	60 mL
½ tsp	dry mustard powder	2 mL
½ cup	milk (soy or rice milk can be substituted)	125 mL
3 Tbsp	oil of your choice (hazelnut, pistachio, etc.)	45 mL
¾ cup	sour cream or plain yogurt	180 mL
1	large bag fresh spinach, washed, dried, and chopped	1

Preheat oven to 400°F (200°C). Spread grated cheese over the bottom of the prepared piecrust. In a bowl beat eggs and add garlic, feta, onion, mushrooms, parsley, basil, dry mustard powder, milk, oil, and sour cream together. Mix in spinach. Pour spinach, egg, and cheese mixture into piecrust. Bake for 10 minutes at 400°F (200°C), then reduce heat to 325°F (165°C) and bake until knife comes out of the center clean, approximately 30 minutes. Let cool for 10 minutes before slicing.

Makes 4 servings.

Condiments

EXCELLENT GINGER SAUCE

This is great with rice, Chinese vegetables, chicken, or seafood. You will probably want to double the recipe because this sauce is so good with a variety of dishes.

½ cup	finely chopped onion	125 mL
2 Tbsp	peeled and grated or finely sliced gingerroot	30 mL
3	garlic cloves, minced	3
2 Tbsp	olive oil or hazelnut oil	30 mL
½ cup	organic and wheat-free tamari	125 mL
½ cup	water	125 mL
2 tsp	Omega Apple Cider Vinegar	10 mL
1 Tbsp	cornstarch	15 mL
2 Tbsp	Omega Essential Balance Oil or Udo's Choice Ultimate Oil Blend	30 mL

Frizzle onion, gingerroot, and garlic in olive oil in a saucepan on low heat. Combine tamari, water, Omega Apple Cider Vinegar, and cornstarch. Whisk until mixed well. Add mixture to saucepan and stir until sauce thickens, about three to five minutes. Remove from heat and stir in Omega Essential Balance Oil. Refrigerate in an airtight container.

Makes 2 cups (500 mL).

HOMEMADE TOMATO KETCHUP

3 lbs	tomatoes	1.5 kg
3 Tbsp	sea salt	45 ml
2 cups	Omega Apple Cider Vinegar	500 mL
3 Tbsp	Sucanat (pure cane sugar available from health food stores)	45 mL
2 tsp	dry mustard powder	10 ml
1 tsp	black pepper	5 ml

Blanch tomatoes to make peeling and seeding easier, then chop tomatoes. Sprinkle with sea salt and let stand for at least three hours. Combine all ingredients in a saucepan and bring to a boil. Let simmer for 30 minutes, stirring frequently. When thick and smooth, fill clean bottles and let sit for a few days in the refrigerator before using.

Makes 2 cups (500 mL).

PESTO

While basil is in season, you can make plenty of pesto and freeze it so you can enjoy the summer's best during the winter.

3 cups	packed fresh basil leaves, washed, dried, and with thick stems removed	750 mL
4–6	garlic cloves, peeled	4–6
½ cup	pine nuts	125 mL
½ cup	freshly grated Parmesan cheese	125 mL
½ cup	Omega Essential Balance Oil, or Udo's Choice Ultimate Oil Blend, or hazelnut oil, or flaxseed oil	125 mL

Add basil leaves, garlic, pine nuts, Parmesan cheese and half of the oil to the food processor and blend until ingredients are well mixed. While the processor is still running, pour in the remaining oil. Pesto will become a thick paste. Keep sealed in refrigerator and use within one day or basil will oxidize and turn black. Cook your favorite pasta and serve it dressed with delicious pesto.

VARIATIONS ON BASIL PESTO:
Sun-Dried Tomato Pesto: Replace half of the basil with a 2 oz (60 g) jar of sun-dried tomatoes (oil drained).

Roasted Red Pepper Pesto: Replace half of the basil with two large roasted red peppers. To roast red peppers, place in a 250°F (120°C) oven for 25 minutes. Turn twice during cooking. Remove from oven and leave to cool on a wire rack. When cool, peel skin and remove seeds. Roasted red peppers are excellent as a side dish with a little Omega Garlic-Chili Flax Seed Oil.
Makes 2 cups (500 mL).

TAHINI SAUCE

1 cup	tahini	250 mL
½ cup	freshly squeezed lemon juice	125 mL
½–1 cup	purified water	125–250 mL
4	garlic cloves	4
1 Tbsp	organic and wheat-free tamari	15 mL
4 Tbsp	extra-virgin olive oil	60 mL

Combine all ingredients in a blender and process until smooth. Refrigerate.
Makes 1½ cups (375 mL).

TZATZIKI (CUCUMBER YOGURT) SAUCE

1 cup	plain yogurt	250 mL
½ cup	grated cucumber	125 mL
4 Tbsp	sunflower, flaxseed, or olive oil	60 mL
2 Tbsp	finely minced onion	30 mL
2	garlic cloves, minced	2

Combine all ingredients. Chill for one hour. Serve with falafels (page 385), pita bread, chicken, spanakopita (page 387), or fresh vegetables.

Makes 1½ cups (375 mL).

Desserts

APPLE CRISP

FILLING:

10–12	large organic cooking apples, peeled and sliced (if you are in a hurry you can leave the peel on)	10–12
	juice of one medium lemon	
½ cup	chopped fresh or frozen cranberries	125 mL
1 tsp	cinnamon	5 mL

TOPPING:

2 cups	raw oats	500 mL
½ cup	whole wheat flour	125 mL
1 tsp	cinnamon	5 mL
¼ tsp	nutmeg	1 mL
¼ cup	sweetened coconut	60 mL
⅛ cup	Omega Hi-Lignan Nutri-Flax or Udo's Wholesome Fast Food Blend	30 mL
¼ cup	chopped nuts (pecans are great)	60 mL
½ cup	honey or real maple syrup	125 mL
1 cup	organic fresh (not from concentrate) apple juice, to be poured over apples and topping	250 mL

Preheat oven to 350°F (180°C).

Mix together apples, lemon juice, cranberries, and cinnamon. Put apple mixture into a deep 8 in × 8 in (20 cm × 20 cm) casserole dish.

Mix topping ingredients until well blended and spread on top of filling. Pour apple juice over entire mixture and bake uncovered until apples are soft, for 45–60 minutes.

A mixture of apples, berries, pears, or peaches makes a very special variation for the filling.

Makes 6 servings.

BLUEBERRY MUFFINS

¾ cup	soy or rice milk	180 mL
1 cup	oatmeal	250 mL
1 cup	unrefined whole wheat flour	250 mL
1 tsp	non-alum baking powder	5 mL
½ tsp	baking soda	2 mL
¼ tsp	sea salt	1 ml
1 cup	organic blueberries	250 mL
1	free-range egg or flax egg substitute	1
¼ cup	melted coconut butter	60 mL
⅓ cup	honey	80 mL

Preheat oven to 400°F (200°C). In a medium bowl combine soy milk and oatmeal; soak for 10 minutes. Combine flour, baking powder, baking soda, and sea salt in separate bowl. Fold in blueberries.

Beat egg lightly in medium bowl. Add melted coconut butter and honey to egg and beat. Blend together egg mixture and oatmeal.

Then add moist mixture to dry mixture and stir lightly. Grease muffin tray or use paper muffin liners. Fill to top. Bake for 20 minutes or until toothpick comes out clean.

Makes 12 muffins.

FIBER-RICH CRANBERRY MUFFINS

⅔ cup	plain yogurt	160 mL
1 Tbsp	organic orange rind grated	15 mL
¼ cup	sunflower oil	60 mL
½ cup	honey	60 mL
1	egg, well-beaten	1
1 cup	chopped (fresh or unsweetened frozen) cranberries	250 mL
½ cup	Omega Hi-Lignan Flax or Udo's Choice Wholesome Fast Food Blend	125 mL
¾ cup	whole wheat flour	180 mL
½ cup	wheat germ	125 mL
1 tsp	baking soda	5 mL

Preheat oven to 350°F (180°C). In a medium bowl combine yogurt, orange rind, oil, honey, egg, and cranberries. In a large bowl combine the remaining ingredients. Quickly mix wet ingredients into the dry, stirring lightly. Grease muffin tray or use paper muffin liners. Fill muffin trays and bake for 20 minutes.

Makes 12 muffins.

HEALTHY DATE MUFFINS

1 cup	whole wheat flour	250 mL
1 cup	oat bran	250 mL
¼ cup	wheat germ	60 mL
¼ cup	Omega Hi-Lignan Flax or	60 mL
	Udo's Choice Wholesome Fast Food Blend	
3 tsp	baking powder	15 mL
⅓ cup	sunflower oil	90 mL
1	egg, well-beaten	1
2 Tbsp	molasses	30 mL
2 tsp	vanilla	10 mL
1 cup	buttermilk or runny yogurt	250 mL
1 cup	finely chopped dates	250 mL
6 Tbsp	Omega Hi-Lignan Flax (to keep dates	90 mL
	from sticking to one another)	

Preheat oven to 350°F (180°C). Mix the first five ingredients and set aside. Mix together the oil, egg, molasses, vanilla, and buttermilk and set aside. Mix chopped dates with Omega Hi-Lignan Flax. Combine all the ingredients. Grease muffin tray or use paper muffin liners. Fill muffin tray and bake for 15–20 minutes or until the center springs back and a toothpick comes out clean.

Makes 12 muffins.

MOM'S PIECRUST

I never liked making piecrust with lard or shortening so we just did not eat pies. My family raved at the flaky texture and delicious flavor of this crust.

4 cups	unbleached white flour	900 g
1 tsp	sea salt	5 mL
1½ cups	Omega Coconut Butter	375 mL
2 tsp	Omega Apple Cider Vinegar	10 mL
1 cup	ice water	250 mL

Mix flour and salt in a large bowl. Cut in Omega Coconut Butter with a pastry knife until crumbly. Add vinegar to water. Stir in two-thirds of water and vinegar to flour mixture. Add in the remaining water and vinegar mixture until dough forms a ball and is not sticky. Refrigerate one hour before rolling into a piecrust. (Keeps up to one week in the fridge or freezer). *Makes 2 double-crust pies.*

PARMESAN CHEESE PIECRUST

This is great for spinach quiche (page 400).

1 cup	sifted whole wheat pastry flour	250 mL
½ cup	grated Parmesan cheese	125 mL
¼ cup	hazelnut or almond oil	60 mL
2 Tbsp	water	30 mL
½ cup	sesame seeds	125 mL

Preheat oven to 250°F (120°C).

Mix together flour and Parmesan cheese. Slowly stir in oil with a fork until thoroughly mixed. Stir in enough water to make dough form a ball. Chill for one hour.

Sprinkle sesame seeds on wax paper and place dough on top. Roll out the dough between two pieces of wax paper. Peel off the top paper and discard. Use the remaining piece of wax paper to help place the piecrust (paper side up) in a 9 in (23 cm) pie pan or quiche dish. The sesame seeds will be visible. Remove and discard the second piece of wax paper. Fill piecrust with desired filling. Bake for 10 minutes. Watch the edge—it may burn if the oven temperature is too high. Cover the edge with foil to stop it from browning too quickly.

Makes 1 single 9 in (23 cm) piecrust.

SNICKER SNACKERS

These are instant treats. Because they are not baked, they contain plenty of enzymes, sterols and sterolin. This recipe is a family favorite that is very quick to make, delicious, and nutritious. These are a great alternative to rum balls at Christmas time. We have to pack extras in the lunch bags for friends at school. Adults love them too!

There are so many variations on this original recipe. When we are out of one of the ingredients, we create our own special mixture. Substitute ground pumpkin seeds, almonds, cashews, finely chopped dates, or raisins. A drop of vanilla or a pinch of cinnamon will give these treats a new twist. Choose seeds and nuts that are organic, raw, unsalted, and not roasted.

½ cup	sunflower seeds*	125 mL
½ cup	sesame seeds*	125 mL
⅓–½ cup	honey	80–125 mL

½ cup	nut butter (cashew, pumpkin, peanut, or a mixture of several)	125 mL
½ cup	unsweetened carob powder	125 mL
¼ cup	Omega Hi-Lignan Flax, or Udo's Choice Wholesome Fast Food Blend, or wheat germ, or oat bran	60 mL
¼ cup	unsweetened coconut	60 mL

*If you are feeding these to toddlers and you are not using a food processor, grind the seeds first in your coffee grinder.

Add the ingredients one at a time and blend in a food processor until the mixture forms a ball. Pinch off small amounts and form into bite-size balls. For a special effect, roll in extra sesame seeds or coconut. Store in an air-tight container and refrigerate.

Makes 24 bite-size balls.

Spreads and Egg Replacement

BETTER BUTTER

We all love the taste of butter, but we know that we should cut down on the quantity we consume. Here is a healthier form of butter.

| 1 lb | salted butter | 500 g |
| 1 cup | Omega Essential Balance oil, or Udo's Choice Ultimate Oil Blend | 250 mL |

Cut butter into eight pieces. Put butter and oil into the food processor and blend until smooth. Spoon into covered container and refrigerate. Not only will you have better butter, but it will remain soft in the refrigerator.

Makes 2 cups (500 mL).

COCONUT BUTTER/FLAXSEED OIL SPREAD

| 1 cup | Omega Coconut Butter | 250 mL |
| ½ cup | flaxseed oil | 125 mL |

Place flaxseed oil in freezer for two hours or more. Melt coconut butter on low temperature. Remove from heat. Add frozen flaxseed oil. Blend and keep in refrigerator for up to six weeks. Store in opaque container to prolong life. Not for cooking or baking.

Makes 1½ cups (375 mL) of spread.

FLAX EGG REPLACER

1 Tbsp	Omega Hi-LignanNutri Flax powder	15 mL
3 Tbsp	water	45 mL

Put Omega Hi-LignanNutri Flax powder in a small bowl. Add water and mix. Let sit for 2–3 minutes. Use when thick. Can be used to replace one egg in recipes.

Makes 1 egg replacement.

MAYONNAISE

2	free-range egg yolks at room temperature	2
¼ tsp	dry mustard	1 mL
1 tsp	freshly squeezed lemon juice	5 mL
¼ tsp	salt	1 mL
½ cup	sunflower seed oil	125 mL
½ cup	flaxseed oil, or Omega Essential Balance Oil, or Udo's Choice Ultimate Oil Blend, or Omega Garlic-Chili Flax Seed Oil (for a spicy mayonnaise)	125 mL

Combine egg, mustard, lemon juice, and salt and blend thoroughly in the food processor. While the processor is still running, slowly add oils drop by drop. Mayonnaise will slowly thicken. Adjust salt and lemon juice to taste.

Mayonnaise Variations: Many ingredients can be added to this basic mayonnaise recipe: fresh, finely chopped herbs; dill, parsley, tarragon, and basil work well. You can also add any or a combination of the following:

1 tsp	curry powder	5 mL
1	puréed avocado	1
1 Tbsp	puréed sun-dried tomatoes	1
1 Tbsp	finely chopped green onion	1

Makes 1 cup (250 mL).

REFERENCES

CHAPTER 1

Batmanghelidj, Fereydoon. *Your Body's Many Cries for Water*. Falls Church, VA: Global Health Solutions, Inc., 1997.

Bogdanov, I.G., et al. "Antitumor action of glycopeptides from cell wall of *Lactobacillus bulgaricus.*" *Bull Exp Biol* 84 (1977): 1750.

Dew M.J., B.K. Evans, and J. Rhodes. "Peppermint oil for irritable bowel syndrome: a multicentre trial." *British Journal of Clinical Practice* 38 (1984): 394–98.

Diamond, Harvey and Marilyn Diamond. *Fit for Life*. New York, NY: Warner Books, Inc., 1985.

Elliot, D.E. "Inflammatory Bowel and Celiac Disease." *Autoimmune Disease.* 3rd ed. Baltimore: Academic Press, 1998.

Garrison, Robert H., Jr. and Elizabeth Somer. *The Nutrition Desk Reference.* 2nd ed. New Canaan, CT: Keats Publishing, Inc., 1990.

Grant, I.R., H.J. Ball, and M.T. Rowe. "Inactivation of Mycobacterium paratuberculosis in cow's milk at pasteurization temperatures." *Applied and Environmental Microbiology* 62 (1996): 631–36.

Grave, G. *Antioxidant Nutrients in Inflammatory Bowel Disease*. Crohn's & Colitis Foundation of America physician letter. www.ccfa.org.

Harries, A.D. and R.V. Heatley. "Nutritional disturbances in Crohn's disease." *Postgraduate Medical Journal* 50 (1983): 690–97.

Harvard School of Medicine, "Digestion." *Consumer Information.* www.intelihealth.com (August 31, 1999).

Holt, Stephen "Gastrointestinal Activity Affects Supplement Efficacy: Reassessment of Formulation Strategies," *Herb Clip.* November 22, 2000.

Murray, Michael T. *Encyclopedia of Nutritional Supplements*. Rocklin, CA: Prima Publishing, 1996.

Nanda, R., et al. "Food intolerance and irritable bowel syndrome." *Gut,* 30, Issue 8 (1998): 1099–104.

Shahani, K., et al. "Benefits of Yogurt." *International Journal of Immunotherapy* 9, no. 1 (1993): 65–68.

Shoda A., et al. "Therapeutic efficacy of N–2 polyunsaturated fatty acid in experimental Crohn's disease." *Journal of Gasteroenterology* 30, no. 8 (1995): 98–101.

Thornton, J.R., P.M. Emmett and K.W. Heaton. "Diet and Crohn's Disease: Characteristics of the pre-illness diet." *British Medical Journal* 2 (1998): 762–64.

Vanderhaeghe, Lorna R. and Patrick J.D. Bouic, *The Immune System Cure.* Scarborough, ON: Prentice-Hall Canada Inc., 1999.

Whitaker, Julian. "Dr. Whitaker's Natural Solutions to Diarrhea." *Health & Healing,* www.drwhitaker.com (November 17, 2000).

CHAPTER 2

Baum, Andrew. "Health Psychology: Mapping Biobehavioral Contributions to Health and Illness." *Annual Reviews Psychology* (1999).

Brehm, Barbara A. *Essays on Wellness.* New York, NY: HarperCollins College Publishers, 1993.

Brodsky, M.A., et al. "Magnesium therapy in new-onset atrial fibrillation." *American Journal of Cardiology* 73 (1994): 1227–29.

Garrison, Robert H., Jr. and Elizabeth Somer. *The Nutrition Desk Reference.* 2nd ed. New Canaan, CT: Keats Publishing, Inc., 1990.

Goldberg, Linn and Diane Elliot. *The Healing Power of Exercise.* New York, NY: John Wiley & Sons, Inc., 2000.

Hjermann I. "The metabolic cardiovascular syndrome including Syndrome X, Reaven's syndrome, insulin resistance syndrome, artherthrombogenic syndrome." *Journal Cardiovascular Pharmacology* 20 (supplement) (1992): S5–S10.

Imamura H., et al. "Relationship of cigarette smoking to blood pressure and serum lipids and lipoproteins in men." *Clin Exp Pharmacol Physiol* 23 (1996): 397–402.

Kritz H., P. Schmid, and H. Sinzinger. "Passive smoking and cardiovascular risk." *Arch Intern Med* 155 (1995): 1942–48.

Littarru, G.P. *Energy and Defense, Facts and perspectives on Coenzyme Q10 in biology and medicine.* Roma, Italy: Casa Editrice Scientifica Internazionale, 1995.

Longnecker, M.P. "Do trans fatty acids in margarine and other foods increase the risk of coronary heart disease?" *Epidemiology* 4 (1993): 492.

Merck Website, *Consumer Health Information www.merck.com.*

Muller, M.M., et al. "The relationship between habitual anger, coping strategies and serum lipid and lipoprotein concentrations." *Biol Psychol* 41 (1995): 69–82.

Murray, M.T. *Heart Disease and High Blood Pressure.* Rocklin, CA: Prima Publishing, 1997.

Natural Medicine Online. "Patients taking prescription drugs need to be nutrition–conscious." www.nat-med.com/archives/nutritiontable.htm (March 2000).

Nityanand, S., et al. "Clinical trials with Gugulipid, a new hypolipidaemic agent." *Journal of Associated Physicians of India* 37 (1989): 321–28.

Pelton, R. and J. LaValle. *The Nutritional Cost of Prescription Drugs.* Englewood, CO: Morton Publishing Company, 2000.

Scanu, A.M. and G.M. Fless. "Lipoprotein (a), A genetic risk factor for premature coronary heart disease." *JAMA* 267 (1992): 3326–29.

Stanto, J.L. and D.R. Keast. "Serum cholesterol, fat intake, and breakfast consumption in the United States adult population." *Journal of the American College of Nutrition* 8 (1989): 567–72.

Vahouny, G.V. and D. Kritchevsky. "Plant and marine sterols and cholesterol metabolism." *Nutritional Pharmacology* 4 (1981): 31–72.

Weiss, Decker. "Cardiovascular Disease: Statistics, Pathophysiology and Treatment According to the Natural Paradigm." *Natural Medicine Online.* www.nat–med.com (November 2000).

CHAPTER 3

Alm, J.S., et al. "Atopy in children of families with anthroposophic lifestyle." *Lancet* 353 (May 1, 1999): 1485.

Becker, Wayne and David Deamer, *The World of the Cell.* 2nd ed., Redwood City, CA: The Benjamin/Cummings Publishing Company, Inc., 1991.

Bigazzi, P.E. "Autoimmunity Caused by Xenobiotics." *Toxicology* 119 (1997): 1–21.

Bland, Jeffrey. *Medical Applications of Clinical Nutrition.* New Canaan, CT: Keats Publishing, 1983.

Bouic, P.J.D. "Sterols/Sterolins, The Natural, Non-toxic Immunomodulators and Their Role in the Control of Rheumatoid Arthritis." 1998 preliminary research results paper.

Buhl, R, et al. "Systemic glutathione deficiency in symptom-free HIV-seropositive individuals." *Lancet* 2 (1989): 1294–97.

Carpenter, Siri. "Modern Hygiene's Dirty Tricks." *Science News* 156, no. 7 (October 30, 2000): 108.

Cohen, S. and B.S. Rabin. "Psychological Stress, Immunity and Cancer." *Journal of the National Cancer Institute* 90 (1998): 3–4.

Diodati, Catherine. *Immunization, History, Ethics, Law and Health.* Windsor, ON: Integral Aspects, Inc., 1999. (See additional reference in excerpted section from her book.)

Germano, Carl and William Cabot, *The Osteoporosis Solution.* New York, NY: Kensington Books, 1999.

Granville, D., et al. "Apoptosis: molecular aspects of cell death and disease." *Lab Invest* 78 (1998): 893–913.

Grimble, R.F. "Nutritional modulation of cytokine biology." *Nutrition* 14, no. 7 (1998): 634–40.

Jefferies, William, McK. *Safe Uses of Cortisol.* 2nd ed. Springfield, IL: Charles C. Thomas Publishers, 1996.

Mackay, Ian R. "Tolerance and Autoimmunity." *British Medical Journal* 321 (July 8, 2000): 93-96.

Marshall, E. "A shadow falls on Hepatitis B vaccination effort." *Science* 281 (1998): 630–31.

Meydani, S.N., et al. "Vitamin B-6 deficiency impairs interleukin-2 production and lymphocyte proliferation in elderly adults." *American Journal of Clinical Nutrition* 53 (1991): 1275–80.

Meydani, S.N., et al. "Vitamin supplementation enhances cell-mediated immunity in healthy elderly subjects." *American Journal of Clinical Nutrition* 52 (1990): 557–63.

Newmark, Thomas and Paul Schulick, *Beyond Aspirin.* Prescott, AZ: Hohm Press, 2000.

Nordlink K. "Toxic metals and immune function." *International Clinical Nutrition Review* 9, no. 4 (1989): 175–81.

Peakman, Mark and Diego Vergani, *Basic and Clinical Immunology.* New York, NY: Churchill Livingstone, 1997.

Prasher, Deepak. "Traffic noise increases stress by driving up cortisol." *Lancet Interactiv, www.lancet.com* (October 10, 1998).

Rasmussen, A.F., Jr. "Emotions and Immunity." *Annals of the New York Academy of Sciences* 164, no. 2 (1969): 458–62.

Ropper, A.H. and M. Victor. "Influenza vaccination and the Guillain–Barre syndrome." *New England Journal of Medicine* 339 (1998): 1845–46.

Rose, Noel R. and Ian R. Mackay, eds. *The Autoimmune Diseases.* San Diego, CA: Academic Press, 1998.

Sanchez, A., et al. "Role of sugars in human neutrophilic phagocytosis." *American Journal of Clinical Nutrition* 26 (1973): 180.

Sapse, A.T. "Cortisol, high cortisol diseases and anticortisol therapy." *Psychoneuoendocrinology* 22 (September 1997): S3.

Shoenfeld, Y. and A. Aron-Maor. "Vaccination and Autoimmunity—'Vaccinosis': A Dangerous Liaison?" *Journal of Autoimmunity* 14, no. 1 (February 2000): 1–10.

Soloman, G.F. "Emotions, Stress, the Central Nervous System and Immunity." *Annals of the New York Academy of Sciences* 164, no. 2 (1969): 335–43.

Sompayrac, Lauren. *How the Immune System Works*. Malden, MA: Blackwell Science, Inc., 1999.

Steen, V.D., et al. "D-penicillamine therapy in progressive systemic scleroderma. A retrospective analysis." *Annals of Internal Medicine* 97 (1982): 652–59.

Tashiro, Tsuguhiko, et al. "N-3 versus N-6 polyunsaturated fatty acids in critical illness." *Nutrition* 14, no. 6 (1998): 551–53.

Tortora, Gerard J. and Nichola P. Anagnostakos. *Principles of Anatomy and Physiology*. 6th ed. New York, NY: Harper & Row, 1990.

Vanderhaeghe, Lorna R. and Patrick J.D. Bouic. *The Immune System Cure*. Scarborough, ON: Prentice-Hall Canada Inc., 1999.

Werbach, Melvyn R. *Nutritional Influences on Illness*. Tarzana, CA: Third Line Press, 1993.

CHAPTER 4

American Council on Science and Health. *Endocrine Disrupters: A Scientific Perspective*. New York, NY: American Council on Science and Health, 1999.

Aviram, M. and K. Eigs. "Dietary Olive Oil Reduces Low-Density Lipoprotein Uptake by Macrophages and Decreases the Susceptibility of the Lipoprotein to Undergo Lipid Peroxidation." *Annals of Nutrition and Metabolism* 37 (1995): 75–89.

Babal, K. "Food as Medicine: Maitake mushroom fights cancer." *Health Store News* 4 (January/February 1999).

Balch, James F. and Phyllis A. Balch. *Prescription for Dietary Wellness*. Greenfield, IN: PAB Books, Inc., 1992.

Barone, J., J.R. Hebert, and M.M. Reddy. "Dietary Fat and Natural Killer Cell Activity." *American Journal of Clinical Nutrition* 50 (1989): 861–67.

Batmanghelidj, Fereydoon. *Your Body's Many Cries for Water*. Falls Church, VA: Global Health Solutions, Inc., 1997.

Beck, Leslie. *The Complete Idiot's Guide to Total Nutrition for Canadians*. Scarborough, ON: Prentice Hall Canada, 2000.

Bianchi-Salvadori, B. and R. Vesely. "Lactic Acid Bacteria and Intestinal Microflora." *Microecology and Therapy* 25 (1995): 247–55.

Block, G. "Vitamin C and Cancer Prevention: The Epidemiologic Evidence." *American Journal of Clinical Nutrition* 53 (1991): 270–82.

Calomme, M., et al. "Seleno-Lactobacillus: An Organic Selenium Source." *Biological Trace Element Research* 47 (1995): 379–83.

Carper, J. *Food, Your Miracle Medicine*. New York, NY: Harper Perennial, 1993.

Caygill, C.P., et al. "Fat, fish, fish oil and cancer." *British Journal of Cancer* 74 (1996): 159–64.

Challem, J. "Soy Isoflavones for Women's Health." *Nutrition Science News* 3, no. 9 (1998).

Challem, J. "The Paleolithic Diet Versus Modern Diet: You Are What Your Ancestors Ate." *The Nutrition Reporter* 9 (1998): 1.

Chisaka, T. *Chemical and Pharmaceutical Bulletin* (1988). Cited in: "Green Tea." *The Cancer Solution*. Boca Raton, FL: Peltec Publishing, 1994, p. 75.

DeStefani, E., et al. "Dietary Fiber and Risk of Breast Cancer." *Nutrition and Cancer* 28 (1997): 14–19.

Diamond, Harvey and Marilyn Diamond. *Fit for Life*. New York, NY: Warner Books, Inc., 1985.

Diamond, W. John, W. Lee Cowden, and Burton Goldberg, *Definitive Guide to Cancer*. Tiburon, CA: Future Medicine Publishing, Inc., 1997.

Easterbrook, Kimberly. "Water: Nature's Internal Bath." *Alive Magazine* (March 2001).

Eaton S.B., S.B. Eaton III, and M.J. Konner. "Paleolithic Nutrition Revisited: a Twelve–year Restrospective on its Nature and Implications." *European Journal of Clinical Nutrition* 51 (1997): 207–16.

Erasmus, Udo. *Fats that Heal, Fats that Kill*. Burnaby, BC: Alive Books, 1997.

Erasmus, Udo. *Press Releases: Harvard School of Public Health*. www.fatsthatheal.com.

Ernst, E. "Can Allium Vegetables Prevent Cancer?" *Phytomedicine* 4 (1997): 79–83.

Franceschi, S., et al. "Intake of Macronutrients and Risk of Breast Cancer." *The Lancet* 347 (1996): 1351.

Francheschi, S., et al. "Tomatoes and Risk of Digestive Tract Cancers. *International Journal of Cancer* 59 (1994): 181–84.

Gao, Y.T., et al. "Reduced Risk of Esophageal Cancer Associated with Green Tea Consumption." *Journal of the National Cancer Institute* 86 (1994): 855–58.

Garewal, H. "Antioxidants in Oral Cancer Prevention." *American Journal of Clinical Nutrition* (1995) 62: 1410S–1416S.

Gerhauser, C., et al. "Cancer Chemoprevention Potential of Sulforamate, a Novel Analogue of Sulforaphane that Induces Phase 2 Drug Metabolizing Enzymes." *Cancer Research* 57 (1997): 272–78.

Germano, Carl and William Cabot. *The Osteoporosis Solution*. New York, NY: Kensington Books, 1999.

Getchell, K. "The Role of Soy Products in Reducing Risk of Cancer." *Journal of the National Cancer Institute* 83 (1991): 8.

Gould, G.G. "Absorbability of Beta–Sitosterol." *The New York Academy of Sciences* 18 (1955): 129–34.

Graci, S. *The Power of Superfoods*. Toronto, ON: Prentice Hall, 1997.

Haddad, J.G., et al. "Circulating Phytosterols in Normal Females, Lactating Mothers and Breast Cancer Patients." *Clinical Endocrinology* 30 (1970): 174–80.

Haggans, C.J., et al. "Effects of flaxseed consumption on urinary estrogen metabolites in postmenopausal women." *Nutrition and Cancer* 33 (1999).

Hannigan, B. "Diet and Immune Function." *British Journal of Biomedical Sciences* 51 (1994): 252–59.

Herman, Robin. "Higher Intake of Dairy Products May Be Linked to Prostate Cancer Risk." *Harvard School of Public Health Press Release* (April 4, 2000).

Howe, G. R., et al. "Dietary Factors and Risk of Breast Cancer. Combined analysis of 12 Case Control Studies." *Journal of the National Cancer Institute* 82 (1990): 561–69.

Jankun, J., et al. "Why Drinking Green Tea Could Prevent Cancer." *Nature* 387 (1997): 501.

Keuneke, Robin. *Total Breast Health*. New York, NY: Kensington Books, 1998.

Kinsella, J. and B. Lokesh. "Dietary Lipids, Eicosanoids, and the Immune System." *Critical Care Medicine* 18 (1990): 1.

Klaunig, J.E. "Chemopreventive Effects of Green Tea Components on Hepatic Carcinogenesis." *Preventative Medicine* 21 (1992): 510–19.

Konno, Sensuke. "Maitake D-Fraction: Apoptosis Inducer and Immune Enhancer." *Natural Medicine Online.* www.nat–med.com (October 2000).

Kristal, A., J. Cohen, and J. Stanford. "Veggies may cut by half risk of prostate cancer." *Seattle Times* (January 4, 2000).

La Vecchia, C., et al. "Olive Oil and Breast Cancer Risk in Italy." *Nutrition Research Newsletter* 15 (1996): 12.

Li, G., et al. "Anti-proliferative Effects of Garlic Constituents in Cultured Human Breast Cancer Cells." *Oncology Reports* 2 (1995): 787–91.

"Latest Research Reveals Outstanding Properties of Natural Tomato Lycopene." www.lycopene.com. (2000).

Martin-Moreno, J.M., et al. "Dietary fat, Olive Oil Intake and Breast Cancer Risk." *International Journal of Cancer* 58 (1994): 774–80.

Mead, Nathaniel. *Udder Nonsense: Why Milk Is No Longer Required or Recommended.* New York, NY: Avery Publishing Group, 1995.

Mizuno T. "Shiitake Lentinus edodes: Functional properties for medicinal and food purposes." *Food Rev Int* 11 (1995): 111–28.

Nair, P.P., et al. "Diet, Nutrition Intake and Metabolism in Populations at High and Low Risk for Colon Cancer." *The American Journal of Clinical Nutrition* 40 (1984): 927–30.

Nanba, H., et al. "The chemical structure of an antitumor polysaccharide in fruit bodies of Grifola frondosa (maitake)." *Chem Pharm Bull* 35 (1987): 1162–68.

Newberne, P.M. "Dietary Fat, Immunological Response and Cancer in Rats." *Cancer Research* 41 (1981): 3783–85.

Newmark, Thomas M. and Paul Schulick. *Beyond Aspirin.* Prescott, AZ: Hohm Press, 2000.

Pauling, L. *How to Live Longer and Feel Better.* New York, NY: W.H. Freeman & Company, 1986.

Pegel, K.H. "The Importance of Sitosterol and Sitosterolin in Human and Animal Nutrition." *South African Journal of Science* 93 (1997): 263–68.

Pelton, Ross and James LaValle. *The Nutritional Cost of Prescription Drugs.* Englewood, CO: Morton Publishing Company, 2000.

Quillan, P. and N. Quillan. *Beating Cancer with Nutrition.* Tulsa, OK: Nutrition Times Press, 1994.

Ringsdorf, W.R., Jr., E. Cheraskin, and R.R. Ramsay, Jr. "Sucrose, Neutrophilic Phagocytosis and Resistance to Disease." *Dental Survey* 52 (1976): 46–48.

Rogers, Sherry. A. *Tired or Toxic,* Syracuse, NY: Prestige Publishers, 1990.

Salen, G., et al. "Metabolism of b–sitosterol in Man." *J Clin Invest* 49 (1970): 952–67.

Schuler, I., et al. "Soybean Phosphatidylcholine Vesicles Containing Plant Sterols: a Fluorescence Anisotropy Study." *Biochimica et Biophysica Acta* 1028 (1990): 82–88.

Shahani K., et al. "Anticarcinogenic and Immunological Properties of Dietary Lactobacilli." *Journal of Food Protection* 53 (1990): 704–10.

Shahani, K., et al. "Benefits of Yogurt." *International Journal of Immunotherapy* 9, no. 1 (1993): 65–68.

Shao, Z.M., et al. "Genistein exerts multiple suppressive effects on human breast carcinoma cells." *Cancer Research* 58 (1998).

Stimpel, M., et al. "Macrophage Activation and Induction of Macrophage Cytotoxicity by Purified Polysaccharide Fraction from the Plant Echinaceae Purpurea." *Infection and Immunity* 46 (1984): 845–49.

Teas, J. "The Consumption of Seaweed as a Protective Factor in the Etiology of Breast Cancer." *Medical Hypotheses* 7 (1981): 601–13.

Thresiamma, K., et al. "Protective Effect of Curcumin, Ellagic Acid and Bixin on radiation-induced toxicity." *Indian Journal of Experimental Biology* 34 (1996): 845–47.

Vanderhaeghe, Lorna R. and Patrick J.D. Bouic. *The Immune System Cure.* Scarborough, ON: Prentice Hall Canada Inc., 1999.

Verhoeven, D.T., et al. "Epidemiological Studies on Brassica Vegetables and Cancer Risk." *Cancer Epidemiological Biomarkers* 5 (1996): 733–747.

Wade, Michael. *Human Health and Exposure to Chemicals which Disrupt Estrogen, Androgen and Thyroid Hormone Physiology.* Environmental Health Directive, Health Protection Branch, Health Canada.

Wang, C., et al. "Lignans and Flavonoids Inhibit Aromatase Enzyme in Human Preadipocytes." *Journal of Steroid Biochemistry and Molecular Biology* 50 (1994): 205–12.

Weihrauch, J.L. and J.M. Gardner. "Sterol Content of Foods of Plant Origin." *Journal of The American Dietetic Association* 73 (1978): 39–47.

Whitaker, Julian. "Research Roundup: Green Tea." *Health & Healing* 10, no. 9 (September 2000).

Whitaker, Julian. "Drink More Water!" *Health & Healing* 10, no. 8 (August 2000).

Wolfson, Richard. "Biotech News." *Alive Magazine* (March 2001).

Wong, J.L. "Cancer and Chemicals and Vegetables." *Chemtech* 16 (1986): 100–07.

Wright, J.V. and J. Morgenthaler. *Natural Hormone Replacement for Women over 45.* Petaluma, CA: Smart Publications, 1997.

Wright, Jonathan V. *Is Estrogen Carcinogenic?* Petaluma, CA: Smart Publications, 2000.

Yip, I., et al. "Nutritional Approaches to the Prevention of Prostate Cancer Progression." *Advances in Experimental Medicine and Biology* 399 (1996): 173–81.

Yu, T.G., et al. "Reduced Risk of Esophageal Cancer Associated with Green Tea Consumption." *Journal of the National Cancer Institute* 86 (1994): 855–58.

Yudkin, J. *Sweet and Dangerous.* New York, NY: Peter H. Wyden Publishers, 1972.

Zava, D.T. and G. Euwe. "Estrogenic and Antiproliferative Properties of Genistein and Other Flavonoids in Human Breast Cancer Cells in Vitro." *Nutrition and Cancer* 27 (1997): 31–40.

Zheng, W., et al. "Retinol, Antioxidant Vitamins, and Cancers of the Upper Digestive Tract in a Prospective Cohort Study of Postmenopausal Women." *American Journal of Epidemiology* 142 (1995): 955–60.

Zheng, W., et al. "Tea Consumption and Cancer incidence in a prospective cohort study of postmenopausal women." *American Journal of Epidemiology* 144 (1996): 175–82.

CHAPTER 5

Ali, Elvis, et al. *Natural Remedies and Supplements.* Niagara Falls, NY: AGES Publications, 2000.

Alschuler, L. "Milk thistle: goals and objectives." *International Journal of Integrative Medicine* 1, no. 1 (1999): 29–34.

American Institute for Cancer Research, "Selenium: High in Prevention Potential," *AICR Research News.* www.aicr.org (1999).

Andrews, E. "In Germany, Humble Herb is Rival to Prozac." *New York Times.* (September 9, 1997).

Bates, Charles. *Essential Fatty Acids and Immunity in Mental Health.* Tacoma, WA: Life Sciences Press, 1987.

Beck, Leslie. *Managing Menopause.* Toronto, ON: Prentice Hall, 2000.

Bendich, A. "Carotenoids and the Immune Response." *Journal of Nutrition* 119 (1989): 112–15.

Berges, R.R., et al. "Randomized placebo-controlled, double-blind clinical trial of B-sitosterol in patients with benign prostatic hyperplasia." *Lancet* 345 (1995): 1529–32.

Blumenthal, Mark, A. Goldberg, and J. Brinckman. *Herbal Medicine: Expanded Commission E Monographs*. Newton, MA: Integrative Communications, 2000.

Bouic, P.J.D. "Immunomodulation in HIV/AIDS: The Tygerberg/Stellenbosch University Experience." *AIDS Bulletin* 6 (1997): 18–20.

Bouic, P.J.D. "Sterols/Sterolins, the natural, nontoxic immunomodulators and their role in the control of rheumatoid arthritis." *Arthritis Trust of America Newsletter* (Summer 1998).

Bouic, P.J.D., et al. "The effects of B-sitosterol (BSS) and B-sitosterol glucoside (BSSG) mixture on selected immune parameters of marathon runners: Inhibition of post marathon immune suppression and inflammtion." *Int J Sp Med* 20 (1999): 258–62.

Bouic, P.J.D., R.W. Etsebeth and, C.F. Liebenberg. "Beta-sitosterol and beta-sitosterol glucoside stimulate human peripheral blood lymphocyte proliferation: implications for their use a an immunomodulatory vitamin combination." *Int J. Immunopharmac* 18 (1996): 693–700.

Bradlow, H.L., et al. "Indole-3-carbinol. A novel approach to breast cancer prevention." *Ann N Y Acad Sci* 768 (1995): 180–200.

Braverman, Eric R. and Carl C. Pfeiffer. *The Healing Nutrients Within*. New Canaan, CT: Keats Publishing, Inc., 1987.

Bray, T.M. and C.G. Taylor. "Enhancement of tissue glutathione for antioxidant and immune functions in malnutrition." *Biochemical Pharmacology* (1994).

Buhl, R., et al. "Systemic glutathione deficiency in symptom-free HIV-seropositive individuals." *Lancet* 2 (1989): 1294–97.

Bum, M.K., et al. "Association of vitamin B6 status with parameters of immune function in early HIV infection." *J AIDS* (1991).

Burger, R.A., A.R. Torres, and R.P. Warren. "Echinacea-induced cytokine production by human macrophages." *International Journal of Immunopharmacology* 19, no. 7 (1997): 371–79.

Callahan, L.F., J. Rao and, M. Boutaugh. "Arthritis and Women's Health: Prevalence, Impact and Prevention." *Am J Pre Med* 12, no. 5 (1996): 401–09.

Campbell, S.S. and R.J. Broughton, "Rapid decline in body temperature before sleep: fluffing the physiological pillow?" *Chronobiol Int* 11 (1994): 126–31.

Carbin, B.E., B. Larson, and O. Lindake. "Treatment of benign prostatic hyperplasia with phytosterols." *B J Urol* 66 (1990): 629–41.

Challem, Jack, "Zinc supplements can boost immunity, improve sense of taste some of the time." *The Nutrition Reporter* 9, no. 10 (1998).

Challem, Jack. "NAC: The Best Cold and Flu Remedy Yet?" *The Nutrition Reporter™*, www.thenutritionreporter.com (2000).

Chantre, P., et al. "Efficacy and tolerance of *Harpagophytum procumbens* versus diacerhein in treatment of osteoarthritis." *Phytomedicine* 7, no. 3, (2000): 177–83.

Cleary, J.P. "The NAD Deficiency Diseases." *Journal of Orthomolecular Psychiatry* (1989): 149–57.

Cuccinelli, Janet, "Alternative Medicine: Echinacea." *Clinician Reviews* (September 1999).

Deodhar, S.D., et al. "Preliminary studies on anti-rheumatic activity of curcumin." *Ind J Med Res* 71 (1980): 633.

Diamond, W. John, W. Lee Cowden, and Burton Goldberg. *Definitive Guide to Cancer*. Tiburon, CA: Future Medicine Publishing, Inc., 1997.

Duda, R.B., et al. "American ginseng and breast cancer therapeutic agents synergistically inhibit MCF-7 breast cancer cell growth." *Journal of Surgical Oncology* 72 (1999): 230–39.

Eby, G.A., et al. "Reduction in duration of the common cold by zinc gluconate lozenges in a double-blind study." *Antimicrobial Agents Chemotherapy*. 1984.

Ewan, C., et al. "Ascorbic Acid and Cancer: A Review." *Cancer Research* 39 (1979): 663–81.

Farmer, J.A. and A.M. Gotto, Jr. "Currently available hypolipidaemic drugs and future therapeutic developments." *Baillieres Clin Endocrinol Metab* 9 (1995): 825–47.

Finnegan, John. *The Facts About Fats*; A Consumer's Guide to Good Oils. Berkelely, CA: Celestial Arts, 1993.

Fishman, J., et al. "Increased estrogen-16 alpha–hydroxylase activity in women with breast and endometrial cancer." *J Steroid Biochem* 20, no. 4B (1984): 1077–81.

Folkers, K., et al. "Increase in levels of IgG in serum of patients treated with coenzyme Q10." *Res Commun Chem Pathol Pharmacol* 1982.

Fortes, C. "Aging, zinc, and cell-mediated immune responses." *Aging Clinical and Experimental Research* 7 (1995): 75–76.

Franceschi, S., et al. "Tomatoes and Risk of Digestive Tract Cancers." *International Journal of Cancer* 59 (1994): 181–84.

Garewal, H.S. "Antioxidants in Oral Cancer Prevention." *American Journal of Clinical Nutrition* 62 Supplement (1995).

Ge, X., et al. "3,3'-Diindolylmethane induces apoptosis in human cancer cells." *Biochemical and Biophysical Research Communications* 228 (1996): 153–65.

Germano, Carl and William Cabot. *The Osteoporosis Solution*. New York, NY: Kensington Books, 1999.

Geusens, P., et al. "Long-term effect of omega-3 fatty acid supplementation in active rheumatoid arthritis. A 12-month, double-blind, controlled study." *Arthritis Rheum* 37, no. 6 (1994): 824–29.

Goldberg, Burton and editors. *Alternative Medicine Guide to Women's Health 2*. Tiburon, CA: Future Medicine Publishing, Inc., 1998.

Head, Kathleen A. "Inositol Hexaniacinate: A Safer Alternative to Niacin." *Townsend Letter for Doctors and Patients* (April 2000): 88–92.

Health Sciences Institute. "Free Yourself from Chronic Fatigue with 'Nature's All-day High'." *Members Alert* 4, no. 8, (February 2000).

Hemila, H. "Does Vitamin C Alleviate the Symptoms of the Common Cold. A Review of Current Evidence." *Scandianavian Journal of Infectious Diseases* 26 (1994): 4–5.

Heuser, G. and A. Vojdani. "Enhancement of natural killer cell activity and T and B cell function by buffered vitamin C in patients exposed to toxic chemicals: The role of protein Kinase C." *Immunopharmacology and Immunotoxicology* (1997).

Holman, Ralph, Susan Johnson, and Paul Ogburn. "Deficiency of essential fatty acids and membrane fluidity during pregnancy and lactation." *Biochemistry*, Proceedings of the National Academy of Science. Vol. 88 (June 1991): 4835–39.

Ivorra, M.D., et al. "Anti-hyperglycemic and insulin releasing effects of beta-sitosterol, 3-B-D glucoside and its aglycone Beta-sitosterolin." *Arch Int Pharmacodyn Ther* 296 (1988): 224–31.

Jacob, Stanley W., Ronald M. Lawrence, and Martin Zucker. *The Miracle of MSM: The Natural Solution for Pain.* New York, NY: Penguin Putnam, Inc., 1999.

Jeng, Kee-Ching G., et al. "Supplementation with vitamin C and E enhances cytokine production by peripheral blood mononuclear cells in healthy adults." *American Journal of Clinical Nutrition* (1996).

Jolly, P., et al. "Vitamin A deficiency in HIV infection and AIDS." *AIDS* (1996).

Julius, M., et al. "Glutathione and morbidity in a community-based sample of elderly." *Journal of Clinical Epidemiology* (1994).

Kiremidijian-schumacher, L., et al. "Supplementation with Selenium and Human Immune Cell Function. Its Effect on Cytotoxic Lymphocytes and Natural Killer Cells." *Biological Trace Element Research* 41 (1994): 115–27.

Knekt, P., et al. "Serum Vitamin E Level and Risk of Female Cancers." *International Journal of Epidemiology* 17 (1988): 281–86.

Korpan, M.I. and V. Fialka, "Wobenzym and diuretic therapy in lymphedema after breast operation." *Wien Med Wochenschr* 146, no. 4 (1996): 67–72 [in Zelig].

Lawrence, R.M. "Methylsulfonylmethane (MSM): A double-blind study of its use in degenerative arthritis." *International Journal of Anti-Aging Medicine* 1, no. 1 (Summer 1998): 50.

Levander, O. and M. Beck. "Selenium deficiency results in viral virulence." *Journal of the American College of Nutrition* (1996).

Li, M., et al. "Clinical observation of the therapeutic effect of ginkgo leaf concentrated oral liquor on bronchial asthma." *CJIM* 3 (1997): 264–67.

Lockwood, K., et al. "Partial and complete regression of breast cancer in patients in relation to dosage of coenzyme Q10." *Biochemical and Biophysical Research Communications* 1999 (1994): 1504–08.

Mara, J,. et al. "Glutathione and Morbidity in a Community-based Sample of Elderly." *Journal of Clinical Epidemiology* 47 (1994): 1021–36.

Messina, M. and S. Barnes. "The Role of Soy Products in Reducing Risk of Cancer." *Journal of the National Cancer Institute* 83 (1991): 541–42.

Moghadasian, M.H. and J.J. Frohlich. "Effects of dietary phytosterols on cholesterol metabolism and atherosclerosis: Clinical and experimental evidence." *American Journal of Medicine* 107 (2000): 588–94.

Morreale, P., et al. "Comparison of the anti-inflammatory efficacy of chondroitin sulfate and diclofenac sodium in patients with knee osteoarthritis." *J Rheumatol* 23, no. 8 (1996): 1285–1391.

Moyers, Bill. *Trade Secrets: A Moyers Report.* Public Affairs Television, Inc. Aired on PBS, March 26, 2001.

Murray, Michael T. *Encyclopedia of Nutritional Supplements.* Rocklin, CA: Prima Publishing, 1996.

Murray, Michael T. *Heart Disease and High Blood Pressure.* Rocklin, CA: Prima Publishing, 1997.

Nityanand, S., J.S. Srivastava, and O.P. Asthana. "Clinical trials with gugulipid, a new hypolipidaemic agent." *J Assoc Phys India* 37 (1989): 321–28.

Oh, W.K., et al. "Activity of the herbal combination, PC SPES, in the treatment of patients with androgen-independent prostate cancer." *Urology* 57, no. 1 (January 2001): 122–26.

Panush, R.S., et al. "Diet therapy for rheumatoid arthritis." *Arthritis Rheumat* 26 (1983): 462–71.

Passwater, Richard A. *All About Selenium.* Garden City Park, NY: Avery Publishing Group, 1999.

Patton, S., et al. "Carotenoids of Human Colostrum." *Lipids* 3 (1990): 159–65.

Pegel, K.H. "The importance of sitosterol and sitosterolin in human and animal nutrition." *S Afr J Sci* 93 (1997): 263–68.

Pettit, Jeremy L. "Alternative Medicine: Melatonin." *Clinician Reviews*. (June 2000).

Pettit, Jeremy L. "Alternative Medicine: Milk Thistle." *Clinician Reviews*. (October 2000).

Pinget, M. and A. Lecomte. "The effects of harpagophytum capsules (Arkocaps) in degenerative rheumatology." *Medecine Actuelle* 12, no. 4 (1985): 65–67.

Prasad, A.S. "Effect of Vitamin E Supplementation on Leukocyte Function." *American Journal of Clinical Nutrition* 33 (1980): 606.

Prasad, A.S. "Zinc: An overview." *Nutrition Reviews* (1995).

Ronneberg, R. and B. Skara. "Essential fatty acids in human colostrum." *Acta Paediatra* 82, no. 10 (1992): 779–83.

Rump, J.A., et al. "Treatment of diarrhea in human immunodeficiency virus-infected patients with immunoglobulins from bone colostrum." *Clin Investig* 70, no. 7 (1992): 588–94.

Sandstead, Harold and Nancy Alcock. "Zinc: An Essential and Unheralded Nutrient." *Journal of Laboratory and Clinical Medicine* (1997).

Sazawal, S., et al., "Zinc supplementation reduces the incidence of acute lower respiratory infections in infants and preschool children: A double-blind, controlled study." *Pediatrics* 102 (1998): 1–5.

Schmid B, et al.: "Analgesic effects of willow bark extract in osteoarthritis: results of a clinical double-blind trial." *Fact* 3 (1998): 3–186.

Schwartz, E.R. "The modulation of osteoarthritis development by Vitamin C and Vitamin E." *Int J Vit Nutr Res* 26 (1984): 141.

See, D.M., et al. "In vitro effects of echinacea and ginseng on natural killer and antibody-dependent cell cytotoxicity in healthy subjects and chronic fatigue syndrome or acquired immunodeficiency syndrome patients." *Immunopharmacology* 35, no. 3 (1997): 229–35.

Shamsuddin, Abul Kalam M., *IP-6: Nature's Revolutionary Cancer Fighter*. New York, NY: Kensington Books, 1998.

Shoskes, D.A. "Use of the bioflavonoid quercetin in patients with longstanding chronic prostatitis." *Journal of the American Nutraceutical Association* 2 (1999): 36–39.

Singh, G.B. and C.K. Atal. "Pharmacology of an extract of salai guggal ex-Bosewellia serrata, a new non-steroidal anti-inflammatory agent." *Agents Action* 18 (1986): 407–12.

Stoff, Jesse, A. and Dallas Clouatre. *The Prostate Miracle, New Natural Therapies That Can Save Your Life!* New York, NY: Kensington Books, 2000.

Straussberg, R., et al. "Phagocytosis-promoting factor in human colostrum." *Biol Neonate* 68, no. 1 (1995): 15–18.

Tacket, C.O., et al. "Efficacy of bovine milk immunoglobulin concentrate in preventing illness after Shigella flexneri challenge." *Am J Trop Med* 47, no. 3 (1992): 276–83.

Tarp, U., et al. "Selenuim treatment in rheumatoid arthritis." *Scand J Rheumatol* (1985).

Thiele, B., I. Brink, and M. Ploch. "Modulation of Cytokine Expression by Hypericum Extract." *Journal of Geriatric Psychiatry and Neurology* 7, Supplement 1 (1994): S60–62.

"St. John's Wort and SAMe: The Mood Menders." *Psychology Today* (March 2000).

"St. John's Wort." *NCCAM Clearinghouse, Publication Z02*. (April 1999).

Van Vollenhoven, R.F., et al. "An open study of dehydroepiandrosterone in systemic lupus erythematosus." *Arthritis and Rheumatism* 37 (1994): 1305–10.

Vuksan, Vladimir, et al. "American Ginseng (Panax quinquefolius L.) reduces post-prandial glycemia in non-diabetic subjects and subjects with Type 2 diabetes mellitus." *Arch Intern Med* 160 (2000): 1009–13.

Wagner, H., et al. "Immunologically active polysaccharides of Echinacea purpurea cell cultures." *Phytochemistry* 27 (1988): 119–26.

Werbach, M.R. *Nutritional Influences on Illness. A Sourcebook of Clinical Research*, 2nd ed. Tarzana, CA: Third Line Press, 1993.

Whitaker, Julian. "Prostate Cancer—Treatments You Can Live With." *Health & Healing* 10, no. 9 (2000).

Whitaker, Julian. *The Whitaker Wellness Program: Part 3*. Potomac, MD: Phillips Publishing, Inc., 1999.

Yu, S.Y., et al. "Regional Variation of Cancer Mortality Incidence and its Relation to Selenium Levels in China." *Biological Trace Element Research* 7 (1985): 21–29.

Zeligs, M.A. "Diet and estrogen status: the cruciferous connection." *J Med Foods* 1, no. 2 (1998): 67–82.

Zisapel, N. "The use of melatonin for the treatment of insomnia." *Bio/Signals Recept* 8 (1999): 84–89.

CHAPTER 6

Ader, R., D.L. Felton, and N. Cohen. *Psychoneuroimmunology*. 2nd ed. San Diego, CA: Academic Press, 1991.

Birkenhager-Gillesse, E.G., et al. "Dehydroepiandrosterone Sulphate (DHEAS) in the Oldest Old, Aged 85 and Over." *Annals of the New York Academy of Science* 719 (1994): 543–52.

Bouic, P.J.D., et al. "Beta-Sitosterol and Beta-sitosterol Glucoside Stimulate Human Peripheral Blood Lymphocyte Proliferation: Implications for their Use as an Immunomodulatory Vitamin Combination." *Int. J. Immunopharmacol* 17 (1996): 693–700.

Camus, G., et al. "Are Similar Inflammatory Factors Involved in Strenuous Exercise and Sepsis?" *Intensive Care Medicine* 20 (1994): 602–10.

Clerici, M. and G.M. Shearer. "The TH1-TH2 Hypothesis of HIV Infection, New Insights." *Immunology Today* 15 (1994): 575–81.

Cohen, S., et al. "Types of stressors that increase susceptibility to the common cold in healthy adults." *Health Psychol* 17 (1998): 214–23.

Cohen, S., et al. "Psychological Stress and Susceptibility to the Common Cold." *New England Journal of Medicine* 325 (1991): 606–12.

Cohen, S. and B.S. Rabin. "Psychological Stress, Immunity and Cancer." *Journal of the National Cancer Institute* 90 (1998): 3–4.

Cousins, N. *Anatomy of an Illness*. New York, NY: W.W. Norton, 1979.

Dhabhar, F.S., et al. "Effects of Stress on Immune Cell Distribution: Dynamics and Hormonal Mechanisms." *Journal of Immunology* 154 (1995): 5511–27.

Dillon, K.M., et al. "Positive Emotional States and Enhancement of the Immune System." *International Journal of Psychiatry in Medicine* 15 (1986): 13–17.

Dodge, C.R. and R.H. Kalstoe. "The MMPI in differentiating early multiple sclerosis and conversion hysteria." *Psychol Rep* 29 (1971): 155–59.

Foley, F.W., et al. "Efficacy of stress-inoculation training in coping with multiple sclerosis." *J Consult Clin Psychol* 55 (1987): 919–22.

Foley, F.W., et al. "Psycho remediation of communication skills for cognitively impaired persons with multiple sclerosis." *J Neurol Rehabil* 8 (1994): 165–76.

Foley, F.W., et al. "Stress, multiple sclerosis and everyday functioning: A review of the literature with implications for intervention." *NeuroRehabilitation* 3 (1993): 57–66.

Franklin, G.M., et al. "Stress and its relationship to acute exacerbations in multiple sclerosis." *J Neurol Rehabil* 2 (1988): 7–11.

Gloria, R.M., W. Regelson, and D.A. Padget. "Immune Response Facilitation and Resistance to Viral and Bacterial Infections with DHEA." *The Biological Role of Dehydroepiandrosterone (DHEA)*. M. Kalimi and W. Regelson, eds, New York, NY: Walter de Gruyter, 1990.

Goldberb, Linn and Diane Elliot. *The Healing Power of Exercise*. New York, NY: John Wiley & Sons, Inc., 2000.

Grant, I., et al. "Severely threatening events and marked life difficulties preceding onset or exacerbation of multiple sclerosis." *J Neurol Neurosurg Psychiatry* 52 (1989): 8–13.

Hoffman-Goetz, L. and B.K. Pedersen. "Exercise and the Immune System: A Model of the Stress Response." *Immunology Today* 15 (1994): 382–87.

Jefferies, William, McK. *Safe Uses of Cortisol*. 2nd ed. Springfield, IL: Charles C. Thomas Publishers, 1996.

Kalimi, M., et al. "Anti-glucocorticoid Effects of Dehydroepiandrosterone (DHEA)." *Molecular and Cellular Biochemistry* 131 (1994): 99–104.

Kalokerinos, A. *Every Second Child*. New Canaan, CT: Keats Publishing, 1981.

Kasl, S.V., et al. "Psychosocial Risk Factors in the Development of Infectious Mononucleosis." *Psychosomatic Medicine* 41 (1979): 445–66.

Kimyai-Asadi, A. and Adil Usman. "The Role of Psychological Stress in Skin Disease." *Journal of Cutaneous Medicine and Surgery* (February 7, 2001).

Kroencke, D.C. and D.R. Denney. "Stress and coping in multiple sclerosis: Exacerbation, remission, and chronic subgroups." *Multiple Sclerosis* 5 (1999): 89–93.

Lancet Interactive. "Chronic Jet lag, cortisol and memory." www.lancet.com (March 25, 2000).

Lancet Interactive: Deepak Prasher, "Traffic noise increases stress by driving up cortisol." www.lancet.com (October 10,1998).

Lee, Sally, et al. *The Complete Book of Fitness: Mind-Body-Spirit*. New York, NY: Three Rivers Press, 1999.

Leserman, J., et. al. "Impact of stressful life events, depression, social support, coping and cortisol on progression to AIDS." *American Journal of Psychiatry* (August 2000).

Leserman, J., et al. "How multiple types of stressors impact on health." *Psychosom Med* 60 (1998): 175–81.

Marsit, A., et al. "Effects of ascorbic acid on serum cortisol and testosterone: cortisol ratio in junior elite weightlifters." *J. Strength Cond. Res* 12 (1998): 179.

McCain, G.A., et al. "A controlled trial of the effects of a supervised cardiovascular fitness training program on the manifestations of primary fibromyalgia." *Arthritis Rheum* 31 (1988): 1135–41.

McEwen, B.S. "Protective and damaging effects of stress mediators." *New England Journal of Medicine* 338 (1998): 171–79.

McKay, D.A. "Stress, Illness and the Physician." *Archives of Family Medicine* 4 (1995): 497–98.

Medman, M.E., et al. "Low Sulpho-conjugated Steroid Hormone Levels in Systemic Lupus Erythematosus (SLE)." *Clin. Exp. Rheumatology* 7 (1989): 583–88.

Mohr, D.C., et al. "Stress is associated with the subsequent development of new brain lesions in multiple sclerosis [abstract]." *Ann Behav Med* 20 (1998): S42.

Newcomer, J.W., et al. "Decreased memory performance in healthy humans induced by stress-level cortisol treatment." *Archives of General Psychiatry* 56, no. 6 (1999): 527–33.

Newsholme, E.A. "Biochemical Mechanisms to Explain Immunosuppression in Well-trained and Over-trained Athletes." *International Journal of Sports Medicine* 15 (1994): 142–47.

Nieman, D.C. "Exercise, Infection and Immunity." *International Journal of Sports Medicine* 15 (1994): 131–41.

Nieman, D.C. "Exercise, Upper Respiratory Tract Infections, and the Immune System." *Medicine and Science in Sports and Exercise* 26 (1994): 128–39.

Northoff, H., C. Weinstock, and A. Berg. "The Cytokine Response to Strenuous Exercise." *Int. J. Sports* 15 (1994): 167–71.

Orentreich, N.J., et al. "Age Changes and Sex Differences in Serum Dehydroepiandrosterone Sulfate Concentrations Throughout Adulthood." *J. Clin. Endocrinol. Metab* 56 (1987): 551–55.

Padgett, D.A. and R.M. Loria. "In Vitro Potentiation of Lymphocyte Activation by Dehydroepiandrosterone, Androstenediol, and Androstenetriol." *Journal Immunology* 153 (1994): 1544–51.

Pennebaker, J.W., et al. "Lack of Control as a Determinant of Perceived Physical Symptoms." *Journal of Personal Social Psychology* 35, no. 3 (1977): 167–74.

Peters, E.M., et al. "Vitamin C Supplementation Reduces the Incidence of Post Race Symptoms of Upper Respiratory-Tract Infection in Ultra Marathon Runners." *American Journal of Clinical Nutrition* 57 (1993): 170–74.

Regelson, W., R. Loria, and M. Kalimi. "Dehydroepiandrosterone (DHEA)—The Mother Steroid." *Annals New York Academy of Sciences* 121 (1994): 553–63.

Rook, G.A.W., et al. "Hormones, Peripherally Activated Prohormones, and the Regulation of the TH1/TH2 Balance." *Immunology Today* 15 (1994): 301–303.

Sachs, B.C. "Coping with Stress." *Stress Medicine* 7 (1991): 61–63.

Sapse, A.T. "Cortisol, high cortisol diseases and anticortisol therapy." *Psychoneuoendocrinology* 22 (September 1997): S3.

Schwartz, C.E. "Teaching coping skills enhances quality of life more than peer support: Results of a randomized trial with multiple sclerosis patients." *Health Psychol* 18, no. 3 (1999): 211–20.

Shepard, R.J. and P.N. Shek. "Infectious Diseases in Athletes: New Interest for an Old Problem." *Journal of Sports Medicine and Physical Fitness* 34 (1994): 11–22.

Soloman, G.F. "Emotions, Stress, the Central Nervous System and Immunity." *Annals of the New York Academy of Sciences* 164, no. 2 (1969): 335–43.

Sparling, P.B., D.C. Nieman, and P.J. O'Connor. "Selected Scientific Aspects of Marathon Racing. An Update on Fluid Replacement, Immune Function, Psychological Factors and the Gender Difference." *Sports Medicine* 15 (1993): 116–32.

Stowe, R.P., et al. "Stress-induced reactivation of Epstein Barr virus in astronauts." *Neuroimmunomodulation* 8, no. 2 (2000): 51–58.

Taniguchi, Ataru, et al. "Effect of Physcial Training on Insulin Sensitivity in Japanese Type II Diabetic Patients." *Diabetes Care* (June 2000).

Turner, R.J. and B. Wheaton. "Checklist measurement of stressful life events." *Measuring Stress: A Guide for Health and Social Scientists*. S. Cohen, R.C. Kessler, and L.U. Gordon, eds. New York, NY: Oxford University Press, 1995.

Turner-Cobb, J.M., et al. "Social support and salivary cortisol in women with metastatic breast cancer." *Psychosom Med* 62, no. 3 (2000): 337–45.

Vanninen, E., et al. "Habitual physical activity aerobic capacity and metabolic control in patients with newly-diagnosed type 2 (non-insulin dependent) diabetes mellitus: effect of 1-year diet and exercise intervention." *Diabetologia* 35 (1992): 340–46.

Warren, S., K.G. Warren, and R. Cockrill. "Emotional stress and coping in multiple sclerosis exacerbations." *J Psychosom Res* 33 (1991): 37–47.

Weigl, B.A. "The significance of stress hormones for eruptions and spontaneous remission phases in psoriasis." *Int J. Dermatol* 39, no. 9 (2000): 678–88.

Whitaker, Julian. "Research Roundup: Did You Know?" *Health & Healing* 10 (October 2000).

Winsor, Mari and Mark Laska, *The Pilates Powerhouse*. New York, NY: Perseus Books, 1999.

Wood, B., et al. "Salivary cortisol profiles in chronic fatigue syndrome." *Neuropsychobiology* 37, no. 1 (1998): 1–4.

CHAPTER 7

Adderly, Brenda. "New hope for chronic fatigue sufferers." *Better Nutrition* (April 2000).

Agency for Toxic Substances and Disease Registry. "DDT, DDE and DDD." *Public Health Statement*. www.atsdr.cdc.gov (December 1989).

Ako, H., A. Cheung, and P. Matsura. "Isolation of a fibrinolysis enzyme activator from commercial bromelain." *Arch Int Pharmacodyn* 254 (1981): 157–67.

Ali, Elvis, et al. *Natural Remedies and Supplements*. Niagara Falls, NY: AGES Publications, 2000.

Allison A.C., J.C. Lee, and E.M. Eugui. "Pharmacological Regulation of the Production of the Pro inflammatory Cytokines TNF-a and IL-1b." *Human Cytokines: Their Role in Disease and Therapy*. B. Aggarwal and R. Puri., eds. Malden, MA: Blackwell Science, 1995.

Allison, J.R. "The relation of HCl and vitamin B complex deficiency in certain skin diseases." *Southern Med J* 38 (1945): 235–41.

American Academy of Family Physicians. "Seasonal Affective Disorder." *American Family Physician* (March 1, 2000).

American Autoimmune Related Diseases Association, Inc. www.aardai.org.

American Cancer Society. "Nausea and Vomiting." *Cancer Resource Center*. www.cancer.org (September 14, 1999).

American Cancer Society. www.cancer.org.

American Diabetes Association. www.diabetes.org.

American Heart Association. www.americanheart.org.

American Lung Association. www.lungusa.org.

American Parkinson Disease Association. www.apdaparkinson.com.

Anderson, David. "RSI can strain the bottom line. (Repetitive Strain Injuries)." *Business & Health* (January 1998).

Aqel, M.B. "Relaxant Effect of the Volatile Oil of Rosmarinus Officinalis on Tracheal Smooth Muscle." *Journal of Ethnopharmacology* 33 (1991): 57–62.

Arfvidsson, B., et al. "Risk factors for venous thromboembolism following prolonged air travel." *Hematol Oncol Clin North Am* 14, no. 2 (2000): 391–400.

Arlt, W., et al. "Dehydroepiandrosterone replacement in women with adrenal insufficiency." *New England Journal of Medicine* 341 (1999): 1013–20.

"Artichoke Extract: Improves Digestion, Liver Function and Cholesterol Levels." *Natural Medicine Online*. www.nat-med.com/archives/artichoke.htm (August/September 1998).

Asher, D.W. "Chronic sore throat: The toothbrush connection." *Cortlandt Forum* 57 (1990): 17–28.

Austin, Steve. "Antioxidants and Chemotherapy—A Rebuttal." *HNR* (Winter 1999): 234–36.

Ayres, S., Jr. and R. Mihan. "Acne vulgaris and lipid peroxidation: New concepts in pathogenesis and treatment." *Int J Dermatology* 17 (1978): 305.

Ayers, S., Jr. and R. Mihan. "Acne vulgaris: Therapy directed at pathophysiologic defects." *Cutis* 28 (1981): 41–42.

Ayres, S., Jr. and R. Mihan. "Leg cramps and 'restless leg' syndrome responsive to vitamin E." *Calif Med* 111 (1969): 87–91.

Badwe, R.A., et al. "Timing of surgery during menstrual cycle and survival of premenopausal women with operable breast cancer." *Lancet* 337, no. 8752 (1991): 1261–64.

Baer, A.N., et al. "Intestinal ulceration and malabsorption syndromes." *Gastroenterology* 79 (1980): 754–65.

Baggio, E., et al. "Italian multicenter study on the safety and efficacy of coenzyme Q10 as adjunctive therapy in heart failure. CoQ10 Drug Surveillance Investigators." *Mol Aspects Med* 15 (Suppl) (1994): S287–294.

Balch, Phyllis A., and James F. Balch. *Prescription for Dietary Wellness*. Greenfield, IN: PAB Books, Inc., 1992.

Balch, Phyllis, and James F. Balch. *Prescription for Nutritional Healing*. 3rd ed. Garden City Park, NY: Avery Publishing Group, Inc., 2000.

Baron, J.A., et al. "Calcium Supplements for the Prevention of Colorectal Adenomas." *The New England Journal of Medicine* 340, no. 2 (1999): 101–107.

Barth, Werner F. "Reactive Arthritis (Reiter's Syndrome)." *American Family Physician*. (August 1999).

Bartolin, R., et al. "Blood cadmium and plasma zinc in hypertensive patients." *Rev. Med. Interne* 6, no. 3 (1985): 280–84.

Bates, Charles. *Essential Fatty Acids and Immunity in Mental Health*. Tacoma, WA: Life Sciences Press, 1987.

Batmanghelidg, Fereydoon. *Your Body's Many Cries for Water*. Falls Church, VA: Global Health Solutions, Inc., 1997.

Bauman, Norman. "Keep an Eye Out for Interstitial Cystitis in Male Patients." *Urology Times*, (March 1998).

Bauman, Norman. "Depression Found in Three-Fourths of IC Patients." *Urology Times*, (March 1998).

Bean, W.B. and R.E. Hodges. "Pantothenic acid deficiency induced in human subjects." *Proc Soc Exp Biol Med* 86 (1954): 693–98.

Beisel, W., et al. "Single-nutrient effects of immunologic functions." *JAMA* 245 (1981): 53–58.

Beisel, W.R. "Single Nutrients and Immunity." *American Journal of Clinical Nutrition*. 53 (1991): 386.

Belaiche, P. "Treatment of vaginal infections of Candida albicans with the essential oil of Melaleuca alternifolia." *Phytotherapie* 15 (1985).

Bendich, A. "Vitamins and Immunity." *Journal of Nutrition* 122 (1992): 601–603.

Bendiner, E. "Disastrous trade-off: Eskimo health for white civilization." *Hosp Pract* 9 (1974): 156–89.

Bennett, R.M., et al. "Symptoms of Raynaud's syndrome in patients with fibromyalgia." *Arthritis and Rheumatism* 34, no. 3 (1991).

Bittiner, S.B., et al. "A Double-blind, Randomised, Placebo-controlled Trial of Fish Oil in Psoriasis." *Lancet* 1, no. 8582 (1988): 378–380.

Bjarnaason, I., et al. "Effect of non-steroidal anti-inflammatory drugs on prostaglandins on the permeability of the human small intestine." *Gut* 27 (1986): 1292–97.

Bland, Jeffrey S. *Health Comm International* 1998 and 2001 audio tapes.

Bliznakov, E.G. and G.L. Hunt. *The Miracle Nutrient: Coenzyme Q10*. New York, NY: Bantam, 1986.

Block, M.T. "Vitamin E in the treatment of diseases of the skin." *Clinical Medicine*, (January 1953): 31–34.

Bogden, J.D. "Micronutrient Nutrition and Immunity: Part 2." *Nutrition Report* 9 (1995): 16–17.

Bologna, R.A., et al. "The Efficacy of Calcium Glycerophosphate in the Prevention of Food-related Flares in Interstitial Cystitis," *Interstitial Cystitis and Bladder Research*, (October 19, 2000).

Borgman, R.F. "Dietary factors in hypertension." *Prog Food Nutr. Sci* 9 (1985): 109–47.

Bouic P.J.D., et al. "Beta-sitosterol and Beta-sitosterol Glucoside Stimulate Peripheral Blood Lymphocyte Proliferation: Implications for Their Use as an Immunomodulatory Vitamin Combination." *International Journal of Immunopharmacology* 18 (1995): 693–700.

Bouic, P.J.D. "Sterols/Sterolins, the natural, nontoxic immunomodulators and their role in the control of rheumatoid arthritis." *Arthritis Trust of America Newsletter* (Summer 1998).

Bouic, P.J.D., et al. "Beta-sitosterol and beta-sitosterolin glucoside stimulate peripheral blood lymphocyte proliferation: Implications for their use as an immunomodulatory vitamin combination." *The International Journal of Immunopharmacology* 18, no. 12, (1996): 693–700.

Brasitus, T.A. "Parasites and malabsorption." *Clinical Gastroenterology* 12, no. 2 (1983): 495–510.

Brehm, Barbara A. *Essays on Wellness.* New York, NY: HarperCollins College Publishers, 1993.

Breneman, J.C. *Basics of Food Allergy.* Springfield, IL: Charles C. Thomas, 1978.

Brieva, L., et al. "Polyneuropathy caused by vitamin B12 deficiency secondary to chronic atrophic gastritis and giardiasis." *Rev Neurol* 26, no. 154 (1998): 1019–20.

Broadhurst, C. Leigh. *Diabetes: Prevention and Cure.* New York, NY: Kensington Publishing Corp., 1999.

Broadhurst, C. Leigh. *Natural Relief from Asthma.* Burnaby, BC: Alive Books, 2000.

Brodsky, Ruthan. "Warts." *Gale Encyclopedia of Medicine.* New York, NY: Gale Research, 2001.

Brosnan, C.M. and N.F.C. Gowing. "Lesson of the Week: Addison's Disease." *British Medical Journal* 312 (1996): 1085–87.

Broughton, K.S., et al. "Reduced Asthma Symptoms with n-3 Fatty Acid Ingestion Are Related to 5-series Leukotriene Production." *American Journal of Clinical Nutrition* 65 (1997): 1011–17.

Brox, A., K. Howson-jan, and A.A. Fauser. "Successful Treatment of Immune Thrombocytopenia with Ascorbic Acid." *Immunohematology* (1988).

Bullock, C. "Chronic infectious sinusitis linked to allergies." *Med Trib* (December 1995).

Bullogh, B., et al. "Methylxanthines and fibrocystic breast disease: A study of correlations." *Nurse Pract* 14, no. 2 (1989): 36–37.

Butland, B.K., A.M. Fehily, and P.C. Elwood. "Diet, lung function, and lung function decline in a cohort of 2512 middle-aged men." *Thorax* 55 (2000): 102–108.

Buttram, V., Jr. and R. Reiter. "Uterine leiomyomata: Etiology, symptomatology and management." *Fertil Steril* 36 (1981): 433–45.

Canadian Cancer Society, www.cancer.ca.

Canadian Heart and Stroke Foundation, www.heartandstroke.ca.

Canadian Lung Association website, www.lung.ca.

Capron, J.P., et al. "Meal frequency and duration of overnight fast: A role in gall-stone formation?" *British Medical Journal* 283 (1981): 1435.

Carey, I.M., D.P. Strachan, and D.G. Cook. "Effects of changes in fresh fruit consumption on ventilatory function in healthy British adults." *Am J Respir Crit Care Med* 158 (1998): 728–733.

Carson-DeWitt, Rosalyn S. "Systemic lupus erythematosus." *Gale Encyclopedia of Medicine*, Minnesota: Gale Research Group, 1999.

Catalona, W.J., et al. "Measurement of prostate specific antigen in serum as a screening test for prostate cancer." *New England Journal of Medicine* 324 (1991): 1156–61.

Catalona, W.J., et al. "Prostate cancer detection in men with serum PSA concentrations of 2.6–4.0 ng/ml and benign prostate examinations." *Journal of the American Medical Association* 277 (1997): 1452–55.

Celiac Support Group web page. *Celiac.com*, www.celiac.com.

Challem, J., B. Berkson, and M.D. Smith. *Syndrome X*. New York, NY: John Wiley & Sons, Inc., 2000.

Challem, Jack. "NAC: The Best Cold and Flu Remedy Yet?" *The Nutrition Reporter™*. www.thenutritionreporter.com (2000).

Chapel, H., et al. *Essentials of Clinical Immunology*. 4th ed. Malden, MA: Blackwell Science, 1999.

Charbonneau, Nicolle. "Tooth Troubles Linked to Severe Stress." *Health Scout*. www.healthscout.com (March 16, 2000).

Childs, Nathan D. "Could Lyme Vaccine Trigger Autoimmune Arthritis?" *Pediatric News* 33, no. 6 (1999): 20.

Christensen, Damaris. "Is Snoring a DiZZZease?" *Science News* (March 11, 2000).

Cichoke, Anthony J. "Natural Relief for Autoimmune Disorders." *Better Nutrition* (June 2000).

Clark, Hulda Regehr. *The Cure for all Cancers*. San Diego, CA: ProMotion Publishing, 1993.

Clerici, M. and G.M. Shearer. "A Th-1 to Th-2 Switch is a Critical Step in the Etiology of HIV Infection." *Immunology Today* 14 (1993): 107–111.

Cohen, B.I., et al. "The Effect of Dietary Bile Acids, Cholesterol and B sitosterol Upon Formation of Coprostanol and 7-dehydroxylation of Bile Acids in the Rat." *Lipids* 9 (1974): 1027–29.

Cohen, H.A., et al. "Blocking Effect of Vitamin C in Exercise Induced Asthma." *Archives of Pediatric Adolescent Medicine* 151 (1997): 367–70.

Colgan, Michael. "Protect Your Prostate." *Colgan Chronicles* 3, no. 1 (1999).

Cooper, J.C., Jr. "Health and Nutrition Examination Survey of 1971–75: Part II. Tinnitus, subjective hearing loss, and well-being." *J Am Acad Audiol* 5, no. 1 (1994): 37–43.

Crohn's and Colitis Foundation of America, www.ccfa.org.

Crompton, D.W.T. *Parasites and People*. London, England: Macmillan Publishers Ltd., 1984.

Crook, William. *The Yeast Connection: A Medical Breakthrough*. New York, NY: Vintage Books, 1986.

Crook, William. *The Yeast Connection Handbook*. Jackson, TN: Professional Books, Inc., 2000.

Cunningham, Anthony L. "The Management of Postherpetic Neuralgia: If early treatment fails, then patients should be referred to pain clinics." *British Medical Journal* (September 30, 2000).

Custovic A., et al. "Allergen avoidance in the treatment of asthma and atopic disorders." *Thorax* 53 (1998): 63–72.

Dagnelie, C.F., et al. "Do patients with sore throat benefit from penicillin? A randomized double-blind, placebo controlled clinical trial with penicillin in general practice." *Br J Gen Pract* 46 (1996): 589–93.

Dawson, Earl B. "Third-Trimester Amniotic Fluid Metal Levels Associated with Preeclampsia." *Archives of Environmental Health* (November 1999).

Day, E.A., et al. "Tumor sterols." *Metabolism* 18 (1969): 646–51.

Daynes, R.A., et al. "Altered Regulation of IL-6 Production With Normal Aging." *The Journal of Immunology* 150 (1993): 5219–30.

De Marco, Carolyn. *Take Charge of Your Body*. Aurora, ON: The Well Women Press, 1997.

Delport, R., et al. "Vitamin B_6 Nutritional Status in Asthma: The Effect of Theophylline Therapy on Plasma Pyridoxal-5-Phosphate and Pyridoxal Levels." *Int J Vitam Nutr Res* 58, no. 1 (1988): 67–72.

Denning, D.W., et al. "Fungal Nail Disease: A Guide to Good Practice." *British Medical Journal* 311 (1995): 1277–81.

Deodhar, S.D., et al. "Preliminary studies on anti-rheumatic activity of curcumin." *Ind J Med Res* 71 (1980): 633.

DeRoin, Dee Ann. "Adult Health Supervisor: Diverticulosis." *Clinical Reference Systems*. www.realage.com (1998).

Deuster, P. "A novel treatment for fibromyalgia improves clinical outcomes in a community-based study." *Serammune Physicians Lab* (1996).

Dew, M.J., B.K. Evans, and J. Rhodes. "Peppermint oil for irritable bowel syndrome: a multicentre trial." *British Journal of Clinical Practice* 38 (1984): 394–98.

Diamond, W. John, W. Lee Cowden, and Burton Goldberg. *Definitive Guide to Cancer*. Tiburon, CA: Future Medicine Publishing, Inc., 1997.

Dicke, W.K., H.A. Weijers, and J.H. van de Knamer. "Coeliac disease: II. The presence in wheat of a factor having a deleterious effect in cases of coeliac disease." *Acta Paediatr. Scand.* 42 (1996): 34–41.

Diehm C., et al. "Comparison of leg compression stockings and oral horse chestnut seed extract therapy in patients with chronic venous insufficiency." *Lancet* 347 (1996): 292–94.

Dolby, Victoria. "Chronic fatigue syndrome: getting to the root of the problem." *Better Nutrition* (July 1998).

Donovan, P. "Bowel Toxemia, Permeability and Disease—New Information to Support an Old Concept" *A Textbook of Natural Medicine*. J.E. Pizzorno and M.T. Murray, eds. Seattle, WA: John Bastyr College Publications, 1989.

Douglas, B.R., et al. "Coffee stimulation of cholecystokinin release and gallbladder contraction in humans." *American Journal of Clinical Nutrition* 52 (1990): 553–56.

Droste, J.H.J., et al. "Does the use of antibiotics in early childhood increase the risk of asthma and allergic disease?" *Clinical and Experimental Allergy* 30 (2000): 1547–53.

Dubey, M.P., et al. "Pharmacological studies on coleono, a hypotensive diterpene from Coleus forskohlii." *J. Ethnopharmacol* 3 (1981): 1–13.

Duda, R.B., et al. "American ginseng and breast cancer therapeutic agents synergistically inhibit MCF-7 breast cancer cell growth." *Journal of Surgical Oncology* 72 (1999): 230–39.

Edelson, Edward. "Gum Trouble Doesn't Increase Heart Risk." *Health Scout*. www.healthscout.com (September 19, 2000).

Eisenbarth, G.S. and R.A. Jackson. "Immunogenetics of polyglandular failure and related diseases." *HLA in Endocrine and Metabolic Disorders*. N. Farid, ed. New York, NY: Academic Press, 1981.

Elizabeth Glaser Pediatrics AIDS Foundation, www.pedaids.org.

Enders, U., et al. "The spectrum of immune responses to *Campylobacter jejuni* and glycoconjugates in Guillain-Barré syndrome and in other neuroimmunological disorders." *Ann Neurol* 34 (1993): 136–44.

Erasmus, Udo. *Fats that Heal, Fats that Kill.* Burnaby, BC: Alive Books, 1997.

Fabender, H.M., et al. "Glucosamine sulfate compared to ibuprofen in osteoarthritis of the knee." *Osteoarthritis and Cartilage* 2, no. 1 (1994): 61–69.

Fendrick, A.M. and J.M. Scheiman. "Helicobacter pylori and NSAID Gastropathy: An Ambiguous Association." *Curr Rheumatol Rep* 3, no. 2 (2001): 107–111.

Finnegan, John. *The Facts About Fats.* Berkeley, California: Celestial Arts, 1993.

Fischer-Rasmussen, W., et al., "Ginger treatment of hyperemesis gravidarum." *Eur J Obstet Gynecol Reprod Biol* 38 (1990): 19–24.

Folkers, K., et al. "Biochemical evidence for a deficiency of vitamin B_6 in the carpal tunnel syndrome based on a crossover clinical study." *Proc Natl Acad Sci* 75, no. 7 (1978): 3410–12.

Folkers, K., et al. "Bioenergetics in clinical medicine. Reduction of hypertension in patients with coenzyme Q10." *Res Commun Chem Pathol Pharmacol* 31 (1981): 129.

Folmer, R.I., S.E. Griest, and W.H. Martin. "Chronic tinnitus as phantom auditory pain." *Otolaryngol Head Neck Surg* 124, no. 4 (2001): 394–400.

Forsyth, L., et al. "Therapeutic effects oral NADH on the symptoms of patients with chronic fatigue syndrome." *Annals of Allergy, Asthma & Immunology* 82 (1999): 185–91.

Fujita, T., et al. "Cytokines and osteoporosis." *Ann NY Acad Sci* 5 (1990): 587.

Furlan, R., et al. "Modifications of cardiac autonomic profile associated with a shift schedule of work." *Circulation* 102, no. 16 (2000): 1912–16.

Gaby, A.R. "The Role of Coenzyme Q10 in Clinical Medicine." *Alternative Medicine Review* 1 (1996): 12.

Gadsby, Patricia. "Fear of Flu Pandemic Influenza Outbreaks." *Discover* (January 1999).

Galland, L. "Increased Requirements For Essential Fatty Acids in Atopic Individuals, A Review with Clinical Descriptions." *American Journal of Clinical Nutrition* 5 (1986): 213–28.

Garfinkel, Marian, et al. "Yoga-based Intervention for Carpal Tunnel Syndrome: A Randomized Trial." *Journal of the American Medical Association* (November 11, 1998).

Garg, Rekha, et al. "Niacin treatment increases plasma homocysteine levels." *American Heart Journal* 138 (1999): 1082–87.

Garrison, Robert H., Jr. and Elizabeth Somer. *The Nutrition Desk Reference.* 2nd ed. New Canaan, CT: Keats Publishing, Inc., 1990.

Gately, C.A. and N.J. Blundred. "Drug Points: Alopecia and Breast Disease." *British Medical Journal* 314 (1997): 481.

Gately, Gary. "Study Links Gum Disease, Premature Births." *Health Scout.* www.healthscout.com (June 29, 2000).

Genco, R., et al. "Periodontal disease and risk for myocardial infarction and cardiovascular disease." *CVR&R* (March 1998): 34–40.

Germano, C. and W. Cabot. *Nature's Pain Killers.* New York, NY: Kensington Books, 1999.

Germano, Carl and William Cabot. *The Osteoporosis Solution.* New York, NY: Kensington Books, 1999.

Geusens, P., et al. "Long-term effect of omega-3 fatty acid supplementation in active rheumatoid arthritis. A 12-month, double-blind, controlled study." *Arthritis Rheum* 37, no. 6 (1994): 824–29.

Giorgi, A., et al. "Muscular strength, body composition and health responses to the use of testosterone: a double-blind study." *J Sci Med Sport* 3, no. 4 (1999): 341–55.

Giovanucci, E., et al., "Intake of carotenoids and retinal in relation to risk of prostate cancer." *J Nat Can Inst* 87 (1995): 1767–76.

Gittleman, Ann Louise. *Guess What Came to Dinner: Parasites and Your Health,* Garden City, NY; Avery Publishing, 1993.

Gleicher, N., et al. "Is endometriosis an autoimmune disease?" *Obstet Gynecol* 70 (1987): 115–22.

Gloth, F.M., III, W. Alam, and B. Hollis. "Vitamin D vs. broad spectrum phototherapy in the treatment of seasonal affective disorder." *J Nutr Health Aging* 3, no. 1 (1999): 5–7.

Goldberg, Burton, et al. *Alternative Medicine.* Puyallup, WA: Future Medicine Publishing, Inc., 1993.

Goldberg, Burton, et al. *Alternative Medicine Guide to Women's Health 2,* Tiburon, CA: Future Medicine Publishing, Inc., 1998.

Goldberg, Linn and Diane Elliot. *The Healing Power of Exercise.* New York, NY: John Wiley & Sons, Inc., 2000.

Gottschall, E. *Food and the Gut Reaction.* ON: The Kirkton Press, 1986.

Gould, R.G., et al. "Absorbability of B-sitosterol in Humans." *Metabolism* 18 (1969): 652–62.

Grant, I.R., H.J. Ball, and M.T. Rowe. "Inactivation of Mycobacterium paratuberculosis in cow's milk at pasteurization temperatures." *Applied and Environmental Microbiology* 62 (1996): 631–36.

Grant, J.E., M.S. Veldee, and D. Buchwald. "Analysis of dietary intake and selected nutrient concentrations in patients with chronic fatigue syndrome." *J Am Diet Assoc* 96 (1996): 383–86.

Gratacos, E., et al. "Lipid peroxide and vitamin E patterns in pregnant women with different types of hypertension in pregnancy." *Amer J Obstet Gyn* 178 (1998): 1072–76.

Grave, G. "Antioxidant Nutrients in Inflammatory Bowel Disease." *Crohn's & Colitis Foundation of America physician letter.* www.ccfa.org.

Gursche, Siegfried and Zoltan Rona. *The Encyclopedia of Natural Healing.* Burnaby, BC: Alive Publishing, Inc., 1998.

Haddad, J.G., et al. "Circulation Phytosterols in Normal Females, Lactating Mothers and Breast Cancer Patients." *Clinical Endocrinology* 30 (1970): 174–80.

Halme, J. and S. Becker. "Increased activation of pelvic macrophages in infertile women with mild endometriosis." *Am J Obstet Gynecol* 145 (1983): 333–37.

Hamm, R.M., R.J. Hicks, and D.A. Bemben. "Antibiotics and respiratory infections: Are patients more satisfied when expectations are met?" *J Fam Pract* 43, no. 1 (1996): 56–62.

Harries, A.D. and R.V. Heatley. "Nutritional disturbances in Crohn's disease." *Postgraduate Medical Journal* 50 (1983): 690–97.

Hartwell, J.L. "Types of Anticancer Agents Isolated from Plants." *Cancer Treat* 60 (1976): 1031–67.

Harvard School of Medicine. "Anger and Depression Predict Artery-hardening Risks and Behavior." *Consumer Information.* www.intelihealth.com (March 22, 2001).

Harvard School of Medicine. "Gastrointestinal Disorders and Smoking." *Consumer Information.* www.intelihealth.com (August 31, 1999).

Harvard School of Public Health. "Higher Intake of Dairy Products May Be Linked to Prostate Cancer Risk." *Press Release.* www.hsph.harvard.edu (April 4, 2000).

Hathcock, J.N., et al. "Micronutrients and Immune Function." *New York Academy of Science* 587 (1990): 257–258.

Hautanen, A., et al. "Cigarette smoking is associated with elevated adrenal androgen response to adrenocorticotropin." *J Steroid Biochem Mol Biol* 45, no. 2 (1993): 245–51.

Hay, I.C., M. Jamieson, and A.D. Ormerod. "Randomized trial of aromatherapy. Successful treatment of alopecia areata." *Arch Dermatol* 134 (1998): 1349–52.

Hay, Louise L. *Heal Your Body*. Santa Monica, CA: Hay House, 1988.

Health Sciences Institute. "Ancient Chinese Remedy Fights Leukemia: Indirubin Prevents Cancer Cells from Spreading." *Member Alert* 5, no. 2 (2000).

Health Sciences Institute. "Potent Plant Extract Reduces Migraines by 50 Percent." *Members Alert* 5, no. 5 (2000).

Heart and Stroke Foundation of Canada. www.bc.heartandstroke.ca.

Hermon-Taylor, John, et al. "Mycobacterium paratuberculosis Cervical Lymphadenitis followed five years later by terminal ileitis similar to Crohn's Disease." *British Medical Journal* (1998).

Hertog, M.L. and P.H. Hollman. "Potential Health Effects of the Dietary Flavonol Quercetin." *European Journal of Clinical Nutrition* 50 (1996): 63–71.

Hingley, A. "Campylobacter: Low-Profile Bug is Food Poisoning Leader." *US Food and Drug Administration, FDA Consumer.* www.vm.cfsan.fda.gov.

Hodge, L., et al. "Consumption of oily fish and childhood asthma risk." *Medical Journal of Australia* 164 (1996): 137–40.

Horowitz, B., S. Edelson, and L. Lippman. "Sexual Transmission of Candida." *Obstet Gynecol* 69, no. 6 (1987): 883–86.

Hudson, Tori. *Women's Encyclopedia of Natural Medicine: Alternative Therapies and Integrative Medicine.* Lincolnwood, IL: NTC/Contemporary Publishing Group, Inc., 1999.

Hueston, William J. "Acute Bronchitis." *American Family Physician* (March 15, 1998).

Hunt, P.J., et al. "Improvement in mood and fatigue after dehydroepiandrosterone replacement in Addison's disease in a randomized double blind trial." *J Clin Endocrinol Metab* 85 (2000): 4650–56.

Illi, Sabine, et al. "Early childhood infectious diseases and the development of asthma up to school age: a birth cohort study." *British Medical Journal* 322 (2001): 390–95.

Interstitial Cystitis Association. www.ichelp.com (March 1999).

Isenberg, David A. and Carol Black. "ABC of Rheumatology: Raynaud's Phenomenon, Scleroderma and Overlap Syndromes." *British Medical Journal* 310 (1995): 795–98.

Isolauri, E., et al. "Breast Feeding of Allergic Infants." *Pediatrics* 134 (1999): 27–32.

Izaka, K., et al. "Gastrointestinal absorption and anti-inflammatory effect of bromelain." *Jpn J Pharmacol* 22 (1972): 519.

Jacob, Stanley W., Ronald M. Lawrence, and Martin Zucker. *The Miracle of MSM: The Natural Solution for Pain.* New York, NY: Penguin Putnam, Inc., 1999.

Jaffe, Russell. "Autoimmunity and cofactor replacement (Part Two)." *International Journal of Integrative Medicine* 2, no. 3 (2000): 15–19.

Jaffe, Russell. "Immune defense and repair systems in biological medicine I: Autoimmunity. Clinical relevance of biological modifiers in diagnosis, treatment and testing." Health Studies Collegium.

Jarosz, M., et al. "Tobacco smoking and vitamin C concentration in gastric juice in healthy subjects and patients with Helicobacter pylori infection." *Eur J Cancer Prev* 9, no. 6 (2000): 423–28.

Jensen, K. *Menopause*. Toronto, ON: Prentice Hall, 1999.

Jensen, M.N. "Good health requires good gums." *Science News* 153 (1998): 300–301.

Johnson, L.W. "Communal showers and the risk of plantar warts." *J Fam Pract* 40, no. 2 (1995): 136–38.

Jones, Pamela. "The Therapeutic Effect of Calcium Glycerophosphate (Prerelief(r)) in Interstitial Cystitis: A Survey of Interstitial Cystitis Support Group (UK) Members." Unpublished study (January 2000).

Juhlin, L., et al. "Blood glutathione-peroxidase levels in skin diseases: Effect of selenium and vitamin E treatment." *Acta Derm Venereal (Stockh)* 62, no. 3 (1982): 211–14.

Kauffmann, S.H.E. "Immunity to Intracellular Bacteria." *Annual Review of Immunology* 11 (1993): 129–63.

Kaufman, W.F. "The diet and acne." Letter to the Editor. *Arch Dermatology* 119 (1983): 276.

Kaul, R. and W.M. Wenman. "Chlamydia pneumoniae facilitates monocyte adhesion to endothelial and smooth muscle cells." *Microb Pathog* 30 (no. 3 (2001): 149–55.

Kearns, Brenda. "No More Tummy Troubles!" *First for Women*. www.4woman.gov May 1999.

Kellock, B. *The Fiber Man*. Belleville, MI: Lion Publications, 1985.

Keuneke, Robin. *Total Breast Health*. New York, NY: Kensington Books, 1998.

Kidd, P.M. and W. Huber. "Living With The AIDS Virus: A Strategy for Long-term Survival." *HK Biomedical* (1990).

Kiddy, D.S., et al. "Improvement in endocrine and ovarian function during dietary treatment of obese women with polycystic ovary syndrome." *Clin Endocrinol* 36, no. 1 (1992): 105–11.

Kiechl, S., et al. "Insulin sensitivity and regular alcohol consumption." *British Medical Journal* 313, no. 7064 (1996): 1040–44.

Kirchner, Jeffrey T. "Diagnostic Evaluation of Patients with Palpitations." *American Family Physician* (September 1, 1998).

Kirchner, Jeffrey T. "Strategies for Detecting UTIs in Young Febrile Girls." *American Family Physician* (October 2000)

Kjellberg, L., et al. "Smoking, diet, pregnancy and oral contraceptive use as risk factors for cervical intra-epithelial neoplasia in relation to human papillomavirus infection." *Br J Cancer* 82, no. 7 (2000): 1332–38.

Kleine, M.W., G.M. Stauder, and E.W. Beese. "The intestinal absorption of orally administered hydrolytic enzymes and their effects in the treatment of acute herpes zoster as compared with those of oral acyclovir therapy." *Phytomedicine* 2 (1995): 7–15.

Kovacs, S.O. "Vitiligo." *Journal of the American Academy of Dermatology* 38, no. 5 (1998): 647–68.

Kulnis, Randall, et al. "Cephalometric Assessment of Snoring and Nonsnoring Children" *Chest* 118, no. 3 (2000): 596–603.

Kuroki, S., et al. "*Campylobacter jejuni* strains from patients with Guillain-Barré syndrome belong mostly to Penner serogroup 19 and contain beta-N-acetyl-glucosamine residues." *Ann Neurol* 33 (1993): 243–247.

Kuvaeva, I., et al. "The microecology of the gastrointestinal tract and the immunological status under food allergy." *Nahrung* 28 (1984): 689–93. In *Nutritional Influences on Illness*. New Canaan, Connecticut: Keats Publishing, 1987.

Langer, Stephen and James F. Scheer. *Pocket Guide to Natural Health*. New York, NY: Twin Stream Keats Publishing Corp., 2001.

Larkin, Marilyn. "Loud Snoring Should Be Taken Seriously." *Lancet* 353, no. 9157 (1999).

Lee, John R., Jesse Hanley, and Virginia Hopkins. *What Your Doctor May Not Tell You about Premenopause*. New York, NY: Warner Books, 1999.

Lee, John R. *Natural Progesterone The Multiple Roles of a Remarkable Hormone*. New York: BLL Publishing, 1997.

Leinonen, K., K. Poutanen, and H. Mykkanen. "Rye Bread Decreases Serum Cholesterol Levels in Hypercholesterolemic Men." *Journal of Nutrition* 130 (2000): 164–70.

Leslie, D. and M. Gheorghiade. "Is there a role for thiamine supplementation in the management of heart failure?" *Am Heart J* 131 (1996): 1248–50.

Leu, S., et al. "Immune-inflammatory markers in patients with seasonal affective disorder: Effects of light therapy." *J Affect Disord* 63, nos. 1–3 (2001): 27–34.

Levy, S.B. *The Antibiotic Paradox: How Miracle Drugs Are Destroying The Miracle*. New York: Plenum Publishers, 1992.

Li, M., et al. "Clinical observation of the therapeutic effect of ginkgo leaf concentrated oral liquor on bronchial asthma." *CJIM* 3 (1997): 264–67.

Lichtenstein, L.M. "Allergy and the Immune System." *Scientific American* (September 1993): 116–24.

Liddle, G.W. "The Adrenals." *Textbook of Endocrinology*. 6th ed. Philadelphia, PA: WB Saunders, 1981.

Lindberg, Eva, et al. "Snoring and Hypertension: A 10-year follow-up." *Eur Resp J* 11, no. 4 (1998): 884–89.

Ling, W.H. and P.J.H. Jones. "Dietary Phytosterols: A Review of Metabolism, Benefits and Side Effects." *Life Sciences* 57 (1995): 195–206.

Loes, M. and D. Steinman. *The Aspirin Alternative*. Topanga, CA: Freedom Press, 1999.

Loes, Michael. "Irritable Bowel Syndrome: A Review of Natural Medicines." *Natural Medicine Online*. www.nat-med.com (September 2000).

Long, P.J., et al. *Nutrition: An Inquiry into the Issues*. Englewood Cliffs, NJ: Prentice Hall, 1983.

Longnecker, M.P. "Do trans fatty acids in margarine and other foods increase the risk of coronary heart disease?" *Epidemiology* 4 (1993): 492.

Lotufo, P.A., et al. "Male pattern baldness and coronary heart disease: the Physician's Health Study." *Arch Intern Med* 160, no. 2 (2000): 165–71.

Lupus Foundation of America. www.lupus.org.

Lutgen, N., et al. "Prevalence and treatment of *Helicobacter pylori* in gastroduodenal ulcers. An experience in Liege." *Rev Med Liege* 56, no. 1 (2001): 25–30.

Lyon, Michael. "Attention Deficit Disorder: Effective Alternatives to Worrisome Drugs." *Consumer Health Organization of Canada Newsletter* 23, no. 11 (2000).

Mackenzie, G.D., et al. "Inflammatory Response to Parasites." *Parasitology* 94 (1987): 9–10.

Marklund, Marie. "The effect of a mandibular advancement device on apneas and sleep in patients with obstructive sleep apnea." *Chest* (March 1998).

Matricardi, P.M., et al. "Exposure to food-borne and orofecal microbes versus airborne viruses in relation to atopy and allergic asthma: epidemiological study." *British Medical Journal* 320 (2000): 412–17.

Mayer, Emeran. "IC and GI Disturbances: What's Your Gut Feeling?" *ICA Update* (December 2000).

McCarty, M. "High chromium yeast for acne?" *Med Hypothesis* 14 (1984): 307–10.

McMillan, Robert. "Therapy for Adults with Refractory Chronic Immune Thrombocytopenic Purpura." *Annals of Internal Medicine* 126 (1997): 307–314.

Meilles, M.J., et al. "Phytosterols and Cholesterol in Malignant and Benign Breast Tumors." *Cancer Research*. 27 (1977): 3034.

Meittinen, T.A. and S. Tarpila. "Fecal B-sitosterol in Patients with Diverticular Disease of the Colon in Vegetarians." *Scandinavian Journal of Gastroenerology* 13 (1978): 573–76.

Merck Manual of Medical Information. West Point, PA: Merck Research Laboratories, 1997.

Mian, E., et al. "Anthocyanidinosides and the walls of microvessels: further aspects of the mechanism of action of their protective effect in syndromes due to abnormal capillary fragility." *Minerva Med* 68, no. 52 (1977): 3565–81.

Michaelsson, G., et al. "A double-blind study of the effect of zinc and oxytetracycline in acne vulgaris." *Brit J Dermatology* 97 (1977): 561.

Michaelsson, G., et al. "Erythrocyte glutathione peroxidase activity in acne vulgaris and the effect of selenium and vitamin E treatment." *Acta Derm Venereol* (Stockholm) 64, no. 1 (1984): 9–14. In *Nutritional Influences on Illness.* Melvyn R. Werbach. New Canaan, CT: Keats Publishing.

Mims, C.A. *The Pathogenesis of Infectious Disease.* San Diego, CA: Academic Press, 1987.

Mittman, P. "Randomized double-blind study of freeze-dried Urtica dioica in the treatment of allergic rhinitis." *Planta Med* 56 (1990): 44–47.

Morisco, C., B. Trimarco, and M. Condorelli. "Effect of Coenzyme Q10 therapy in patients with congestive heart failure: A long term multicentre randomized study." *Clin Invest* 71, no. 8 (1993): 134–36.

Morreale, P., et al. "Comparison of the anti-inflammatory efficacy of chondroitin sulfate and diclofenac sodium in patients with knee osteoarthritis." *J Rheumatol* 23, no. 8 (1996): 1285–1391.

Moyers, Bill. *Trade Secrets: A Moyers Report.* Public Affairs Television, Inc. www.pbs.org. Aired on PBS, March 26, 2001.

Mullins, R., et al. "Identification of thyroid stimulating hormone receptor-specific T cells in Graves' disease thyroid using autoantigen-transfected Epstein Barr virus-transformed B cell lines." *J Clin Invest* 96 (1995): 30–37.

Multiple Risk Factor Intervention Trial Research Group, "Baseline rest electrocardiographic abnormalities, antihypertensive treatment, and mortality in the Multiple Risk Factor Intervention Trial." *American Journal of Cardiology* 55 (1985): 1–15.

Multiple Sclerosis Society of Canada. www.mssociety.ca.

Murray, Gloria and Kathe A. Gabel. "Licorice Root: Helpful or Harmful?" *Topics in Clinical Nutrition* 15, no. 3 (2000): 59–65.

Murray, Michael T. *Encyclopedia of Nutritional Supplements.* Rocklin, CA: Prima Publishing, 1996.

Murray, Michael T. *Heart Disease and High Blood Pressure.* Rocklin, CA: Prima Publishing, 1997.

Murray, Michael T. "Horse Chestnut Seed Extract in Chronic Vein Insufficiency." *Natural Medicine Online.* www.nat-med.com (July 1999).

Murray, Michael T. and J. Pizzorno. *Encyclopedia of Natural Medicine.* Revised 2nd ed. Rocklin, CA: Prima Health, 1998.

Murray, Michael T. and M.R. Werbach. *Botanical Influences on Illness.* Tarzana, CA: Third Line Press, 1994.

Muscato, J., et al. "Sperm phagocytosis by human peritoneal macrophages: a possible cause of infertility in endometriosis." *Am J Obstet Gynecol* 144 (1982): 503–10.

Nair, P.P., et al. "Diet, Nutrition Intake and Metabolism in Populations at High and Low Risk for Colon Cancer." *The American Journal of Clinical Nutrition* 40 (1984): 927–30.

Nanda, R., et al. "Food intolerance and irritable bowel syndrome." *Gut* 30, no. 8 1998: 1099–1104.

Nassauto, G., et al. "Effect of silybin on Biliary lipid composition. Experimental and clinical study." *J Hepatol* 12 (1991): 290–295.

National Diabetes Information Clearinghouse. "Hypoglycemia." www.wellnessweb.com.

National Psoriasis Foundation. www.psoriasis.org.

Nervi, F., et al. "Influence of legume intake on Biliary lipids and cholesterol saturation in young Chilean men." *Gastroenterology* 96, no. 3 (1989): 825–30.

Neuman, I., H. Nahum, and A. Ben-Amotz. "Reduction of exercise-induced asthma oxidative stress by lycopene a natural antioxidant." *Allergy* 55 (2000): 1184–89.

Newmark, Thomas M. and Paul Schlulick. *Beyond Aspirin.* Prescott, AZ: Hohm Press, 2000.

Nityanand, S., et al. "Clinical trials with Gugulipid, a new hypolipidaemic agent." *Journal of Associated Physicians of India* 37 (1989): 321–28.

Nobile-Orazio, E., et al. "Guillain-Barré syndrome associated with high titers of anti-GM1 antibodies." *J Neurol Sci* 109 (1992): 200–206.

O'Garra, A. "Interleukins and the Immune System One." *Lancet* (April 29, 1989): 943–47.

O'Garra, A. "Interleukins and the Immune System Two." *Lancet* (May 6, 1989): 1003–1005.

Older, S.A., et al. "Can immunization precipitate connective tissue disease? Report of five cases of systemic lupus erythematosus and review of the literature." *Semin Arthritis Rheum* 29, no. 3 (1999): 131–39.

Passwater, Richard A. *All About Selenium.* Garden City Park, NY: Avery Publishing Group, 1999.

Patterson, Eric. "Banishing blemishes: fed up with antibiotics and drying creams? Try a natural approach instead." *Vegetarian Times* (June 1996).

Paul, R.H., et al. "Quality of life and well-being of patients with myasthenia gravis." *Muscle Nerve* 24, no. 4 (2001): 512–16.

Paul, W.E.. "Infectious Diseases and the Immune System." *Scientific American* (September 1993): 90–97.

Pavlidis, N.A., J. Karsh, and H.M. Moutsopoulos. "The clinical picture of primary Sjogren's syndrome: A retrospective study." *J Rheumatology* 9 (1982): 685–690.

Pellerier, X., et al. "A diet moderately enriched in phytosterols lowers plasma cholesterol concentrations in normocholesterolemic humans." *Annals of Nutrition Metabolism* 39 (1995): 291–295.

Peltier, J.Y., et al. "Frequency and prognostic importance of thrombocytopenia in symptom-free HIV-infected individual: A 5-year prospective study." *AIDS* 5 (1991): 381.

Pelton, Ross and James B. LaValle. *The Nutritional Cost of Prescription Drugs.* Englewood, CO: Morton Publishing Company, 2000.

Perlmutter, D. "Functional Therapeutics in Neurodegenerative Disease." *Journal of Applied Nutrition* 51, no. 1 (1999): 3–13.

Perros, P., et al. "Prevalence of pernicious anaemia in patients with Type I diabetes mellitus and autoimmune thyroid disease." *Diabet Med* 17, no. 10 (2000): 749–51.

Petri, Michelle, et al. "Plasma homocysteine as a risk factor for atherothrombotic events in systemic lupus erythematosus." *Lancet* 348 (October 26, 1996): 1120–24.

Phillips, R.L. "Role of Life-style and Dietary Habits in Risk of Cancer Among Seventh-Day Adventists." *Cancer Research* (1975) 3513–22.

Pinget M. and A. Lecomte. "The effects of harpagophytum capsules in degenerative rheumatology." *J Medecine Actuelle* 12, no. 4 (1985): 65–67.

Platelet Disorder Support Association. www.itppeople.com.

Plioplys, A.V. and S. Plioplys. "Amantadine and L-carnitine treatment of chronic fatigue syndrome." *Neuropsycholbiol* 35, no. 1 (1997): 6–23.

Polsdorfer, J. Ricker. "Intestinal Polyps." *Gale Encyclopedia of Medicine.* Gale Research. www.findarticles.com (January 1, 2001).

Polsdorfer, J. Ricker. "Vocal Cord Nodules and Polyps." *Gale Encyclopedia of Medicine.* Gale Research. www.findarticles.com (January 1, 2001).

Poole, M.D. "Antimicrobial therapy for sinusitis." *Otolaryngol Clin North Am* 30 (1997): 331–39.

Porikos, K.P. and T.B. van Itallie. "Diet-induced changes in serum transaminase and triglyceride levels in healthy adult men. Role of sucrose and excess calories." *American Journal of Medicine* 75 (1983): 624.

Powell, Pauline, et al. "Randomised controlled trial of patient education to encourage graded exercise in chronic fatigue syndrome." *British Medical Journal* (February 17, 2001).

Pulec, J.L., M.B. Pulec, and I. Mendoza. "Progressive sensorineural hearing loss, subjective tinnitus and vertigo caused by elevated blood lipids." *Ear Nose Throat J* 76, no. 10 (1997): 716–20, 725–26.

Quatrini, M., et al. "Helicobacter pylori prevalence in patients with diabetes and its relationship to dyspeptic symptoms." *J Clin Gastroenterol* 32, no. 3 (2001): 215–17.

Quillan, Patrick. "Nutrients as Biological Response Modifiers." *Natural Medicine Online.* www.nat-med.com (December 1998).

Raicht, R.F., et al. "Protective Effect of Plant Sterols Against Chemically Induced Colon Tumors in Rats." *Cancer Research* 40 (1980): 403–405.

Raloff, Janet. "Magnesium: We don't appear to be getting enough." *Science News* (August 29, 1998).

Rappaport, E.M. "Achlorhydria: Associated symptoms and response to hydrochloric acid." *New England Journal of Medicine* 252, no. 19 (1955): 802–805.

Raynaud's and Scleroderma Foundation. www.raynauds.demon.co.uk.

Rea, W.J. and C.W. Suits. "Cardiovascular disease triggered by foods and chemicals." *Food Allergy: New Perspectives.* J.W. Gerrard, ed. Springfield, IL: Charles C. Thomas, 1980.

Rice, J. "Cranberry juice may combat ulcers, *E. coli*, gum disease." *Beverage Online.* www.beverageonline.com. (September 20, 2000).

Robertson, D., et al. "Caffeine and hypertension." *Am J Med* 77, no. 1 (1984): 54–60.

Robertson, I.D., et al. "The role of companion animals in the emergence of parasitic zoonoses." *Int J Parasitol* 30, nos. 12–13 (2000): 1369–77.

Robinson, Richard. "Myasthenia gravis." *Gale Encyclopedia of Medicine.* Gale Research Group. www.findarticles.com (1999).

Rochlitz, S. *Allergies and Candida.* New York, NY: Human Ecology Balancing Sciences, Inc., 1991.

Rogers, S. *No More Heartburn.* New York, NY: Kensington Health Books, 2000.

Rogers, Sherry. *Tired or Toxic? A Blueprint for Health.* Syracuse, NY: Prestige Publishing, 1990.

Rose, D., et al. "Effect of a low-fat diet on hormone levels in women with cystic breast disease. I. Serum steroids and gonadotropins." *J JCK* 78, no. 4, (1987): 623–26.

Rose, Noel R. and Ian R. Mackay, ed. *The Autoimmune Diseases.* San Diego, CA: Academic Press, 1998.

Rosenbaum, M. and Susser, M. *Solving the Puzzle of Chronic Fatigue Syndrome.* Tacoma, WA: Life Sciences Press, 1992.

Ross, Jonathan H. and Robert Kay. "Urinary Tract Infections in Children." *American Family Physician* (March 15, 1999).

Rossi, G., et al. "Prevalence, clinical and laboratory features of thrombocytopenia among HIV-infected individuals." *AIDS Res Hum Retroviruses* 6 (1990): 261.

Rothwell, P.M. "Seasonality of birth in children with diabetes in Europe: Multicentre cohort study." *British Medical Journal* (October 2, 1999).

Runcie, C.J., C.G. Semple, and S.D. Slater. "Addison's disease without pigmentation." *Scott Med J* 31 (1986): 111–12.

Rushton, D.H. "Management of hair loss in women." *Dermatol Clin* 11, no. 1 (1993): 47–53.

Ryan, R. "A double-blind, clinical evaluation of bromelain in treatment of acute sinusitis." *Headache* 7 (1967): 13–17.

Sanchez, A., et al. "Role of sugars in human neutrophilic phagocytosis." *Am J Clin Nutr* 26 (1973): 1180–84.

Savage, C.O.S. "Vasculitis: ABC of Arterial and Vascular Disease." *British Medical Journal* 320 (May 13, 2000): 1325–28.

Schmid, B.,et al. "Analgesic effects of willow bark extract in osteoarthritis: results of a clinical double-blind trial." *Fact* 3 (1998): 186.

Schwartz, A.G. and L.L. Pashko. "Cancer Chemoprevention with the Adrenocortical Steroid Dehydroepiandrosterone and Structural Analogs." *Journal of Cellular Biochemistry* 17 (1993): 73–79.

Schwartz, E.R. "The modulation of osteoarthritis development by Vitamin C and Vitamin E." *Int J Vit Nutr Res* 26 (1984): 141.

Scleroderma Foundation. www.scleroderma.org.

Scott, Donald W. "The linking pathogen in neuro-systemic diseases chronic fatigue, Alzheimer's, Parkinson's and multiple sclerosis." *Consumer Health Newsletter*, Consumer Health Organization of Canada, 23, no. 6 (June 2000).

Scott, F.W. "Cow milk and insulin-dependent diabetes mellitus: Is there a relationship?" *Am J Clin Nutr* 51 (1990): 489–91.

Seelig, Mildred and William J. Rea. *Science News* 133 (June 4, 1988).

Seppa, Nathan. "Snoring impedes blood flow in brain: Air passage obstruction that causes snoring can also increase the risk of stroke." *Science News* (January 31, 1998).

"Serum cholesterol, fat intake, and breakfast consumption in the United States adult population." *Journal of the American College of Nutrition* 8 (1989): 567–72.

Shahani, K., et al. "Benefits of Yogurt." *International Journal of Immunotherapy* 9, no. 1 (1993): 65–68.

Shamsuddin, AbulKalam M. *IP6: Nature's Revolutionary Cancer-fighter.* New York, NY: Kensington Books, 1998.

Sheldon, T. "Link between pollution and asthma uncovered." *British Medical Journal.* www.bmj.com (March 20, 1999).

Sher, A. and R.L. Coffman. "Regulation of Immunity to Parasites by T Cells and T Cell-derived Cytokines." *Annual Review of Immunology.* 10 (1992): 385–409.

Shi, F.D., et al. "Natural killer cells determine the outcome of B cell-mediated autoimmunity." *Nature Immunology* 1, no. 3 (2000): 245–51.

Shoda, A., et al. "Therapeutic efficacy of N-2 polyunsaturated fatty acid in experimental Crohn's disease." *Journal of Gasteroenterology.* 30, supplement 8 (1995): 98–101.

Shoenfeld, Y. and A. Aron-Maor. "Vaccination and Autoimmunity—'Vaccinosis': A Dangerous Liaison. *Journal of Autoimmunity* 14 (2000): 1–10.

Shoskes, Daniel A. "Use of the Bioflavonoid Quercetin in Patients with Longstanding Chronic Prostatitis." *Journal of the American Nutraceutical Association* 2 (1999): 36–39.

Signorello, L.B., et al. "Hormones and hair patterning in men: A role for insulin-like growth factor-1?" *J Am Acad Dermatol* 40, no. 2 (1999): 200–203.

Simone, C.B. *Cancer and Nutrition.* Garden City Park, NY: Avery Publishing Group, 1992.

Sinard, Robert J. "The Aging Voice: How to Differentiate Disease From Normal Changes." *Geriatrics* (July 1998).

Singer, Sydney Ross, and Soma Grismaijer. *Dressed to Kill: The Link Between Breast Cancer and Bras.* Garden City Park, NY: Avery Publishing Group, 1995.

Singh, G.B. and C.K. Atal. "Pharmacology of an extract of salai guggal ex-Bosewellia serrata, a new non-steroidal anti-inflammatory agent." *Agents Action* 18 (1986): 407–12.

Sjogren's Syndrome Foundation, Inc. www.sjogrens.com.

Slatosky, John. "Thyroiditis: Differential Diagnosis and Management." *American Family Physician* (February 15, 2000).

Smith, C.M. "Congenital Neonatal Thyrotoxicosis and Previous Maternal Radio iodine Therapy." *British Medical Journal* (May 6, 2000).

"Smoking and Drinking May Foster Polyps." *USA Today Magazine* (February 2000).

Sobota, A.E. "Inhibition of bacterial adherence by cranberry juice: Potential use for the treatment of urinary tract infections." *J Urology* 131 (1984): 1013–16.

Stankus, Seth John. "Management of Herpes Zoster (Shingles) and Postherpetic Neuralgia." *American Family Physician* (April 15, 2000).

Stengler, Mark. *The Natural Physician: Your Health Guide to Common Ailments.* Burnaby, BC: Alive Books, 1997.

Strong, A.M.M., et al. "The effect of oral linoleic acid and gamma-linolenic acid (Efamol)." *British Journal of Clinical Practice* (November/December 1985): 444.

Sun, D., H.S. Courtney, and E. Beachey. "Berberine sulfate blocks adherence of streptococcus pyogenes to epithelial cells." *Antimicrobial Agents and Chemotherapy* 32 (1988): 1370–74.

Sussex Publishers, Inc., "DHA: The Good Fat." *Psychology Today* (March 1999).

Swab, J.H. "Suppression of the Immune Response by Microorganism." *Bacteriol Review.* 39 (1975): 121.

Syrjanen, K.J. "Spontaneous evolution of intraepithelial lesions according to the grade and type of the implicated human papillomavirus (HPV)." *Eur J Obstet Gynecol Reprod Biol* 65, no. 1 (1996): 45–53.

The Arthritis Foundation. www.arthritis.org.

The Multiple Sclerosis Foundation, Inc. www.msfacts.org.

Thomson, G.T., et al. "Post–Salmonella reactive arthritis: Late clinical sequelae in a point source cohort." *American Journal of Medicine* 98 (1995): 13–21.

Tomer, Y. and T.F. Davies. "Infection, thyroid disease and autoimmunity. *Endocr Rev* 14 (1993): 107–21.

Truss, C.O. "The role of candida albicans in human illness." *J Orthomol Psychiatry* 10 (1981): 228–38.

Tymchuk, C.N., et al. "Effects of diet and exercise on insulin, sex hormone-binding globulin, and prostate specific antigen." *Nutr Cancer* 31, no. 3 (1998): 127–31.

University of Manitoba Dental Hygiene Program. "The Wisdom Tooth" *Outreach.* www.umanitoba.ca/outreach/wisdomtooth.

Vahouny, G.V. and D. Kritchevsky. "Plant and marine sterols and cholesterol metabolism." *Nutritional Pharmacology* 4 (1981): 31–72.

Van Vollenhoven, R.F., et al. "An open study of dehydroepiandrosterone in systemic lupus erythematosus." *Arthritis and Rheumatism* 37 (1994): 1305–10.

Vanderhaeghe, Lorna R. and Patric J.D. Bouic. *The Immune System Cure.* Scarborough, ON: Prentice-Hall Canada Inc., 1999.

Verhoeven, D.T., et al. "Epidemiological Studies on Brassica Vegetables and Cancer Risk." *Cancer Epidemiological, Biomarkers and Prevention* 5 (1996): 733–47.

Vinson, D.C. and L.J. Lutz. "The effect of parental expectations on treatment of children with a cough: a report from ASPN." *J Fam Pract* 37, no. 1 (1993): 23–27.

Voelker, R. "Ames agrees with mom's advice: Eat your fruits and vegetables." *The Journal of the American Medical Association* 273, no. 14 (1995): 1077–78.

Vutyananich, T., S. Wongrangan, and R. Rung-aroon. "Pyridoxine for nausea and vomiting of pregnancy: A randomized, double-blind, placebo-controlled trial." *Am J Obstet Gynecol* 173 (1995): 881–84.

Wallace, D.J., et al. "Fibromyalgia, Cytokines, Fatigue Syndromes and Immune Regulation." *Advances in Pain Research and Therapy.* J. R. Fricton and E. Awad, eds. New York, NY: Raven Press, 1990.

Walling, Anne D. "Treatment of Patients with Nasal Polyps." *American Family Physician* (May 1, 2000).

Walpert, Naomi. "The Eyes Have It." *American Family Physician* (February 2000).

Walpert, Naomi. "The Highs and Lows of Autoimmune Thyroid Disease." *Nursing* (December 1998).

Warburg, Otto. "On the Origin of Cancer Cells." *Science* 123 (1956): 309–315.

Watson, J. and D. Mochizuki. "Interleukin 2: A Class of T Cell Growth Factors." *Immunology Review* 51 (1980): 257–78.

Weijl, N.I., F.J. Cleton, and S. Osanto. "Free radicals and antioxidants in chemotherapy-induced toxicity." *Cancer Treatment Reviews* 23 (1997): 209–40.

Werbach, M.R. and M.T. Murray. *Botanical Influences on Illness.* Tarzana, CA: Third Line Press, 1994.

Werbach, Melvyn R. *Healing Through Nutrition.* New York, NY: HarperCollins Publishers, 1993.

Werbach, Melvyn R. *Nutritional Influences on Illness. A Sourcebook of Clinical Research.* 2nd ed. Tarzana, CA: Third Line Press, 1990.

Whitaker, Julian. *Health & Healing* 10, no. 8 (August 2000).

Whitaker, Julian. *Health & Healing* 10, no. 9 (September 2000).

Whitaker, Julian. *Health & Healing* 10, no. 11 (November 2000).

Whitaker, Julian. *Health & Healing* 11, No. 1 (January 2001).

Williams, D.E., et al. "Frequent salad vegetable consumption is associated with a reduction in the risk of diabetes mellitus." *J Clin Epidemiol* 52, no. 4 (1999): 329–35.

Wilson, P.W.F. "High-density lipoprotein, low-density lipoprotein and coronary artery disease." *American Journal of Cardiology* 66 (1990): 7A–10A.

Wilson, T., et al. "Decreased natural killer cell activity in endometriosis patients: relationship to disease pathogenesis." *Fertil Steril* 62, no. 5 (1994): 1086–88.

Winsa, B., et al. "Stressful life events and Graves' disease." *Lancet* 338 (1991): 1475–79.

Wooston, Joseph. "Case Study: Missed diagnosis and mistreatment of unrecognized comorbid Graves' disease." *Journal of the American Academy of Child and Adolescent Psychiatry* (July 1999).

World Headache Alliance, "Latest news for the public about headaches and migraines." www.w-h-s.org.

Worman, Howard J. "Autoimmune Hepatitis." *Columbia University Gastroenterology Web*. www.cpmcnet.columbia.edu/dept/gi/autoimmune.html.

Yamada H., et al. "Effects of Phytosterols on Anticomplementary Activity." *Chemical Pharmacy Bulletin* 35, no. 12 (1987): 4851–55.

Yamagami T., et al. "Bioenergetics in clinical medicine. Studies on coenzyme Q10 and essential hypertension." *Res. Commun. Chem. Pathol. Pharmacol* 11 (1975): 273.

Yannick, P. and E.J. Gosselin. "Audiologic and metabolic findings in 90 patients with fluctuant hearing loss." *J Am Audiol Soc* 2, no. 1 (1976): 15–18.

Yarnell, Eric. "Southwestern and Asian Botanical Agents for Diabetes Mellitus." *Alternative & Complimentary Therapies* (February 2000): 7–11.

Yoshimoto, T., et al. "Flavonoids: Potent Inhibitors of Arachidonate-5-lipoxygenase." *Biochemical Biophysiolgical Research Communication* 116 (1983): 612–18.

Zacharias, Yvonne. "The risks of eating sushi." *The Vancouver Sun* (April 27, 2001).

Zajicek, G. "A New Cancer Hypothesis." *Medical Hypotheses* 47 (1996): 111–15.

Zhu J., et al. "Prospective study of pathogen burden and risk of myocardial infarction or death." *Circulation* 103, no. 1 (2001): 45–51.

INDEX